Imperial College London

AF572499

Understanding Evidence-Based Rheumatology

Hasan Yazici • Yusuf Yazici • Emmanuel Lesaffre
Editors

Understanding Evidence-Based Rheumatology

A Guide to Interpreting Criteria, Drugs, Trials, Registries, and Ethics

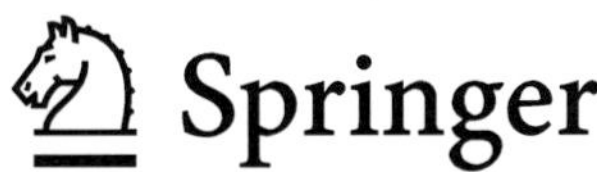

Editors
Hasan Yazici, MD
Istanbul University
Beyazit, Istanbul
Turkey

Yusuf Yazici, MD
New York University School of Medicine
NYU Hospital for Joint Diseases
New York, NY, USA

Emmanuel Lesaffre, PhD
Department of Biostatistics, Erasmus MC
Rotterdam, The Netherlands

L-Biostat, KU Leuven, Leuven, Belgium

ISBN 978-3-319-08373-5 ISBN 978-3-319-08374-2 (eBook)
DOI 10.1007/978-3-319-08374-2
Springer Cham Heidelberg New York Dordrecht London

Library of Congress Control Number: 2014948050

Printed on acid-free paper

Springer is part of Springer Science+Business Media (www.springer.com)

Preface

What Should the Reader Expect from This Book?

The background for this book is a series of almost-parallel conferences on clinical research methodology organized by the senior and junior Yazici, in either Bodrum or Istanbul by the senior and in New York by Yusuf Yazici. However, it was Emmanuel Lesaffre, our third coeditor and several times a speaker in these conferences, who came up with the idea of this book. These annual conferences have been held since 2006 as a single-day or weekend courses. The audiences have been, we like to think, purposefully small with around 40–50 people, to encourage interactive discussion. The full texts of the majority of the presentations for the New York courses are available on PubMed as manuscripts derived from the lectures, free to download at the web page of *Bulletin of the Hospital for Joint Diseases* (www.nyuhjdbulletin.org). It should therefore not come as a surprise to the reader that most of the contributors to this book have been speakers at these conferences.

We acknowledge that an excellent text and source book on similar topics as in this book has been available, namely, *Evidence-Based Rheumatology* by Peter Tugwell, also a speaker in our methodology conferences, since 2004. However, we reasoned that there still was an unmet need for our book for several reasons. A decade has passed since the publication of the volume by Tugwell et al. Ten years is a long period, and we believed that many things in rheumatology have significantly changed in quantity, direction, and quality. Furthermore, *Evidence-Based Rheumatology* has been almost an official guidebook of the Cochrane Foundation and its extension, the OMERACT (Outcome Measures in Rheumatology) group. Finally, a continuous and critical appraisal of the evidence for what we do or should do is to us the very essence of evidence-based medicine. With our book, we attempt to stand up to this challenge, both recommended and perceived.

We begin with an account of the birth of evidence-based medicine or, perhaps more correctly, "new evidence-based medicine," as we like to call it. Being particular about evidence in medical practice has surely been around ever since Enlightenment. On the other hand, it surely needed a boost toward the end of the last century with the tremendous increase in our understanding of, and the remedies to, many diseases. We argue that there were several important considerations for the emergence of evidence-based medicine. First, the biomedical model, most successful in explaining and managing acute illness, was surely not that successful in chronic diseases. Rather, a biopsychosocial model was more promising. The new evidence-based medicine was needed both to guide the practicing physician away from explaining the entirety of the multisystem disease of unknown etiology by the biomedical model and to check the science in the biopsychosocial model. The unnecessary medical services, especially in the light of ever-rising costs of medical care, were another main reason behind the new evidence-based medicine.

The chapter titled "Evidence-based medicine in rheumatology: how does it differ from other diseases?" also reminds us that the birth of rheumatology, as a separate subspecialty of internal medicine, is contemporary with the new evidence-based medicine. The idea and the scientific methodology of evidence-based medicine were surely most welcome in that "the multisystem disease of unknown etiology" has been and is the main preoccupation of our still relatively young discipline.

After all this rationalizing and theorizing, the chapter titled "A review of statistical approaches for the analysis of data in rheumatology" abruptly and intentionally brings us to the reality of numbers. With specific instructions to stay away from the integral sign, something that still makes most clinicians uncomfortable, the author makes a serious attempt to explain to the reader the arithmetic, both what is and what ought to be, behind evidence-based rheumatology. We like to think that the data-driven approach the author utilizes will help to explain the common, descriptive statistical approaches currently in use. His main focus is on the intuitive ideas behind the methods rather than on their technical aspects. Practical guidelines are also present throughout this chapter. Finally, the reader is also introduced to Bayesian methods that are becoming more and more popular.

The third chapter begins by emphasizing the importance of disease criteria in rheumatology since many of the rheumatologic diseases are, yet, constructs. In addition, the authors propose that our current separation of criteria as diagnostic or classification, although having an aura of practical or scientific sophistication, is ill founded. They underline that the cerebral exercise behind the two is the same. The thought barriers to this unhelpful bi-labeling are discussed while proposals for preparing more useful diagnostic/classification criteria are provided.

The chapter titled "Biomarkers, genetic association, and genomic studies" on biomarkers, including those of the genetic kind, is an assiduous account of our tribulations, accomplishments, hopes, and not uncommon wishful thinking around how to improve our laboratory capabilities to diagnose and monitor rheumatologic diseases. We like to think that this chapter, by using rheumatoid arthritis (RA) as a case example, shows how demanding, be it biochemical or genetic, it is to come up with a sensitive, specific, or more importantly a clinically useful disease marker.

The ensuing chapter "Outcome measures in rheumatoid arthritis" is on outcome measures in RA. While what happens to the patient at the end of what the physicians do or fail to do is the primary concern of medicine, it is rather surprising that we have not made a sincere effort to this end until recently. We used to think that we physicians, with our laboratory tests and imaging gadgetry, always knew better than the patients themselves how they fared. Well, we now know this is not the case, and this chapter is all about how this recent realization relates particularly to RA.

The chapter titled "Issues in setting up a study and data collection" is a handy manual on both how to go about a research project and, while doing or interpreting that, avoid a *biomedical bestiary* of biases.

The following two chapters are detailed accounts of the randomized clinical trial (RCT), most certainly the flagship of evidence-based medicine, especially the new evidence-based medicine ever since the groundbreaking MRC streptomycin tuberculosis trial of 1948. Over 65 years have passed since the first-ever scientific application of this very important research tool. As expected, there are many finer points and caveats concerning the many forms of RCT now available dealing with the study design, its analysis, and most importantly the fit of the one with the other. The Bayesian RCT, which is more popular in our age of haste, is also introduced.

The following chapter by Ted Pincus is a healthy and critical discussion of perhaps the undue importance we give to the RCT as our golden measure of evidence. He gives in-depth examples to document his concern. One cannot help thinking that perhaps it is not only the undue importance the researcher, the practitioner, and the health authorities gave to this tool but rather its more recent abuse that justifies many of Ted Pincus' concerns.

Whatever their causes, issues with the RCTs have recently led the medical community to put increasing faith in observational studies. One reason for this turn is our current ability to electronically collect and interpret vast amounts of data in a very short time. An additional reason for the recent popularity of observational data might be the contemporary interest in the inductive scientific approach.

Keeping up with our general and hopefully useful critical approach, Marie Hudson and Samy Suissa give us an expert overview of the many pitfalls in observational studies, especially in those studies that stem from data based on large patient repositories, such as administrative databases. A clear account of how to best recognize and avoid them is provided with special emphasis on data collection time–related biases in which the authors are leading experts.

With RCT struggling to maintain its flagship status in the face of many whips and arrows, recent years quietly put another mode of research into the pinnacle of evidence in evidence-based medicine. Meta-analysis is the science of reanalyzing the outcomes of different studies on a same subject by amalgamating individual research reports. Its most popular approach is to combine the experience from the RCTs. The Achilles heel of this approach is to put apples and oranges together in such analyses. We believe the authors of this relatively short chapter "Systematic reviews and meta-analyses in rheumatology" give a very useful account of how not to do this.

Our penultimate chapter is "Ethical issues in study design and reporting." Any talk about ethics has the danger of being either too dry or too juicy. In this chapter, we have tried to avoid a discourse on the Helsinki declaration or provide particular examples of physician or industry misconduct which everybody knows and recognizes either from boring texts or daily tabloids. We have attempted to better describe what is not readily recognized not only by the public but many a time by the medical profession itself. This we like to call the cerebral form of ethics, as distinct from the pudendal form of the tabloids. The cerebral form, we propose, is perhaps more pertinent to many things we do not like about the science and practice of medicine today.

Our final chapter is "Future directions." It is our sincere hope that the readers of this book will have formulated their own priorities once they have gone this far in our book.

We extend our appreciation and many thanks to the other invited speakers in the New York and Bodrum/Istanbul conferences over the years, who have contributed immensely to the ideas presented in this book. They include (in alphabetical order) Nurullah Akkoc, Anca Askanase, Martin Bergman, Maarten Boers, Hermann Brenner, Isabel Castrejon, David Cella, Jeffrey Curtis, Ayhan Dinc, Haner Direskeneli, Maxime Dougados, Anders Ekbom, Onder Ergonul, Brian Feldman, Jeffrey Greenberg, Ahmet Gul, Vedat Hamuryudan, Tom Huizinga, Murat Inanc, John Ioannidis, Hilal Maradit Kremers, Alfred Mahr, Fredrick Naftolin, Cem Ozesen, Salih Pay, Alan Silman, Richard Smith, Tuulikki Sokka-Isler, Samy Suissa, Necdet Sut, Koray Tascilar, Peter Tugwell, and Nathan Vastesaeger.

Finally and surely we also much thank our Springer editors for their expert help in putting all this together.

Istanbul, Turkey — Hasan Yazici, MD
New York, NY, USA — Yusuf Yazici, MD
Rotterdam, The Netherlands — Emmanuel Lesaffre, Dr. Sc.

Contents

Evidence-Based Medicine in Rheumatology: How Does It Differ from Other Diseases? 1
Theodore Pincus and Hasan Yazici

A Review of Statistical Approaches for the Analysis of Data in Rheumatology 13
Emmanuel Lesaffre and Jolanda Luime

Disease Classification/Diagnosis Criteria 65
Hasan Yazici and Yusuf Yazici

Biomarkers, Genetic Association, and Genomic Studies 79
Mehmet Tevfik Dorak and Yusuf Yazici

Outcome Measures in Rheumatoid Arthritis 127
Yusuf Yazici and Hilal Maradit Kremers

Issues in Setting Up a Study and Data Collection 141
Hilal Maradit Kremers and Banu Çakir

The Randomized Controlled Trial: Methodological Perspectives 159
Emmanuel Lesaffre

Limitations of Traditional Randomized Controlled Clinical Trials in Rheumatology 179
Theodore Pincus

Methodological Issues Relevant to Observational Studies, Registries, and Administrative Health Databases in Rheumatology 209
Marie Hudson and Samy Suissa

Systematic Reviews and Meta-analyses in Rheumatology 229
Theo Stijnen and Gulen Hatemi

Ethical Issues in Study Design and Reporting 247
Hasan Yazici, Emmanuel Lesaffre, and Yusuf Yazici

Future Directions 265
Hasan Yazici, Yusuf Yazici, and Emmanuel Lesaffre

Index 269

Contributors

Banu Çakir, MD, MPH, PhD Department of Public Health, Hacettepe University Faculty of Medicine, Ankara, Turkey

Mehmet Tevfik Dorak, MD, PhD School of Health Sciences, Liverpool Hope University, Liverpool, UK

Gulen Hatemi, MD Division of Rheumatology, Department of Internal Medicine, Cerrahpasa Tip Fakultesi, Cerrahpasa Medical School, Istanbul University, Aksaray, Istanbul, Turkey

Marie Hudson, MD, MPH Division of Rheumatology, Department of Medicine, Centre for Clinical Epidemiology, Jewish General Hospital, McGill University, Montreal, QC, Canada

Hilal Maradit Kremers, MD Department of Health Science Research and Orthopedic Surgery, Mayo Clinic, Rochester, MN, USA

Emmanuel Lesaffre, Dr. Sc. Department of Biostatistics, Erasmus MC, Rotterdam, The Netherlands

L-Biostat, KU Leuven, Leuven, Belgium

Jolanda Luime, PhD Department of Rheumatology, Erasmus MC, Rotterdam, The Netherlands

Theodore Pincus, MD Division of Rheumatology, New York University Hospital for Joint Diseases, New York, NY, USA

Theo Stijnen, MSc, PhD Department of Medical Statistics and Bioinformatics, Leiden University Medical Center, Leiden, The Netherlands

Samy Suissa, PhD Division of Rheumatology, Department of Medicine, Centre for Clinical Epidemiology, Jewish General Hospital, McGill University, Montreal, QC, Canada

Hasan Yazici, MD Division of Rheumatology, Department of Medicine, Cerrahpasa Medical Faculty, Cerrahpasa Hospital, University of Istanbul, Istanbul, Turkey

Yusuf Yazici, MD Division of Rheumatology, Department of Medicine, Seligman Center for Advanced Therapeutics and Behcet's Syndrome Center, NYU Hospital for Joint Diseases, New York University School of Medicine, New York University, New York, NY, USA

Evidence-Based Medicine in Rheumatology: How Does It Differ from Other Diseases?

Theodore Pincus and Hasan Yazici

The Absence of a "Gold Standard" in Rheumatic Diseases

The authors are now sufficiently senior to recall the early 1970s, at which time rheumatologists were considered elite members of the medical community in their zealous search for evidence in clinical care. Rheumatology fellows were using terms such as "sensitivity," "specificity," "true negatives" and "false positives" more than trainees in other fields. This emphasis may have resulted from an important difference in rheumatic diseases versus many other diseases – the absence of a single "gold standard" measure for diagnosis, prognosis, management and assessment of outcomes in each individual patient with a given diagnosis. Trainees in cardiology, endocrinology, nephrology and other fields had a lesser interest in complexities of clinical measures as they often had a definitive "gold standard," such as sustained elevated blood pressure in hypertension, sustained elevated glucose in diabetes mellitus, or a definitive biopsy in lymphoma, to guide clinical care.

The discovery in 1948 of rheumatoid factor [1] and the LE cell phenomenon [2] gave hope that a single gold standard biomarker would be available similarly for diagnosis, prognosis, management and assessment of outcomes in rheumatoid arthritis (RA) or systemic lupus erythematosus (SLE), the two most common inflammatory rheumatic diseases. However, despite extensive clinical research, that hope has not been met. Rheumatoid factor was described as present in 70 % of patients seen with RA in the initial report of Rose, Ragan *et al.* [1],

T. Pincus, MD (✉)
Division of Rheumatology, Rush University Medical Center, 1611 West Harrison Street, Chicago, IL 60612, USA

H. Yazici, MD (✉)
Division of Rheumatology, Department of Medicine, Cerrahpasa Medical Faculty, University of Istanbul, Istanbul, Turkey (retired)

H. Yazici et al. (eds.), *Understanding Evidence-Based Rheumatology*,
DOI 10.1007/978-3-319-08374-2_1

virtually identical to 69 % in a recent meta-analysis [3]. Furthermore, rheumatoid factor is found in about 5–10 % of people in the general population [3], including patients with chronic infections and no apparent disease at all. Antibodies to citrullinated proteins (anti-CCP or ACPA) show increased specificity for RA, as they are seen in fewer than 5 % of individuals in the normal population; however, these antibodies are found in only 67 % of RA patients [3], quite comparable to rheumatoid factor.

Further biomarkers have been sought in RA based on the erythrocyte sedimentation rate (ESR) or C-reactive protein (CRP). As with rheumatoid factor and ACPA, these measures are abnormal in the majority of patients. However, at this time, at least 40 % of patients do not show elevated values [4], although this proportion has declined from about 80 % in the early 80s to approximately 55 % in recent years [5], as RA patient clinical status has been improving [6]. The absence of a gold standard laboratory biomarker such as serum glucose, cholesterol, creatinine, hemoglobin or hemoglobin A1c, therefore, distinguishes rheumatic diseases from many chronic diseases for clinical trials, other clinical research and routine clinical care.

Pooled Indices as Quantitative Measures of Clinical Status in Rheumatic Diseases.

In the absence of "gold standard" laboratory tests or other quantitative biomarkers such as blood pressure or bone densitometry scores, pooled indices are required to assess quantitatively clinical status and responses to therapy in individual patients with a rheumatic diagnosis. The most successful pooled indices are seen in RA, based on a core data set of 7 measures: 3 recorded by a physician from a physical examination, *i.e.*, tender joint count, swollen joint count, and physician global estimate of status; 3 based on a patient self-report questionnaire – physical function, pain, and patient global estimate of status; and only 1 laboratory test, ESR or CRP [7]. Patients who may have many swollen joints and low pain levels, or a reciprocal pattern, are assessed according to an identical quantitative index. The core data set has been used for more than 2 decades and may be regarded as one of the major advances in rheumatology, prerequisite for the better status of patients at this time compared with previous decades [6].

The most prominent traditional index for RA has been the disease activity score (DAS) [8] and DAS28 [9], based on 4 measures: tender joint count, swollen joint count, ESR or CRP, and patient global estimate of status. The limitations of the DAS28 include a need for a laboratory test [ESR or CRP], which often is not available at the time of the visit, and is normal in up to 40 % of patients [4], and complex calculations, although easily accomplished at an excellent website. These limitations are overcome by the clinical disease activity index (CDAI) [10], which is simply a total of 4 measures: 28 tender joint count, 28 swollen joint count, and physician and patient global estimates 10 cm visual analog scales (VAS), total 0–76. An index of only the 3 patient self-report measures, known as routine assessment of patient index data (RAPID3), includes three 0–10 scales for physical function, pain and patient estimate of global status, total 0–30 [11]. Levels have been established for high, moderate, low activity or severity of each index [12]; an index of only patient measures is not as specific to assess disease activity, since it might be sensitive to joint damage and chronic pain, but the other indices also are affected, though less so [13].

In analyses of clinical trials, essentially any 3 or 4 core data set measures will give very similar results, as was shown in analyses to establish remission criteria for RA [14]. Some rheumatologists support use of the simplest measure, RAPID3, as the patient does 95 % of the work and measurement involves the same single observer – the patient – at all visits. At the same time, other rheumatologists, particularly outside the USA, feel uncomfortable with only patient measures and include a CDAI or a DAS28.

Indices for Other Rheumatic Diseases

Indices exist for many other rheumatic diseases. In general, all include at least one measure from a physical examination and from patient self-report questionnaire, as well as a laboratory test. All are more complex than a "gold standard" measure. However, it also is possible that clinical decisions based on a gold standard measure may oversimplify what is needed for optimal patient care in chronic diseases. For example, functional status is as significant as ejection fraction to predict 3-year hospitalizations and deaths in congestive heart failure [15], CD4/CD8 ratios and other AIDS-specific measures to predict 3-year mortality in AIDS [16], and physiologic data and comorbidities to predict 1-year mortality in hospitalized elder patients [17]. Therefore, the importance of these measures may extend beyond rheumatology.

Some indices in rheumatology may be insensitive to clinical changes, which may account in part for some of the limitations in clinical trials. If an index includes, say, 10 measures, only 2 of which may change substantially and the others not at all, the index may indicate no change when an important clinical change has occurred in the 2 measures. Ironically, criteria for psychometric validation of indices based on statistical tools such as Cronbach's alpha and convergent validity generally may reduce sensitivity to change. Such sensitivity often is greatest with simple 10 cm visual analog scales (VAS). Nonetheless, it is essential to have an index for diseases in which certain clinical manifestations may vary widely and be prominent in some patients and absent in others, as noted for joint swelling and pain for RA.

Prominence of Patient History and Physical Examination in Clinical Decisions in Rheumatology

A survey was conducted in which 313 physicians, approximately half of whom were rheumatologists and half non-rheumatologists, estimated the relative importance of 5 elements of the clinical encounter – vital signs, patient history, physical examination, laboratory tests and ancillary studies (imaging, biopsy, endoscopy, etc.) – in clinical decisions in 8 chronic diseases: congestive heart failure (CHF), diabetes mellitus, hypercholesterolemia, hypertension, lymphoma, pulmonary fibrosis, rheumatoid arthritis, and ulcerative colitis. The response options were 1–100 % in 5 equally divided intervals [18].

As expected, vital signs were most prominent in hypertension; laboratory tests were most prominent for diabetes and hyperlipidemia; and ancillary studies were most prominent for lymphoma, pulmonary fibrosis, ulcerative colitis, and congestive heart failure (Figure 1) [18]. RA was the only one of the 8 chronic conditions in which a patient history and physical examination accounted for more than 50 % of the information required for diagnosis and management (the total could be higher than 100 % due to "ties") [18]. These data provide evidence that the clinical encounter in rheumatology practice differs substantially from that in other subspecialties.

The results of this survey are reflected in the 7 items of the RA core data set, which includes 3 items from a patient questionnaire, 3 from a physical examination, and 1 laboratory test. A patient self-report questionnaire may be regarded as providing information for the patient history as quantitative data rather than narrative non-quantitative descriptions. A formal joint count may be regarded as providing information from the physical examination as quantitative data rather than narrative non-quantitative descriptions. The RA indices therefore reflect patient history and physical examination in contrast to gold standard biomarkers, which are most prominent in clinical decisions in many other chronic diseases.

Limitations of Laboratory Findings

As noted above, when rheumatoid factor was discovered in 1948, it was initially thought that this autoantibody might be both causative and diagnostic, as with antinuclear antibodies in 1960 for SLE, HLA B27 in ankylosing spondylitis, and mutant gene associations in FMF and MEFV [19]. However, the information from the laboratory is relatively limited in rheumatic diseases, compared to lab tests in other subspecialties of internal medicine, such as hemoglobin A1c or serum glucose. Of course, laboratory markers are important in groups and as clues to pathogenesis and development of treatments. For example, the development of biological therapy for RA may be traced directly to identification of rheumatoid factor with subsequent recognition of cytokines.

Laboratory markers are not positive in 30–50 % of all patients with RA [20]. Furthermore, they are "abnormal" (false positive) in some individuals in the normal population who have other diseases or no disease whatsoever, unlike measures such as sustained hypertension or elevated glucose over time.

There is value in calculating the sensitivity and specificity and predictive value of different tests, for the probability of a certain disease being present in a patient. However, the individual patient who may not have any positive tests but has pathognomonic clinical features of a disease has a 100 % probability of having the disease, regardless of the test results. A test that is positive in only 70 % of patients has limited utility in daily practice, although most rheumatologists are not aware of this problem. It is sobering to remember that information from the laboratory in rheumatology is not pathognomic as in other diseases.

Limitations of Imaging

Structural changes are prominent in many rheumatic diseases, which might suggest an expectation that imaging would be most informative in diagnosis and management. Magnetic resonance imaging (MRI) and ultrasound certainly have improved sensitivity compared to plain radiographs. However, these new imaging modalities have not improved specificity. It is also worth remembering that the severe outcomes of RA such as work disability and premature death are predicted at far higher levels of significance by physical function on a patient questionnaire and by comorbidities than by hand radiographs [21].

Ironically, one possible limitation of studies to analyze radiographs as prognostic of severe outcomes may be that radiographic data are derived from the hand, whereas work disability and death are far more prominently influenced by large joints, particularly knees, but also hips and shoulders. For example, the initial series reported on mortality in RA indicated that 6 joints, 2 shoulders, 2 hips and 2 knees could predict mortality as effectively as all joints [22].

Furthermore, radiographic findings and clinical symptoms are often highly dissociated. For example, joint tenderness and radiographic findings have no correlation whatsoever [23]. Many people who may have 4+ osteoarthritis of the knee report no pain [24].

Limitations of Histopathology

Rheumatic diseases may include biopsies in an effort to establish or feel more secure about a given diagnosis. However, many findings have little tissue specificity, such as the synovitis in RA which can be seen in many forms of inflammatory arthritis. While tissue specificity is seen in immune complexes in the kidneys or dermoepidermal junction in SLE, uric acid crystals in synovial fluid or tophi in gout, giant cells and in the vessel wall in giant cell arteritis and in Takayasu disease, lymphocyte infiltration in salivary gland biopsies in Sjogren's syndrome, and bacilli in the intestinal wall in Whipple's disease; it is difficult to further expand the scope of histopathology in rheumatic disease.

Table 1 Comparison of "biomedical model" and "biopsychosocial model" of disease

	Biomedical Model	Biopsychosocial Model
Cause	Each disease has a single "cause"	Disease etiology is multifactorial: external pathogens, toxins, and internal host milieu, genes, behavior, social support
Diagnosis	Identified primarily through laboratory tests, radiographs, scans; information from patients of value primarily to suggest appropriate tests	A patient medical history provides 50%–90% of the information needed to make many, perhaps most, diagnoses
Prognosis	Also established most accurately based on information from high-technology sources, rather than from a patient	Information provided by a patient often is the most valuable data to establish a prognosis
Treatment	Involves only actions of health professionals, eg, medications, surgery	Must involve patient, family, social structure
Role of health professionals and patients in general health and disease outcomes	Health and disease outcomes are determined primarily by decisions and actions of health professionals	Health and outcomes of chronic diseases are determined as much by actions of individual patient as by health professionals

Rheumatology Assessment as a Challenge to the Biomedical Model

The major paradigm for advances in medical care over the last two centuries is a "biomedical model," in which clinical observations are translated into quantitative high-technology data from laboratory tests and ancillary studies. Early examples include bacterial cultures and quantitative laboratory measures of organ function (e.g., liver, kidney function tests), which can be used to guide care as "gold standard' measures for diagnosis, management, prognosis and assessment of outcomes in individual patients.

Over the last few decades there has been growing awareness that the traditional biomedical model, while spectacularly effective in acute disease and acute aspects of many chronic diseases, includes some significant limitations, particularly for chronic diseases. A classical statement was provided by George Engel, in a widely-read article in *Science* in 1978 [25]:

> "I contend that all medicine is in crisis and, further, that medicine's crisis derives from … adherence to a model of disease no longer adequate for its scientific tasks and social responsibilities…The biomedical model embraces both reductionism, the philosophic view that complex phenomena are ultimately derived from a single primary principle, and mind-body dualism, the doctrine that separates the mental from the somatic."

We may contrast the classical biomedical model with a biopsychosocial model of disease, which appears relevant to rheumatic diseases as complementary to a biomedical model (Table 1).

Some important differences between the biomedical and the biopsychosocial models are summarized in Table 1 [26].

The Biopsychosocial Model in Rheumatic and Other Diseases

Some essential elements to the biopsychosocial model (interestingly, without actually calling it as such) as it applies to rheumatology have been masterfully explained and discussed by H. Holman in his 1994 article "Thought Barriers to Understanding Rheumatic Diseases" [27]. Holman asserted that the main problem with the practice and the science of rheumatology is that "the prevailing conceptual base of our investigation is incommensurate with the rheumatic disease problems which we confront." He gives two main reasons:

1. While most rheumatologic diseases are chronic, the traditional medical teaching put the emphasis on acute pathology.
2. There is the prevailing notion of a "single cause" for a single disease. This, of course, has its roots in medicine's spectacular success in handling the infectious diseases. This reductionism is common in research, where we tend to overlook interactive biological pathways, common in many of our diseases.

As we note, Holman does not give a formal reference to the biopsychosocial model in this article. Perhaps he might have decided to underplay the psychological and social components of said model.

Nonetheless, the Vernon Riley experiment he relates in detail in this paper actually provides a brilliant example of the inadequacy of the biomedical model. The experiment concerned breast cancer in C3H mice [28]. This cancer, seen in C3H mice, is both genetic and environmental. The tumor appears around 1 year of age only among those mice that have been infected with a specific virus during suckling. All the cross-experiments of the biomedical dictum confirm these genetic and environmental components.

Riley introduced a third dimension, a psychosocial dimension if you will, to this model. He randomized C3H female offspring into 2 groups: one under usual experimental conditions of crowded cages and frequent blood samples, and the other in spacious cages and little if any bleeding. The outcome was that the latter group developed the expected tumor a median of almost 200 days later.

Limitations of EBM as Randomized Trials in Application to Clinical Care

The randomized controlled clinical trial may be considered a development in the tradition of the biomedical model. It is designed to mimic a laboratory experiment, in isolating a single variable that tests therapy while keeping all the other variables constant [29]. The clinical trial is most successful in acute infectious disease in which the outcome may be known within a week or two. A trial becomes progressively more limited over time in chronic diseases, as discussed in detail in the chapter concerning limitations of randomized controlled clinical trials (see chapter "Limitations of traditional randomized controlled clinical trials in rheumatology"). Nonetheless, in these introductory comments, we recognize that even proponents of evidence-based medicine (EBM) as clinical-based trials recognize some limitations in application of results to clinical care.

Any evidence, in the last analysis, can be considered as a tool to convince either oneself or somebody else of the strength of a "truth" under consideration. More simply, evidence is what makes an object or a concept "evident" to us or to others. Verbose as it is, this definition – unlike its standard dictionary versions – has the advantage of emphasizing that the quality of evidence is quite dependent on ***a)*** who is to be convinced and ***b)*** the circumstances under which "the convincing" takes place. To convince your 3-year-old child that his plate is hot, you would never resort to the most direct evidence, the "gold standard" as the jargon goes, that he should touch it briefly and see for himself. However, for his mother, and if you are occasionally brave, this direct evidence might be used!

One example of some limitations of application of randomized controlled clinical trials to clinical care recognized by a leading proponent of EBM may be found in the introduction to the book *Philosophy of Evidence Based Medicine* by Dr. Jeremy Howick [30]. Here the author takes a direct quote from Dr. Chalmers, who saw many children with measles who also were malnourished and in general poor health, while working as a young doctor in a Palestinian refugee camp in the Gaza Strip. Unless there was clear evidence of superinfection he refrained from prescribing antibiotics, as he had been taught in medical school.

However, mortality among his patients was considerably higher than among those of his Palestinian colleague who routinely prescribed prophylactic antibiotics. Chalmers observed: "This clinical impression was very sobering. It made me wonder whether what I had been taught at medical school might have been lethally wrong, at least in the circumstances in which I was working, and precipitated a now incurable 'septicemia' about authoritarian therapeutic prescriptions and prescriptions unsupported by trustworthy empirical evidence" [30].

The catch line here is, of course, "…in the circumstances in which I was working…." The "evidence" about not starting prophylactic antibiotics in managing measles might have been true for the more fortunate locations where Chalmers' professors resided, but not for the Gaza strip. This business of "to whom" and "under which circumstances" – or the *external validity* (in the jargon) – is an important and often neglected aspect of EBM.

All evidence can either be direct or indirect. Some good examples of direct evidence as it concerns our discipline are: a wedge-shaped crushed vertebral body on a radiograph in osteoporosis; finding sodium mono urate crystals in the synovial fluid (making a diagnosis of gout); colchicine preventing attacks of familial Mediterranean fever (management); or anti-Ro antibodies sitting in the cardiac conduction system causing heart block in neonates (understanding disease mechanisms). Examples of such similar direct evidence from other disciplines are tell-tale EKG findings in a myocardial infarction, massive proteinuria in nephrotic syndrome, or antibodies to acetylcholine receptors in myasthenia gravis. Much more common in our field is indirect evidence, as seen in the biopsychosocial model (Table 1). Here our young discipline differs substantially from other specialties, as noted above.

EBM as a Long-Standing Tradition

EBM surely did not surely begin abruptly in 1992 when it was publicly announced, nor did the Enlightenment and Industrialization bypass evidence in medicine. As early as the 17th century, Francis Bacon, the scientist and the philosopher, severely criticized Hippocrates for the anecdotal nature of his (as the name openly says) "aphorisms" [31]. A century later, the eminent English physician Francis Clifton made a strong plea for a meticulous tabulation of disease occurrence in English towns by sex, race, age and the type of illness [31]. The 19th century gave us much more objective tools for observation like the stethoscope and the microscope. Again in the 19th century, mankind began to benefit from scientifically powerful medicines for prevention: the smallpox vaccine, and antisera to treat diphtheria and tetanus. Medicine became much more scientific in the 20th century, not only with new and effective drugs and vaccines, but with spectacular advances in imaging and surgery. Moreover arithmetic, statistics, probability and randomness began to be taken seriously, discussed and also required by the physician practitioner and the medical scientist alike.

In 1948 the first properly randomized clinical trial [32] was conducted, and showed that the new drug streptomycin was superior in treating patients with tuberculosis compared to the available "standard of care," bed rest. Many other, similarly well-conducted trials in many other diseases followed. So what was wrong with prior EBM that made its founders declare the *new* EBM in 1992?

Possibly at least four, and somewhat related, reasons were behind the emergence of the new EBM as based on randomized controlled clinical trials.

The first was that the new EBM advocates wanted to give to the proponents of unconventional remedies one additional blow. This was surely timely, especially in the light of ever-rising medical costs in the setting of limited resources. Nothing more needs to be said here.

A second important issue behind the emergence of the new EBM was that, although the science of medicine had progressed substantially, this progression was often not translated into usual clinical care. In other words, the application was not commensurate with the level of science.

A third driving force may have been the relative inability of the biomedical model to address common, as well as less common, ills – as aptly exemplified both in Dr. Chalmers' story in the Gaza strip and in Riley's rats. It was that the traditional *science* of medicine fell short of explaining our ills and how to prevent or handle them to our satisfaction, and this is surely related to the second issue just discussed. However, when EBM is regarded as exclusively based on randomized controlled clinical trials, it does not give much headway to the biopsychosocial model. It mimics a laboratory experiment with a reductionist focus on a single variable, attempting to control all other variables through randomization. Instead it does something else and this, perhaps, leads us to the fourth issue.

The new EBM with its authors, journals, books, governments and surely the drug control agencies like FDA considered that the medical field and profession needed many degrees and levels of central control – and, as in the first issue, the limited money/resource concern was the main reason. To put it another way, for the new EBM what was more important was the correct implementation of existing science rather than promoting science, and the monetary concern was also dominant. One effort toward control was placement of meta-analysis at the top of the hierarchy of evidence-based medicine (Figure 2) [28]. However, a meta-analysis is only as informative as its component clinical trials, and limitations of clinical trials such as patient selection, short-term time frame in chronic diseases, and reporting of data only in groups, may render a meta-analysis less accurate concerning clinical care than observational studies.

It must also be brought up here that this justified concern for money led to a central control that, ironically, kindled more money and resource problems – after the drug industry began to use this central control, in many instances, to their financial interests [33, 34]. It is as if medicine has learned little from the economists and business administrators that central control of business, in the long run, almost always takes a bigger chunk out of public money than private enterprise.

Over the last few years, some of the limitations of regarding evidence-based medicine only as clinical trials, invariably superior to other sources of clinical evidence, have gained increasing recognition. A more up-to-date view of "evidence-based medicine" is expressed by the Oxford Centre for Evidence-Based Medicine [35]: "While they are simple and easy to use, early hierarchies that placed randomized trials categorically above observational studies were criticized [28] for being simplistic [36]. In some cases, observational studies give us the 'best' evidence [28]. For example, there is a growing recognition that observational studies – even case-series [37] *and anecdotes* [38] can sometimes provide definitive evidence." Nevertheless, the principles of "evidence-based medicine" continue to evolve, hopefully leading to improved patient care and outcomes.

References

1. Rose HM, Ragan C, Pearce E, Lipman MO. Differential agglutination of normal and sensitized sheep erythrocytes by sera of patients with rheumatoid arthritis. Proc Soc Exp Biol Med 1948; 68:1–6.
2. Hargraves MM, Richmond H, Morton R. Presentation of two bone marrow elements: The "tart" cell and "L.E." cell. Proc Staff Meet Mayo Clin 1948; 23:25–8.
3. Nishimura K, Sugiyama D, Kogata Y, Tsuji G, Nakazawa T, Kawano S, et al. Meta-analysis: Diagnostic accuracy of anti-cyclic citrullinated peptide antibody and rheumatoid factor for rheumatoid arthritis. Ann Intern Med 2007; 146(11):797–808.
4. Sokka T, Pincus T. Erythrocyte sedimentation rate, C-reactive protein, or rheumatoid factor are normal at presentation in 35 %-45% of patients with rheumatoid arthritis seen between 1980 and 2004: analyses from Finland and the United States. J Rheumatol 2009; 36(7):1387–90.

5. Abelson B, Sokka T, Pincus T. Declines in erythrocyte sedimentation rates in patients with rheumatoid arthritis over the second half of the 20th century. J Rheumatol 2009; 36(8):1596–9.
6. Pincus T, Sokka T, Kautiainen H. Patients seen for standard rheumatoid arthritis care have significantly better articular, radiographic, laboratory, and functional status in 2000 than in 1985. Arthritis Rheum 2005; 52:1009–19.
7. Felson DT, Anderson JJ, Boers M, Bombardier C, Chernoff M, Fried B, et al. The American College of Rheumatology preliminary core set of disease activity measures for rheumatoid arthritis clinical trials. Arthritis Rheum 1993; 36:729–40.
8. van der Heijde DMFM, van't Hof M, van Riel PLCM, van de Putte LBA. Development of a disease activity score based on judgment in clinical practice by rheumatologists. J Rheumatol 1993; 20:579–81.
9. Prevoo MLL, van't Hof MA, Kuper HH, van Leeuwen MA, van de Putte LBA, van Riel PLCM. Modified disease activity scores that include twenty-eight-joint counts: Development and validation in a prospective longitudinal study of patients with rheumatoid arthritis. Arthritis Rheum 1995; 38:44–8.
10. Aletaha D, Smolen J. The simplified disease activity index (SDAI) and the clinical disease activity index (CDAI): a review of their usefulness and validity in rheumatoid arthritis. Clin Exp Rheumatol 2005; 23:S100-S108.
11. Pincus T, Swearingen CJ, Bergman MJ, Colglazier CL, Kaell A, Kunath A, et al. RAPID3 on an MDHAQ is correlated significantly with activity levels of DAS28 and CDAI, but scored in 5 versus more than 90 seconds. Arthritis Care Res 2010; 62(2):181–9.
12. Pincus T, Hines P, Bergman MJ, Yazici Y, Rosenblatt LC, Maclean R. Proposed severity and response criteria for Routine Assessment of Patient Index Data (RAPID3): results for categories of disease activity and response criteria in abatacept clinical trials. J Rheumatol 2011; 38(12):2565–71.
13. Pincus T, Yazici Y, Bergman MJ. RAPID3, an index to assess and monitor patients with rheumatoid arthritis, without formal joint counts: similar results to DAS28 and CDAI in clinical trials and clinical care. Rheum Dis Clin North Am 2009; 35(4):773–8.
14. Felson DT, Smolen JS, Wells G, Zhang B, van Tuyl LH, Funovits J, et al. American College of Rheumatology/European League Against Rheumatism provisional definition of remission in rheumatoid arthritis for clinical trials. Arthritis Rheum 2011; 63(3):573–86.
15. Konstam V, Salem D, Pouleur H, Kostis J, Gorkin L, Shumaker S, et al. Baseline quality of life as a predictor of mortality and hospitalization in 5,025 patients with congestive heart failure. Am J Cardiol 1996; 78(8):890–5.
16. Justice AC, Aiken LH, Smith HL, Turner BJ. The role of functional status in predicating inpatient mortality with AIDS: A comparison with current predictors. J Clin Epidemiol 1996; 49:193–201.
17. Covinsky KE, Justice AC, Rosenthal GE, Palmer RM, Landefeld S. Measuring prognosis and case mix in hospitalized elders. The importance of functional status. J Gen Intern Med 1997; 12:203–8.
18. Castrejón I, McCollum L, Durusu Tanriover M, Pincus T. Importance of patient history and physical examination in rheumatoid arthritis compared to other chronic diseases: Results of a physician survey. Arthritis Care Res 2012; 64(8):1250–5.
19. Esen F, Celik A, Yazici H. The use of diseased control groups in genetic association studies. Clin Exp Rheumatol 2009; 27(2 Suppl 53):S4-S5.
20. Pincus T, Yazici Y, Sokka T. Complexities in assessment of rheumatoid arthritis: absence of a single gold standard measure. Rheum Dis Clin North Am 2009; 35(4):687–97.
21. Pincus T, Bergman MJ, Maclean R, Yazici Y. Complex measures and indices for clinical research compared with simple patient questionnaires to assess function, pain, and global estimates as rheumatology "vital signs" for usual clinical care. Rheum Dis Clin North Am 2009; 35(4):779–86.

22. Pincus T, Brooks RH, Callahan LF. Prediction of long-term mortality in patients with rheumatoid arthritis according to simple questionnaire and joint count measures. Ann Intern Med 1994; 120:26–34.
23. Fuchs HA, Callahan LF, Kaye JJ, Brooks RH, Nance EP, Pincus T. Radiographic and joint count findings of the hand in rheumatoid arthritis: Related and unrelated findings. Arthritis Rheum 1988; 31:44–51.
24. Hannan MT, Felson DT, Pincus T. Analysis of the discordance between radiographic changes and knee pain in osteoarthritis of the knee. J Rheumatol 2000; 27:1513–7.
25. Engel GL. The biopsychosocial model and the education of health professionals. Ann N Y Acad Sci 1978; 310:169–81.
26. McCollum L, Pincus T. A biopsychosocial model to complement a biomedical model: patient questionnaire data and socioeconomic status usually are more significant than laboratory tests and imaging studies in prognosis of rheumatoid arthritis. Rheum Dis Clin North Am 2009; 35(4):699–712.
27. Holman HR. Thought barriers to understanding rheumatic diseases. Arthritis Rheum 1994; 37:1565–72.2011.
28. Riley V. Mouse mammary tumors: alteration of incidence as apparent function of stress. Science 1975;189(4201):465–7.
29. Feinstein AR. An additional basic science for clinical medicine: II. The limitations of randomized trials. Ann Intern Med 1983; 99:544–50.
30. Howick J. The Philosophy of Evidence-Based Medicine. Oxford: Wiley-Blackwell;
31. Trohler U. An early 18th-century proposal for improving medicine by tabulating and analysing practice. J R Soc Med 2010; 103(9):379–80.
32. MRC Streptomycin in Tuberculosis Trials Committee. Streptomycin treatment of pulmonary tuberculosis. Br Med J 1948; 2(4582):769–82.
33. Hickey S, Roberts H. Tarnished Gold: The Sickness of Evidence Based Medicine. CreateSpace; 2011.
34. Stamatakis E, Weiler R, Ioannidis JP. Undue industry influences that distort healthcare research, strategy, expenditure and practice: a review. Eur J Clin Invest 2013; 43(5):469–75.
35. OCEBM Levels of Evidence Working Group. The Oxford 2011 Levels of Evidence. http://www.cebm.net/index.aspx?o=5653. 2011. Oxford U.K., Oxford Centre for Evidence-Based Medicine
36. Smith GCS, Pell JP. Parachute use to prevent death and major trauma related to gravitational challenge: systematic review of randomised controlled trials. BMJ 2003; 327:1459–61.
37. Glasziou P, Chalmers I, Rawlins M, McCulloch P. When are randomised trials unnecessary? Picking signal from noise. BMJ 2007; 334(7589):349–51.
38. Aronson JK, Hauben M. Anecdotes that provide definitive evidence. BMJ 2006; 333(7581):1267–9.

A Review of Statistical Approaches for the Analysis of Data in Rheumatology

Emmanuel Lesaffre and Jolanda Luime

Introduction

Too often statistics is regarded as a set of rules, even recipes, to end up in a final *P*-value or at best a confidence interval. Good Statistical Practice (GSP) is much more than (even correctly) applying a bunch of statistical tests. In fact, it involves the whole research process from posing the appropriate research questions to writing up the results and drawing the appropriate conclusions. The order in which the statistical techniques are discussed in this chapter somewhat reflects how the statistical analysis of comparative studies is done. We start with descriptive statistics, look at methods to compare two or more treatments, and then discuss correlation and regression techniques to finally review methods for the analysis of follow-up studies. We also briefly discuss multivariate statistical approaches. In addition, we draw the attention to possible pitfalls of the discussed methods to provide guidance in analyzing data. While no clear-cut recipes for GSP can be expected, we hope that this chapter helps the reader in preparing a well-motivated statistical plan and analysis.

The appropriate choice of statistical analysis depends on many factors, such as the type of measurement (continuous, categorical, count, etc.), the research question (comparison of two groups, establishing relationship between one measurement and

E. Lesaffre, Dr. Sc. (✉)
Department of Biostatistics, Erasmus MC, Dr. Molewaterplein, 50-60, Rotterdam 3015 GE, The Netherlands

L-Biostat, KU Leuven, Leuven, Belgium
e-mail: e.lesaffre@erasmusmc.nl

J. Luime, PhD
Department of Rheumatology, Erasmus MC, P.O. Box 2040, Rotterdam 3000 CA, The Netherlands
e-mail: j.luime@erasmusmc.nl

H. Yazici et al. (eds.), *Understanding Evidence-Based Rheumatology*,
DOI 10.1007/978-3-319-08374-2_2

other measurements, etc.), the size of the study, the presence and amount of missing data, outliers in the study, etc. These aspects will be discussed in this chapter.

The statistical techniques are illustrated using the data from two rheumatoid arthritis studies conducted in Erasmus MC in Rotterdam, i.e., the RAPPORT and the tREACH study. Besides these two data sets, fictive data (inspired by the above two data sets) were generated to illustrate some statistical concepts. We used here exclusively the freely available R software [1]; however, software packages like SAS® [2], SPSS® [3], etc. could have also been used. For more elaborate texts on statistics (and some more technical details), many handbooks in the literature can be consulted, e.g., [4] and [5].

Data Sets

RAPPORT Study

The Rheumatoid Arthritis Patients rePort Onset Reactivation study (*RAPPORT study*) [6] was a longitudinal study that aimed to identify an increase in disease activity by self-reported questionnaires in the 3 months preceding the clinical assessment. In this study, 159 patients aged 18 years and older with rheumatoid arthritis (RA) or polyarthritis using disease-modifying antirheumatic drugs (DMARDs) for at least 3 months were recruited. Patient disease activities were evaluated using the Disease Activity Score of 28 joints (DAS28) every 3 months as part of their standard care by a rheumatologist at the clinic. The DAS28 is a composite index [7, 8], which varies between 0 and 10, built up from swollen joint count, tender joint count, a visual analog scale of the patient's assessment of general health, and erythrocyte sedimentation rate at the first hour. A higher score of DAS28 indicates a higher disease activity. Treatment was recommended to be intensified when DAS28 > 3.2 and may be tapered down at DAS28 < 2.6.

In addition, the self-reported instruments consisting of Health Assessment Questionnaires (HAQ), Rheumatoid Arthritis Disease Activity Index (RADAI), a visual analog scale of the patient's global assessment of disease activity (VAS global), and a visual analog scale for fatigue (VAS fatigue), were measured using a web-based form producing patient-reported outcomes (PROs). The HAQ contains eight dimensions of daily functional activities such as dressing, rising, eating, walking, hygiene, reach, and grip, and is scored from 0 to 3 on a Likert scale with 3 corresponding to the worst condition [9]. Further, the RADAI measures the self-reported disease activity and is composed of five items, each varying between 0 and 10 (for items 4 and 5, see [10]): (1) global disease activity during the previous month, (2) disease activity in terms of swollen and tender joints throughout the day, (3) amount of arthritis pain throughout the day, (4) morning stiffness, and (5) self-assessed tender joints. The VAS global was used to estimate the patient's assessment for general health. Note that the VAS global is also a part of the DAS28. Finally, the VAS fatigue measures the severity of the patient's fatigue over the previous week by a similar VAS scale [11].

tREACH Study

The tREACH is a trial within the Rotterdam Early Arthritis CoHort (tREACH) [12, 13]. It is a multicenter, stratified single-blinded trial conducted in eight rheumatology centers in the Netherlands. RA patients older than 18 years, with arthritis in ≥1 joint(s), and symptoms less than 1 year are included. Eligible patients were stratified into three strata (low, intermediate, and high) according to their likelihood of progressing to persistent arthritis (i.e., RA) based on the Visser prediction rule [14], a precursor of the new ACR/EULAR RA 2010 classification criteria [15]. For this chapter we use patients with a high risk who were randomized into one of the following initial treatment strategies: (1) triple DMARD therapy (MTX, sulphasalazine, and hydroxychloroquine with GCs intramuscular), (2) triple DMARD therapy with an oral GC tapering scheme, and (3) MTX with oral GCs as in strategy 2 [12].

Describing the Collected Data

An essential first step in any empirical research is to describe the collected data with numerical values and/or graphical displays. The way this is done depends on the type of data. We consider here: categorical data (ordinal and nominal), counts, and continuous data. *Categorical* data, like adverse events in a drug trial, are typically summarized in tables with frequencies (and proportions or percentages) of each possible outcome as entries. A *bar chart* with these entries displayed as the heights of bars is a common graphical display for such data. When there is ordering in the values of the categorical variable, e.g., severity of the adverse event, one speaks of an *ordinal* variable. For a *nominal* variable, values are not ordered, e.g., for a particular type of adverse event. A special case of a categorical variable is a *binary* or *dichotomous* variable, where there are only two possible values. An example is gender and for this the nominal variable "1" could stand for men and "2" for women. In the RAPPORT study, there are 121 (76 %) men and 38 (24 %) women.

For variables with at least an ordinal character but with too many different values (e.g., DAS28), counts, and *continuous* variables (e.g., weight), the *histogram* provides a better way to graphically summarize the distribution of the data. Now the X-axis is split up into (often equally sized) intervals, and in each interval, the frequency (proportion/percentage) of values is represented as a bar (in another version the area of the bar represents frequencies/proportions/percentages). The histogram not only shows the spread of the collected data but can also spot *outlying values*, which are values that are located remotely from the bulk of the data. Figure 1a, b show the histograms of baseline DAS28 and HAQ values of the RAPPORT study, respectively. The histogram of DAS28 is (roughly) symmetric around its *mean*, defined as $\overline{X} = \frac{1}{n}\sum_{i=1}^{n} X_i$ where X_i represents here the DAS28 value for the ith patient and $n = 159$ is the size of the RAPPORT study. The symbol $\sum_{i=1}^{n}$ signifies that the sum

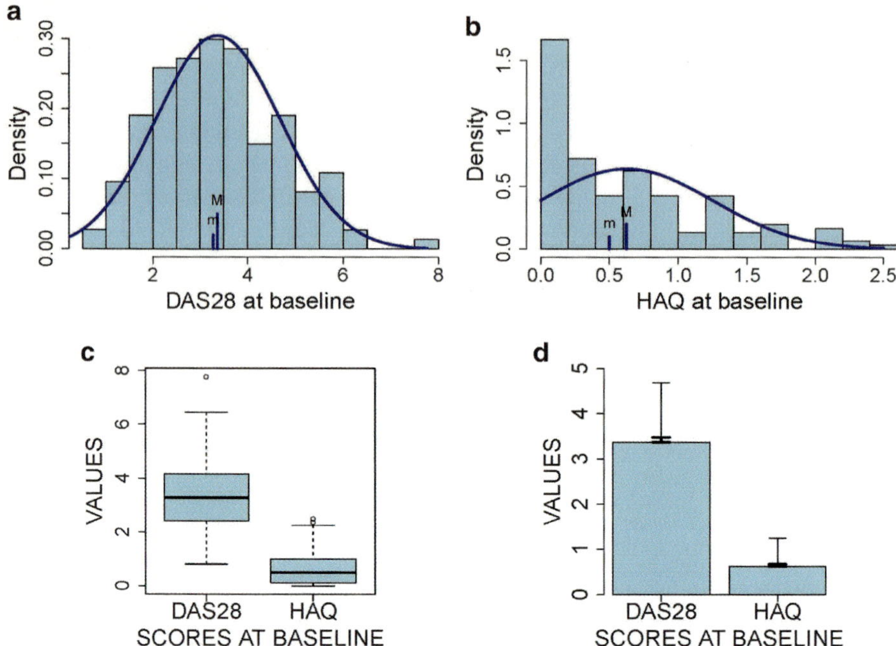

Fig. 1 RAPPORT study: (**a**) histogram of DAS28 at baseline together with the best fitting normal distribution, (**b**) histogram of HAQ at baseline together with the best fitting normal distribution, (**c**) box plots of DAS28 and HAQ at baseline, and (**d**) error bar plots of DAS28 and HAQ at baseline. The histograms have the property that the total area of the bars is equal to one. *M* represents the mean and *m* represents the median. In the error bar plots, the longest bars have length equal to the standard deviation; the shortest bars represent the SEM

is taken of all 159 patients of the RAPPORT study. In contrast, HAQ has a right-*skewed* distribution (with a right tail). The *median* value corresponds to the value such that 50 % of the observations are left to it; it is also referred to as the *50%-ile* and denoted as $Q_{50.}$ While the median can always be interpreted as a central value, this is not necessarily the case for the mean value, see, e.g., Fig. 1b for HAQ. The spread of the collected data around a central value can be expressed in various ways. The *standard deviation* (denoted as *s* or *SD*) is the square root of the *variance* s^2, which is equal to the average squared deviation of the data from their mean, i.e., $s^2 = \frac{1}{n-1}\sum_{i=1}^{n}\left(X_i - \overline{X}\right)^2$. The SD has the advantage over the variance that it is expressed in the original units of the data. For example, since blood pressure is measured in mmHg, the variance is expressed in mmHg^2, while the SD is also expressed in mmHg.

When the SD is greater in treatment arm A than in arm B, we conclude that the variability of the data must be greater in A than in B. However, apart from this interpretation, it is not immediately obvious how the SD relates to the spread of the data. An alternative, easier-to-interpret, measure is the *interquartile range* (*IQR*), defined as $Q_{75} - Q_{25}$, where Q_{25} is the *25 %-ile* and Q_{75} is the *75 %-ile* of the data. The IQR is therefore easily understood as the length of the central interval that contains 50 % of the data. The mean and median are called *summary statistics for location*, while SD and IQR summarize the *variability* of the data. The mean/median (SD/IQR) for DAS28 in Fig. 1a is 3.37/3.28 (SD = 1.31/ IQR = 3.28 − 2.42 = 0.86), while for HAQ (Fig. 1b) we have 0.62/0.50 (SD = 0.63/IQR = 1.00 − 0.125 = 0.875).

It is customary to summarize continuous data in medical publications with *mean ± SD*. While not always understood, this tradition stems from assuming that the interval [mean-SD, mean + SD] contains 68 % of the central data. However, this interpretation only holds when the histogram can be well approximated by the *Gauss curve or distribution*. The Gauss distribution, also called the "*normal*" distribution, is the most used distribution in mathematics and statistics, see, e.g., [4, 5]. It reflects the stochastic behavior of a random measure that is the result of the sum of many independent causative factors. Typical measurements that have a normal distribution in a general population are height and weight. For DAS28 the interval [3.37 − 1.31, 3.37 + 1.31] contains indeed 68 % of the central data. The 68 % CI for HAQ, equal to [0.62 − 0.63, 0.62 + 0.63], contains about 80 % of the data, but more importantly it contains negative values, which is clearly nonsense. In Fig. 1, we observe that the Gauss curve approximates well the histogram of DAS28, but not for HAQ.

The *error bar plot* is a popular way to graphically represent the characteristics of the data. In Fig. 1d we show this plot for DAS28 and HAQ. The height of the rectangle is equal to the mean, while the bar emanating from it has length equal to the SD. Hence, this plot graphically displays the interval [mean, mean + SD]. While popular, this plot cannot reveal a possibly skewed distribution of the data. An alternative graph is the *box (−whisker) plot* shown in Fig. 1c. The edges of the box represent Q_{25} (lower edge) and Q_{75} (upper edge); the horizontal line represents the median. The lines emanating from the box are called *whiskers*. The whiskers give a graphical impression of the skewness of the distribution. The dots indicate *outlying values*. The definition of the whiskers and outliers depend on the software (here, R).

Time-to-event data express the time until the event of interest occurs. This event includes, besides death, also nonterminal events such as remission (DAS < 1.6) in an RA study, a cardiac event in a cardiology study, caries in a dental study, etc. Another term for such data is *survival time*. Typically, survival times have a (right) skewed distribution, and hence the median (and IQR) is here preferred over the mean (and SD). However, most often the exact survival time is not known but is *censored*. A survival time is *right censored* when it is only known that the event hasn't happened during the conduct of the study. *Left censoring* occurs when event happened before the patient entered the study. This may occur in retrospective studies but such patients are excluded in cohort studies where an association between a risk factor and the event is examined. *Interval censoring* is relatively common in clinical studies. A survival time is interval censored when it is only known that the event has occurred between two examinations. In this chapter we consider only right censoring. There are various reasons for (right) censoring. For instance, when patients are recruited rather late in the study, the probability is low that they will experience the event. Other reasons are: a patient leaves the study prior to experiencing the event because he changed medication, because of adverse events, because the patient died, etc. It is important to mention that the time at which censoring occurs must not be correlated with the survival time. For instance, removing patients from the study immediately prior to experiencing an event will bias the results and the conclusions of every survival analysis applied to the time-to-event data.

Classical statistical descriptive and inference techniques are not appropriate for survival data. Indeed, for a right-censored survival time, the true survival is only known to be greater than its recorded value. Hence, the mean (median, SD, histogram, box plot, etc.) of the recorded (censored) survival times cannot provide a good estimate of the mean (median, etc.) of the true survival times. Indeed, dedicated techniques are needed in such a case, such as the *Kaplan–Meier curve*. This curve is a proper estimate of the distribution of the true survival times, called the *survivor function*. In Fig. 2, we show the Kaplan–Meier curve of a fictive RA study where RA patients were followed up from the first time they were in remission until their DAS increased above 1.6. This curve shows for each possible survival time (less than the maximum observed time) the estimated proportion of subjects in remission. The Kaplan–Meier curve provides also an estimate of the median survival time, which here is 1.5 months; see Fig. 2. However, the Kaplan–Meier curve cannot provide other descriptive statistics such as the mean survival and its SD. Note that, in the fictive RA study, we assumed right censoring, while in practice, interval censoring certainly would apply since DAS needs to be determined at examination times by the treating rheumatologist.

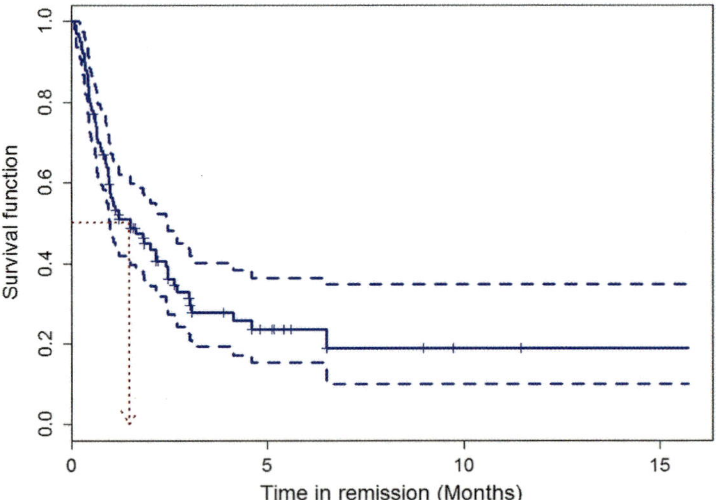

Fig. 2 Fictive study: Kaplan–Meier curve that estimates for each time point the proportion of patients that are still in remission. The symbol "+" indicates when the "survival" time is right censored. The *arrow points* to the estimated median "survival" time. The *dashed lines* correspond to the 95 % CIs at each observed time of "death"

Introduction to Statistical Inference

The Sample and the Population

The goal of drug research is to establish the effect of an experimental medication for all possible eligible patients. These patients constitute the *population*. The population of subjects for whom the drug may apply is to some extent artificial since some of the eligible patients may not have been born yet. For this reason, but also due to practical (financial, time constraints, etc.) considerations, it is almost never possible to examine the whole population of interest, and one must confine to a limited set of subjects.

When the sample is taken in a random manner from the population, probability laws can tell us how the sample characteristics vary around the population characteristics. For instance, when a new DMARD reduces DAS28 after 3 months on the average with 0.5, then this average will fluctuate from study to study around its true mean μ (=0.5). The variability in the study mean is expressed by the *standard error of the mean* (SEM). It is in principle impossible to know SEM since studies are never repeated in exactly the same way. However, from probability laws, we know that it can be estimated from a single study using the formula $\text{SEM} = {}^{s}\!/_{\sqrt{n}}$. This formula shows that when the patient population is homogeneous (small variance) and/or the study is large, there is little variation of the sample mean around the true mean and then taking the study mean for the population mean will not induce a great error. One can also guess the distance between the true and sample mean with the *confidence interval* (*CI*). Namely, the 95 % confidence interval given by $\left[\bar{X} - 2 \times \text{SEM}, \bar{X} + 2 \times \text{SEM}\right]$ contains the true mean with 0.95 probability. Note that the coefficient "2" in the above expression is approximate and varies with the study size, as seen later. Thus, the smaller the 95 % CI, the more precise statement we can make about the true mean. For the RAPPORT study, the SEM of the mean DAS28 at baseline is equal to ${}^{1.31}\!/_{\sqrt{147}} = 0.11$ (for some patients, DAS28 is missing), yielding a 95 % CI equal to [3.15, 3.58]. This implies that we are not sure about the true mean of DAS28, but we believe with 95 % certainty that it is greater than 3.15 and smaller than 3.58. For HAQ at baseline, we obtained an $\text{SEM} = {}^{0.63}\!/_{\sqrt{153}} = 0.05$ and the 95 % CI now becomes [0.52, 0.72]. Bars have been added in Fig. 1 that represent the SEM.

Finally, note that the 95 % CI is most popular, but confidence intervals of any size can be determined. In fact, occasionally one reports the 90 % CI or the 99 % CI.

The above probability properties hold when the sample is taken from the population by random sampling (simple random sampling or a more sophisticated version) mechanism. This is often not possible but rather a *convenience sample* is taken, as with the RAPPORT study. This is a sample that is obtained by simply collecting the information from (consecutive) patients who are available to the investigator.

The problem with a convenience sample is that it is not obvious how the results can be extrapolated to a well-defined population. A similar problem occurs with randomized clinical trials (see chapter "The randomized controlled trial: methodological perspectives").

Basic Tools for Statistical Inference

Statistical inference is the activity to draw conclusions from subjects examined in an experimental or observational study for use in future similar subjects. For example, in the RAPPORT study, we might be interested to know whether the change in average DAS28 (in a 12 months' period) differs between men and women. The average difference (DAS28 at 12 months – DAS28 at baseline) for the 26 men for whom both measurements were recorded is equal to 0.10 (so in fact an increase in disease activity was noticed) and it is −0.052 for the 81 women. The difference in averages is not equal to zero. But our interest lies in the difference of means between men and women for the populations from which the RAPPORT patients were taken, i.e., in the difference between μ_{male} and μ_{female}. The 95 % CI of $\mu_{female} - \mu_{male}$, computed from the patients with a recorded DAS28 value at both examinations, is equal to [−0.69, 0.38]. This interval expresses what we know about the true difference from the patients in the RAPPORT study. Since this interval includes zero, we cannot rule out a zero difference in the true means and we decide that there is no (strong) evidence of a different mean change in DAS28 after 12 months of treatment between men and women. Suppose now that we wish to know whether the mean age of women in the RAPPORT study is different from that of men. The mean age of the 121 women is 51.5 years, while for the 38 men, it is 58.4 years. Again we compute the 95 % CI of $\mu_{female} - \mu_{male}$, where μ now represents the average age, and obtain [−11.60, −2.08] (in years). Now the interval excludes zero; hence, we conclude that there is (strong) evidence that on average women are younger than men in the RAPPORT population.

The confidence interval provides a direct way to draw inference from the study to the population. Yet, a more popular and indirect way of inference is based on the *P-value*. When comparing two (unknown true) means, μ_1 and μ_2, one can distinguish two hypotheses:

$$H_0, \mu_1 = \mu_2 \left(\text{or } \Delta = \mu_1 - \mu_2 = 0\right) \quad \text{and} \quad H_a, \mu_1 \neq \mu_2 \left(\text{or } \Delta = \mu_1 - \mu_2 \neq 0\right)$$

The hypothesis of interest is given by H_a, called the *alternative hypothesis*. To test this hypothesis, one reasons indirectly and questions whether H_0, called the *null hypothesis*, can be rejected. This is done via the *P*-value. To establish the *P*-value, one computes the difference of the two observed means and evaluates the extremeness of this difference if $\Delta = 0$ were true. The *P*-value is the result of a *statistical test* and expresses the probability that the observed difference (or more extreme) could have been obtained under H_0. A P-value is sometimes referred to as a *surprise index*. When the P-value is small, doubt is raised about H_0 and one is inclined to reject it. Classically a P-value less than 0.05 or less than 0.01 is considered a value too small to sustain the null hypothesis. When $P<0.05$, one says that the result is *statistically significant at 0.05*; when $P \geq 0.05$, a *nonsignificant result* is obtained. The value of 0.05 is called the *significance level of the test* (in statistical handbooks denoted as $\alpha=0.05$). The significance level needs to be chosen prior to performing the computations. In this chapter we consider only $\alpha=0.05$, which is the most popular choice but there is in principle nothing against choosing $\alpha=0.01$ or $\alpha=0.10$, or any other value as long as the significance level is specified prior to performing the test. The average decrease in DAS28 in 1 year's time between men and women corresponds to $P=0.57$, which is not smaller than 0.05, and hence we see no (strong) evidence against H_0. The conclusion is then that the two groups are not statistically significantly different at 0.05 (often denoted as *NS*). On the other hand, for the comparison of the average age between men and women, we find $P=0.0052$. This result is now statistically significant at 0.05 (often indicated by *) and we state that H_0 is rejected at 0.05.

The statistical test used above is the *two-sample t-test*, also referred to as the *Student's t-test*. The test consists in computing a standardized difference of the two sample means $\bar{X}_1$ and $\bar{X}_2$, i.e., $T=\left(\bar{X}_1-\bar{X}_2\right)/\mathrm{SE}\left(\bar{X}_1-\bar{X}_2\right)$, whereby $\mathrm{SE}\left(\bar{X}_1-\bar{X}_2\right)$ is the standard error of the difference in means (similar to the SEM of a single mean). This standardized difference T is then compared to a reference distribution, here the *t-distribution* with (n_1+n_2-2) *degrees of freedom* (*df*). This distribution reflects the natural variability of T under the null hypothesis that $\Delta=0$. The degrees of freedom is a parameter that depends on the sample sizes of the groups and determines the particular t-distribution. Note that when df $\geq$30, the t-distribution becomes close to the normal distribution. For the comparison of the change in DAS28 between men and women, df $=26+81-2=105$. Under the null hypothesis one expects that T varies around zero, which translates into a statement that under H_0 there is 95 % chance that T is located between two extreme values roughly equal to −2 and 2 (which change with df). Observed T values outside this central interval thus indicate that the null hypothesis may not be true and correspond to a P-value smaller than 0.05. For the DAS28 comparison, this interval is equal to [−1.983, 1.983]. We obtained $T=-0.577$, which belongs to the above central interval and therefore $P>0.05$. For the comparison of the mean ages between men and women, df $=157$ and the central interval is now [−1.975, 1.975]. Since $T=-2.836$ does not belong to this interval, $P<0.05$.

The two-sample t-test is one of the many statistical tests that were developed over the last century to address the various research questions posed in empirical research. Much of this chapter deals with reviewing a variety of statistical tests. A list of popular statistical tests to compare two groups is given in Table 1 and will be further below discussed in section "Statistical tests to compare two groups."

Table 1 Overview of classical statistical tests to compare two groups

Type of measurement	Distributional assumptions	Large study	Small study
Unpaired			
Continuous	Normal in each group and = variance	Two sample *t*-test	Two sample *t*-test
	Normal in each group and ≠ variance	Welch test	Welch test
Continuous	Not normal and = variance	Two sample *t*-test	Wilcoxon rank-sum or Mann–Whitney test[a]
	Not normal and ≠ variance	Welch test	
Binary		Chi-square test	Chi-square test + correction
			Fisher's exact test
Paired			
Continuous	Difference normally distributed	Paired *t*-test	Paired *t*-test
	Difference not normally distributed	Paired *t*-test	Wilcoxon signed-rank test[a]
Binary		McNemar test	McNemar test + correction
			Binomial test

[a]Can also be used for ordinal data

One-Sided and Two-Sided Confidence Intervals and Tests

The confidence intervals and *P*-values introduced in the previous section are *two sided*. For example, in section "The sample and the population," we have seen that the 95 % CI of the mean DAS28 at baseline is equal to [3.15, 3.58]. This interval is bounded at both sides and contains with 0.95 probability the true value. Further, there is 0.025 probability that the true value is below 3.51 and 0.025 probability that the true value is greater than 3.58. We could, however, also give a *one-sided* interval like [3.15, infinity]. This interval expresses that there is 97.5 % probability that the true value is above 3.15. Most often, though, a 95 % two-sided interval is reported.

The *P*-values reported in the section "Basic tools for statistical inference" above are also two sided and therefore sometimes denoted as *2P*. When comparing two means, this means that the null hypothesis will be rejected when the standardized difference of means is either too large positively or too large negatively. Often in practice we must be able to reject the null hypothesis for large positive and large negative differences. Let's take the following example from drug research: A drug company is primarily interested to discover whether their drug is working better than the control drug. In other words, the prime interest lies in rejecting a difference in favor of the experimental drug. Suppose that in a large study, the standardized difference is equal to 1.69 (value obtained from standard normal table) in favor of the experimental drug. Since under the null hypothesis of equal treatment effects, 5 % of the studies show a better result than 1.68, the one-sided *P*-value is smaller than 0.05. But the threshold for two-sided significance is 1.96, and hence at a two-sided level of 0.05, the result is not significant at 0.05. "One-sided" means that we look only in one direction, here in the direction of a better result for the experimental treatment. On the other hand, suppose that the standardized difference is equal to −3, then the two-sided *P*-value is smaller than 0.01 pointing toward a worse effect of the experimental treatment. However, the one-sided *P*-value in the direction of a beneficial effect of the experimental treatment is greater than 0.999. While there is no evidence for a significantly better result for the experimental treatment, there is also no evidence for a worse effect with the one-sided test because one looks away from worse experimental results. Therefore, regulatory agencies demand to use two-sided tests (except for non-inferiority tests, see chapter "The randomized controlled trial: methodological perspectives").

Type I Error, Type II Error, and the Power of a Test

The fundamental problem in empirical research is that one is never sure about the truth. In fact, if the truth were known then empirical research is obsolete and statistical inference is not needed. Hence, it is upfront never clear whether the null or the alternative hypothesis is true so that every decision based on observed data is prone to two errors. The *Type I error* represents the error when one concludes that the alternative hypothesis is true (e.g., two treatments have a different effect), while the null hypothesis is in fact true (the true treatments have equal effect). But the researcher may also decide that there is no evidence for the alternative hypothesis, while in fact it represents the truth. In the latter case, a *Type II error* is committed and then the researcher fails to see that the two treatments really differ in efficacy. The Type I error is controlled by the construction of the statistical test. Namely, by choosing a significance level of 0.05, one automatically fixes the probability of the Type I error to 0.05, called *Type I error rate*. However, the probability of the Type II error is not fixed in advance and depends on, among other things, the study size. The probability of not committing the Type II error is known as the *power of the test* and is equal to the probability of finding a clinically relevant difference in the two groups, if it exists. Establishing the sample size to achieve a desirable power is a necessity in randomized controlled trials but is also desirable in explorative studies. Such a computation is, however, quite technical (see chapter "The randomized controlled trial: methodological perspectives").

The above reasoning indicates that statistical inference is based on *repeated sampling* ideas. That is, the significance level of 0.05 means that the probability of a Type I error is fixed at 0.05. In other words, (even) if the null hypothesis is true then roughly five out of hundred (independent) statistical tests are significant at 0.05. The practical implication is that, when a large number of statistical tests are performed in a study, say that a few hundred of variables are compared between two groups with about 5 % of them statistically significant at 0.05, then, quite likely, the two groups are not different at all (null hypothesis is probably true). Similarly, the power is also expressed in terms of repeated samplings. Namely, when the power is 0.80 for a clinically relevant different effect, say Δ_a, then we expect in 100 similar studies at least 80 of them with a statistically significant result at 0.05 if the difference is indeed at least Δ_a. Finally, the technical definition of the 95 % CI is that in 95 % of the studies set up in the same way as the current study, the true population value is included in the 95 % CI. But for the current study, the true value is inside or outside that interval. This approach of statistical inference, called the *frequentist approach*, is still most popular in clinical research.

In the frequentist approach, the null hypothesis of equality of group means, proportions, etc. can never be demonstrated. Admitted, such a hypothesis never holds in practice (except when two identical treatments are administered). A nonsignificant result must therefore be interpreted as the "absence of evidence against the null hypothesis" possibly due to a too small study size.

The *Bayesian approach* is an increasingly popular statistical approach for inference but based on quite different principles. In this approach, the role of the *P*-value is taken over by a probability that the hypothesis of interest is true after having done the experiment, called the *posterior probability*. This probability addresses, in contrast to the *P*-value, the research question directly. In section "The Bayesian approach" we will elaborate on this approach.

Choice Between **P**-*Value and Confidence Interval*

The analyses of the RAPPORT study in section "Basic tools for statistical inference" show that zero is inside/outside the 95 % CI of a difference in means when the result is not statistically/statistically significant at 0.05. This is true for most statistical tests. We have:

$P \geq 0.05$ (<0.05) if and only if the 95 % CI of the difference does (not) include zero.

The 95 % CI is, however, more informative than the *P*-value since it also provides the uncertainty with which the true effect is estimated. With the *P*-value, inference is disconnected from the substantive problem and may easily lead to interpretational problems. For instance, there is a long-standing debate in the literature about whether a significant *P*-value weighs more in a large rather than in a small study [16]. Major clinical journals like the *NEJM*, *the Lancet*, etc. now require reporting confidence intervals. For instance, the NEJM guidelines for the authors stipulate: "Measures of uncertainty, such as confidence intervals, should be used consistently, including in figures that present aggregated results." Nevertheless, the *P*-value is still here to stand for some time. However, it will probably not be the only basis for statistical inference in the future.

Use and Misuse of the **P**-*Value*

The *P*-value remains the most used but also the most misused tool for statistical inference. For instance, the *P*-value is often misinterpreted as the probability that the posed hypothesis is correct. This, in fact, is the very probability which clearly interests the researcher most. However, it can only be obtained by the Bayesian approach, as will be seen in section "The Bayesian approach."

Another quite frequent misuse of the *P*-value consists in ignoring the increased risk of committing a Type I error when repeatedly testing for significance. This is called the *multiple testing problem*. An example illustrates the problem. An experimental treatment is compared to a control treatment in two different studies, with a *P*-value of 0.03 in the first study and a *P*-value of 0.06 in the second study, both in favor of the experimental arm. With $\alpha = 0.05$, there is in each study a risk of 5 % to claim that the two treatments are different while they are in fact equally effective. If better performance of the experimental treatment is concluded when at least one of the studies shows a significant result at 0.05, then the total risk under the null hypothesis of committing a Type I error is about 10 % and not 5 %—what we aimed at!

The *Bonferroni correction provides an* easy but somewhat crude way to deal with the multiple testing problem. For two tests, the Bonferroni correction consists in dividing the significance level by two, i.e., $\alpha = 0.5/2 = 0.025$. Significance in each test is then claimed only if $P < 0.025$, reducing the overall risk back to approximately 5 %. In our example the treatments cannot be claimed different in efficacy based on Bonferroni's correction. For k tests, Bonferroni correction consists in dividing the significance level by k, i.e., α/k. For k large, it will then become hard to claim any result significant at 0.05. Equivalent to Bonferroni's correction is multiplying the *P*-value with the number of statistical tests, and check whether the product is lower than α [17]. For example, with 10 tests, $10 \times P$ must be smaller than 0.05 for a test to be called significant at 0.05. In chapter "The randomized controlled trial: methodological perspectives", we will treat more refined ways to correct for multiple testing in controlled clinical trials.

There are several versions of the multiple testing problem. Examples are: two treatments compared in several studies (above example), two treatments compared at several time points or for several variables, more than two treatments compared, etc. In (medical) publications, many statistical tests are often needed to arrive at a sound (clinical) conclusion. Correction for multiple testing may not always be an issue, especially for the exploratory part of the study, as long as one is clear about the nature (exploratory) of the tests. A greater concern is *opportunistic testing*, i.e., searching as long as the tests confirm what you always wanted to prove. This is called *data dredging* and emerges especially with a lot of data but no available scientific theory. Finally, we note that statistical testing does not always make sense. For instance, a significance test that compares the baseline characteristics of treatments in a randomized controlled trial makes no sense since at the start, the treatment groups are by definition sampled from the same population.

Statistical Tests to Compare Two Groups

Factors That Determine the Choice of the Statistical Test

Table 1 contains common statistical tests to compare two groups of subjects. The choice of the appropriate test depends on many factors and here we consider four factors: (1) paired versus unpaired data, (2) continuous or binary data, (3) small versus large study, and (4) whether distributional assumptions are met or not. Statistical tests for counts are not included in the table since they are often analyzed (after transformation) as continuous data. If needed, the reader can check the statistical literature for more appropriate tests.

Examples of *paired* data are two measurements taken on the same subject at two time points or sometimes measurements recorded on siblings. This comes down to two groups of related data, where one group contains the first measurements and the other group the second measurements. With *unpaired* data, there is no (systematic) relationship between the measurements. Two groups of continuous data are most often compared via the difference in means or via whole distributions, depending whether some distributional assumptions are met or not. Two proportions are compared in different ways, depending on the type of study. With two observed proportions p_1 and p_2, the *absolute risk reduction AR* is defined as $p_1 - p_2$. In epidemiological research, it is more customary to work with the *relative risk* $\mathrm{RR} = p_2/p_1$ or the *odds ratio* $\mathrm{OR} = \dfrac{p_2/(1-p_2)}{p_1/(1-p_1)}$.

Another factor is the size of the study. However, we must admit that a general definition of a large study is lacking, since it depends on technical aspects of the statistical test. For instance, two groups of 1,000 subjects certainly qualify for a large study to compare two means, but perhaps not when two proportions of rare events are compared.

Furthermore, in applying certain tests, some distributional assumptions need to be met, like that the data should have a normal distribution or that variances should be equal.

That the choice of a statistical test depends on the above (and even other) conditions is purely technical and depends on probability laws developed under the above-specified conditions; see, e.g., [4, 5]. When the aforementioned conditions are fulfilled, the reported *P*-value and 95 % CI are correct. But these conditions rarely apply exactly in practice. For instance, data are never exactly normally distributed. Usually *simulation studies* are conducted to determine the operational characteristics of these tests under deviations from these conditions. This gives us a hint of when the reported *P*-value and 95 % CI are to be trusted in practice. We say that a statistical test is *robust* against an assumed condition when the reported *P*-value is still correct despite this assumption violated by the data; see the section before, and below "Common statistical tests for the comparison of two groups" below for examples.

In addition to the above, still other factors may play a role in choosing a particular test. For instance, if one is concerned about the impact of outliers on the conclusions of a statistical analysis, a test may be needed that is more robust against such outlying values.

In the next section, we review the statistical tests shown in Table 1. This table can be used as guide when performing simple comparisons between two groups or as a tool to understand better the Materials and Methods part of a clinical paper.

Common Statistical Tests for the Comparison of Two Groups

Continuous Data

The t-test introduced in the section "Basic tools for statistical inference" compares the means of, say, two treatments. This test is appropriate for unpaired data from two groups each having a normal distribution with equal variances. For unequal variances but normal distributions, the *t-test for unequal variances*, also called the *Welch test*, applies. However, the classical t-test also works well in this case when the group sizes are about the same, called the *balanced* case. This was discovered via computer simulation studies. The variance of DAS28 at baseline of men and women in the RAPPORT study is equal to 1.50 and 1.17, respectively. Hence, the Welch test seems at its place here, giving $P=0.54$, but this is basically the same to what is obtained from the classical t-test. Another condition for the unpaired t-test is normality in each group. Computer simulations have shown that the t-test is robust against non-normality in the balanced case. For extremely skewed distributions, it may be prudent, however, to check the outcome of the t-test with a *non-parametric* test. Such a test does not depend on the normality assumption. In fact, for a nonparametric test, the data are replaced by their ranks, and hence the P-value from the test becomes independent of the distribution of the data. A popular non-parametric test is the *Wilcoxon rank-sum test*, also called the *Mann–Whitney U test*. A small fictive example illustrates how the test works. Suppose that the DAS28 scores after one year of treatment for group A are 1.0, 1.7, 2.9, and 4.5 and for group B are 2.1, 3.1, 3.3, and 5.9. To compute the Wilcoxon statistic, these scores are ranked irrespective of their group assignment, but their group membership is secured. The ordered values are then 1.0, 1.7, $\underline{2.1}$, 2.9, $\underline{3.1}$, $\underline{3.3}$, 4.5, and $\underline{5.9}$ with the underlined scores pertaining to group B. In the next step, these ordered values are replaced by their ranks 1, 2, $\underline{3}$, 4, $\underline{5}$, $\underline{6}$, 7, and $\underline{8}$, and the ranks pertaining to A are added to give the Wilcoxon rank-sum test statistic $W=1+3+4+7=15$. The extremeness of the obtained W is established using probability laws with a P-value as result. Here $P=0.484$ demonstrating that there is no evidence that the treatments differ in efficacy after one year. In addition to robustness of deviations from normality, a nonparametric test is less vulnerable to outlying values. A disadvantage of a nonparametric test is that the link with the original data is broken, providing basically only a P-value. Note that Wilcoxon rank-sum test can also be used for ordinal data.

Another way to deal with non-normal distributions is to transform the original data such that the transformed data have a normal histogram. The logarithmic function is a popular choice for right-skewed data but may not work when there are a lot of ties in the data. For the HAQ score at baseline, 38 patients have a zero score in the RAPPORT study. Before applying the log transform, we added 1 to the score but then the 38 log (HAQ+1) scores are equal to zero and thus log (HAQ+1) cannot have a normal distribution. In fact, none of the classical transformations, including the square root, can turn the distribution of HAQ into a normal distribution. Further, in a comparative study, it often happens that a different transformation is needed in each of the groups. In that case, transforming the data is not an option. In addition, an interpretation problem may arise when results are based on transformed data. For instance, when the data are log transformed, the 95 % CI of the difference in the means on log scale translates into a 95 % CI of the ratio of *geometric means* on the original scale. But such a 95 % CI is more difficult to interpret as the geometric mean is not equal to the classical mean.

In the case of paired data, inference is based on the difference between the two related values. A statistical significant result is obtained when the mean difference is remote from zero, taking into account statistical fluctuations under H_0. The classical statistical test is now the *paired t-test*. This test requires that the difference of the two related values has a normal distribution. If we do not wish to assume this, one could apply the nonparametric *Wilcoxon signed-rank test*, which is now based on the ranks of the differences. This test is also appropriate for ordinal data.

Nonparametric statistical tests can be applied to all studies regardless of their size. For large studies, the *t*-test is also applicable even when the data grossly deviate from normality. This is a consequence of *The Central Limit Theorem*, a key result in statistics which allows working with the original data (of any distribution) for large studies. In practice "large" means in the balanced unpaired case, group sizes of about 20 or more depending on the deviation from normality, but large(r) sample sizes may be needed in the unbalanced case.

Binary Data

When the outcome of interest is binary, the comparison of two groups involves contrasting two proportions. For unpaired data and a large sample size, the recommended test is the *chi-square test*. This test essentially evaluates a standardized version of the squared difference of the two proportions under the null hypothesis, which is now that the true proportions π_A and π_B are equal. Suppose the observed proportions under treatments A and B are given by p_A and p_B, respectively, then the chi-square test computes $X^2=(p_A-p_B)^2/SE(p_A-p_B)^2$, with $SE(p_A-p_B)$ the standard error of the difference in proportions under H_0. When X^2 is too large (compared to what is expected under the null hypothesis), H_0 is rejected (at $\alpha=0.05$). For the actual calculation of the *P*-value, the *chi-square distribution with one degree of freedom* is used as reference distribution. Table 2 represents a *2×2 contingency*

Table 2 RAPPORT study: observed and expected frequencies of patients split up according to gender who need a more intensive treatment at month 12

	Observed		Expected	
	DAS28 ≤ 3.2	DAS28 > 3.2	DAS28 ≤ 3.2	DAS28 > 3.2
Men	$a = 17$	$b = 11$	$A = 14.25$	$B = 13.75$
Women	$c = 40$	$d = 44$	$C = 42.75$	$D = 41.25$

table contrasting the frequencies of men and women in the RAPPORT study who require step-up treatment (DAS28 > 3.2). This table is a special case of an $r \times c$ *contingency table* when there are r rows and c columns in the table. In Table 2 the lower case symbols stand for the observed frequencies, while the upper case symbols refer to the expected frequencies, i.e., those that one would expect on average to happen under the null hypothesis. Comparing the observed with the expected frequencies leads to an equivalent expression of X^2 given by

$$X^2 = \frac{(a-A)^2}{A} + \frac{(b-B)^2}{B} + \frac{(c-C)^2}{C} + \frac{(d-D)^2}{D}.$$

The above expression shows that X^2 will be large when the observed frequencies deviate a lot from the expected frequencies. For the data in Table 2, we obtained $X^2 = 1.44$ which corresponds to a P-value of 0.23.

For a small study, the *chi-square test with continuity correction* can be used, but *Fisher's Exact test* is recommended. Both tests give a more accurate *P*-value than the chi-square test for a small study. Now "small" is given by the *Cochrane conditions*, which stipulate that the chi-square test may be used when the expected frequencies all exceed 5 (satisfied in our example). The P-value for the Fisher's Exact test is equal to 0.28.

Instead of applying the chi-square test, which only provides a *P*-value, one could also compute the 95 % CI of the absolute risk reduction $AR = p_A - p_B$, with $p_A = b/(a+b)$ and $p_B = d/(c+d)$. When the 95 % CI of AR does not include 0, the two treatments are statistically significantly different at 0.05. For the relative risk $RR = p_B / p_A$ and the odds ratio $OR = \frac{p_B/(1-p_B)}{p_A/(1-p_A)}$, the value of 1 must not be within the 95 % CI to claim a significant effect. Using the observed frequencies in Table 2, the odds ratio is easily seen to be equal to ad/bc. For the entries in Table 2, we obtained RR = 1.28 with 95 % CI = [0.88, 1.85] and OR = 1.7 with 95 % CI = [0.71, 4.06]. Both intervals do include 1 and hence there is no evidence for a difference in the true proportions between men and women.

For paired binary data, a similar reasoning applies but of course the tests must differ. An example of paired proportions is the proportion of patients that have in the RAPPORT study a DAS28 less than 3.2 or greater than 3.2 at baseline (first proportion) versus this proportion at 12 months (second proportion). For a large study, a *McNemar test* is appropriate, which is a variation of the classical chi-square test. For a small study, a corrected version is used or the *binomial test*.

Survival Times

In section "Describing the collected data," we have introduced survival data and mentioned that censoring complicated the analysis of such data. Only right censoring is considered here, which means that it is only known that the survival time is greater than the one recorded in the study. Figure 2 shows the Kaplan–Meier estimate (+95 % CI) of the survival function. The Kaplan–Meier curve is a nonparametric estimate, i.e., no assumption is made about the distribution of the true survival times. If one is willing to assume that the survival times have, say, a *Weibull* or a *lognormal distribution*, then estimates of the mean survival time, its SD, etc. can be derived. However, in survival analysis, there for no generally accepted distribution. Therefore, one is reluctant to base inference on a particular parametric assumption.

We will defer statistical inference with survival data to section "Cox regression," where the Cox proportional hazards (PH) model is introduced. For now, we will limit ourselves by mentioning that the nonparametric tests, such as the Wilcoxon test, have been generalized to survival analysis, as well.

Statistical Tests to Compare More Than Two Groups

Table 1 is limited to statistical tests for the comparison of two groups. In practice a variety of statistical tests are required to tackle the research questions that pop up in clinical research. In this section we review an extension of some of the techniques seen in section "Statistical tests to compare two groups" to compare more than two groups. We restrict ourselves here to the unpaired case. The paired case involves more complicated statistical techniques suitable for correlated data. Some of these techniques are discussed in section "Models for longitudinal studies."

One-Way Comparisons with Continuous Measurements

One possibility to compare $k \geq 2$ groups is to contrast them two by two and perform for each pair a classical unpaired t-test. For $k = 5$ groups, this means 10 t-tests with each 5 % risk of committing a Type I error. A multiple testing problem arises if no correction (such as Bonferroni) is applied. A popular and better way to control the Type I error rate in this setting is to use an *analysis of variance* (*ANOVA*) *test*.

In an ANOVA test, the between-group variance is compared to the variance of the data within the groups. The standardized ratio of these two variances, called the *F-ratio*, should vary around 1 when the null hypothesis of equal means holds. When the alternative hypothesis is true, the F-ratio will often be greater than 1. To evaluate whether there is more variability of the group means than expected under H_0, one computes its extremeness using an *F-distribution* as reference distribution which now has two kinds of degrees of freedom depending on the number of groups and

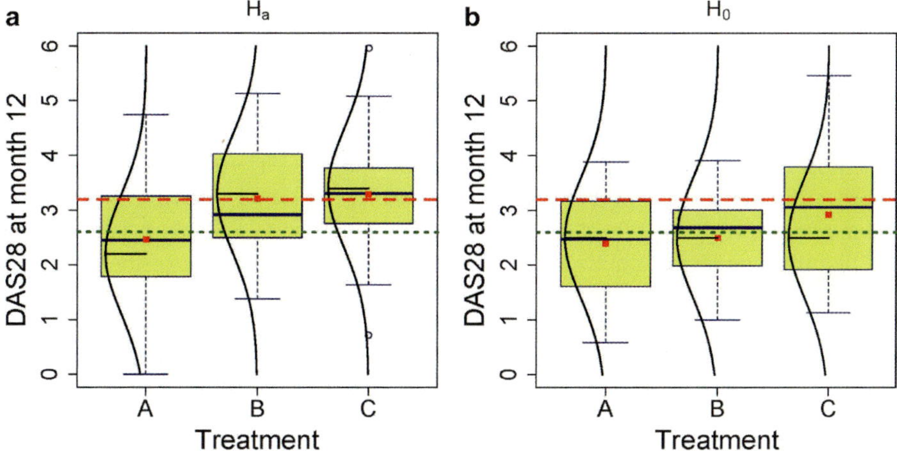

Fig. 3 Fictive study: one-way ANOVA with three treatment groups. (**a**) shows the case of three different true means, while in (**b**) the three groups have equal true means. The box plots are based on each 25 patients drawn from normal populations shown by the curved lines whereby the horizontal lines point to the true means. The observed means are indicated by squares. The *dashed horizontal line* indicates the threshold above which intensified treatment is needed, while below the *dotted horizontal line* indicates that treatment can be reduced

the group sizes. Two fictive studies illustrate the use of the ANOVA test below. This statistical approach is referred to as *one-way ANOVA*, because there is only a single a factor involved in establishing the groups unlike the ANOVA tests reviewed below in section "Two and more way comparisons."

In both panels of Fig. 3, the DAS28 measurements at month 12 are shown. In each of the two experimental treatments (A and B) and the control treatment (C), 25 patients have been included. All data are fictive and were randomly generated using a computer program. In Fig. 3a, it is seen that the true treatment means (indicated by the normal densities and their associated means) are unequal, i.e., 2.2, 3.3, and 3.4. The true standard deviation is for all groups equal to 1.1. An F-ratio equal to 4.20 with $P=0.019$ is obtained. This F-ratio is judged too high to believe that the true means are equal. Because we have generated the data by ourselves, we know that this is the correct decision. In Fig. 3b, it is seen that the true treatment means are all equal to 2.5 with again SD = 1.1. Now an F-ratio of 2.03 is obtained yielding a P-value of $0.14 \geq 0.05$ and we cannot reject the H_a, which is again the correct decision.

The ANOVA test assumes normal distributions with equal variances in all groups, but a violation of these assumptions is not dramatic when the group sizes are roughly equal. When there is gross imbalance, one might need to choose for an alternative approach. There is, however, no commonly used test available that generalizes the Welch test. Another possibility is to use the *Kruskal–Wallis test*, which is a generalization of the Wilcoxon rank-sum test and is based on the same ranking principle. Applied to the same fictive data, we obtained the same qualitative conclusions, but different P-values of course, now equal to 0.029 and 0.24, respectively.

Transformation of the data to normality might sometimes help, but it is in general more difficult to find a transformation that is appropriate for all groups.

The ANOVA F-test only checks whether there is somewhere a difference between the treatment groups but does not give insight which groups are statistically significantly different. In the literature, pairwise t-tests are sometimes applied after a significant F-test, but this may again inflate the Type I error rate. The correct approach is to use so-called multiple comparison tests which penalize the P-value for multiple testing, i.e., the P-value is inflated instead of (equivalently) decreasing the significance level; see also above in section "Use and misuse of the P-value." There are several types of multiple comparison tests, such as *Newman–Keuls*, *Tukey*, *Dunnett*, etc. each with some optimality property. To illustrate their use, we take the first fictive example. The pairwise t-tests without correction for multiplicity result in $P=0.02$ for treatments A and B, and $P=0.011$, $P=0.81$ for treatments A and C, B and C, respectively. With the Tukey multiple comparison test, we obtain (1) $P=0.052$, (2) $P=0.028$, and (3) $P=0.98$, respectively. Hence, by correcting for multiplicity, the first two treatments are not statistically significant anymore. For nonparametric tests, only the approximate Bonferroni correction can be applied or more advanced procedures, which are however not yet supported by common software.

One-Way Comparisons with Categorical Measurements

When DAS28 is categorized into three classes with cutoff points of 2.6 and 3.2, the 3×3 contingency Table 3 is obtained. The research question is now whether the probabilities of belonging to the three disease classes differ in the three treatment groups. When the Cochrane conditions (section "Binary data"), above are fulfilled, we can apply a chi-square test with now 4 degrees of freedom. As for the 2×2 contingency table, this is done by computing X^2, which is again a comparison of observed with expected frequencies. In general, for an $r\times c$ contingency table, the degrees of freedom are $(r-1)\times(c-1)$. For Table 3, $X^2=5.33$ with $P=0.26$. Compare this with the P-value equal to 0.019 obtained from a one-way ANOVA based on the continuous responses. This illustrates that discretizing continuous variables implies a loss of information and hence a decrease in the power of the study. We note that the chi-square test can also be used to test for an association between a row and a factor in an $r\times c$ contingency table. For instance, suppose that in Table 3 the row factor is DAS28 categorized at baseline, then a test for difference in percentages is

Table 3 Fictive study: contingency table of categorized DAS28 at month 12 using 2.4 and 3.2 as cut points (Fig. 3a) together with the row percentages

Treatment	DAS28 ≤ 2.6	2.6 < DAS28 ≤ 3.2	DAS28 > 3.2
1	13 (52 %)	5 (20 %)	7 (28 %)
2	8 (32 %)	6 (24 %)	11 (44 %)
3	6 (24 %)	5 (20 %)	14 (56 %)

actually a test for association between DAS28 at baseline and at month 12. When the Cochrane conditions are not satisfied, then *Exact tests*, which are generalizations of the Fisher's Exact test, are recommended.

In the case of a significant test result in an $r \times c$ table, there is still the question how this significant result came about. For the chi-square test, a significant result can only be obtained when for one or more cells in the contingency table the observed frequency is remote from the corresponding expected frequency. There are advanced statistical approaches to look for the "significant" deviations in the contingency table, but they are beyond the scope of this chapter. Another, but ad hoc, approach is to collapse classes to create 2×2 contingency tables from the $r \times c$ table and to apply the Bonferroni correction afterward to guard ourselves against multiple testing. For instance, from Table 3 one can construct nine 2×2 tables, e.g., left top table with entries 13, 5, 8, and 6 and left bottom table with entries 8, 6, 6, 5, etc. For each of these tables, one can evaluate the association, and the nine P-values are multiplied with nine. If $9 \times P < 0.05$ for a particular subtable, then there is a significant association in that subtable. This was not the case here, however.

Two- and More-Way Comparisons

In one-way ANOVA, the different values of one factor determine the groups. When multiple factors are involved, interest may lie in their joint effect on the response. For instance, suppose that RA patients are treated with either a control treatment C or an experimental treatment E (factor 1), but at the same time concomitant medication c or placebo p (factor 2) are administered. Suppose now that an RCT has been set up randomly allocating patients to the four possible combinations: (1) C and p, (2) E and p, (3) C and c, and (4) E and c. Suppose also that one is interested in the overall effect of the experimental treatment on, say, DAS28 but also in the overall effect of the concomitant treatment and additionally in their joint effect. The overall effect of E is called the *main effect* of E and similarly for the overall effect of c. Suppose that after 12 months of treating the patients with E, the average DAS28 is reduced by 1 unit whether or not concomitant medication is administered. In that case, one speaks of *no interaction* between the two factors. If also the concomitant medication reduces the average DAS28, say by 0.5, then in the absence of interaction, the joint effect of the experimental and concomitant treatment results in a decrease of the average DAS28 by $1 + 0.5 = 1.5$. A *statistical interaction* between the two factors is present when the joint administration does not result in a sum of the individual main effects. In our fictive example, the experimental treatment always reduces the average of DAS28. The interaction is therefore called *quantitative*. On the other hand, when the joint administration would raise DAS28 on average, then we are dealing with a *qualitative interaction*. For a quantitative interaction, adding the concomitant treatment to the experimental treatment does not change our conclusion about the experimental treatment, whereas for a qualitative interaction we must conclude that joint administration of the two treatments here has a negative impact on the patient.

In the above paragraph, we assumed that we knew the true treatment effects. In practice, they need to be estimated from the study at hand. In a second step, they are tested for equality. This is done by a *two-way ANOVA* analysis and it involves now three F-tests, one for each main effect and one for the interaction effect. Each time the null hypothesis corresponds to no effect. Under the assumption of normal distributions with equal variances, the null hypotheses are rejected when the corresponding F-values are judged too large under H_0. Note that we should test first the interaction. If significant, then one explores the main effect of one factor in each level of the other factor. Now follows a fictive example to better explain the practical procedure.

Inspired by the results of the RAPPORT study, we generated 200 DAS28 values (at month 12) from four groups split up according to age less than or more than 55 years (factor 1) and gender (factor 2). Figure 4a shows the generated DAS28 values under no interaction. The F-tests (P-values) are for (1) age (11.44 ($P<0.001$)), (2) gender (8.15 ($P=0.0048$)), and (3) interaction of age with gender (0.021 ($P=0.88$)). Since there is no evidence for interaction, we can estimate the main effects immediately. They are equal to (95 % CI) for gender ((male–female): –0.45 ([–0.75, –0.14])) and for age ((>55 – <55): –0.53 ([–.84, –0.22])). The above 95 % (Tukey) CIs take into account the multiple testing problem. Figure 4b shows the qualitative interaction case. The F-value for the interaction is now 21.68 with $P<0.001$. Now it does not make sense to interpret the main effects for gender and age. In fact, we need to estimate the effect of gender in each of the two age classes and the same holds for age.

Two-way ANOVA can be further generalized to involve more than two factors. In general, such data structures are called *factorial designs*. Factorial designs also

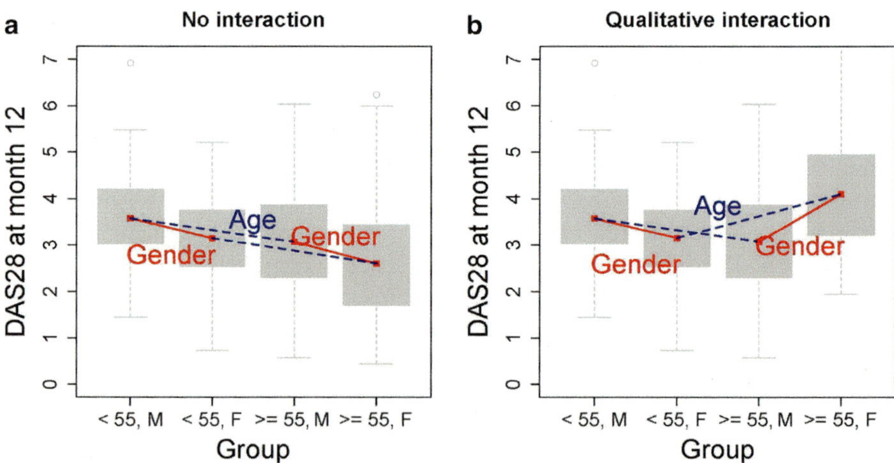

Fig. 4 Fictive study: two-way ANOVA with two factors: age <55 or ≥ 55 and gender. (**a**) shows the case of no interaction between age and gender, while (**b**) shows the case of qualitative interaction. The *solid lines* represent the effect of gender in each of the two classes of age, while the *dashed lines* represent the effect of age in the two gender classes

exist for categorical responses, but these will be treated in section "Regression models" where we look at regression models for binary outcomes.

Measuring and Testing Associations

When two or more measurements are taken on the same subject, it may be of interest to see how much they are related. In this section we consider two situations. In the first case, we look at a general measure for association between two measurements of possibly different nature, so-called correlation measures. In the second case, interest lies in the association of two measurements of the same kind and to know whether they indeed measure the same characteristic. These are called *measures of agreement*. For both cases, continuous, ordinal, and binary data are considered here. We also explain the *Bland–Altman plot* which is a classical tool for continuous measurements often used in medical research to evaluate the dependence of agreement on the level of the measurement.

Association

In the tREACH study, DAS and RADAI (patient-reported outcome of disease activity) are measured at several time points. One would expect that the two measures are positively related, i.e., we expect that when DAS is high, this will be also for RADAI. In Fig. 5a, we notice that when DAS28 is high (or low), then RADAI tends to be also high (or low). A popular measure to evaluate this association is the *Pearson correlation coefficient* r_p. The Pearson correlation r_p is zero, when the two

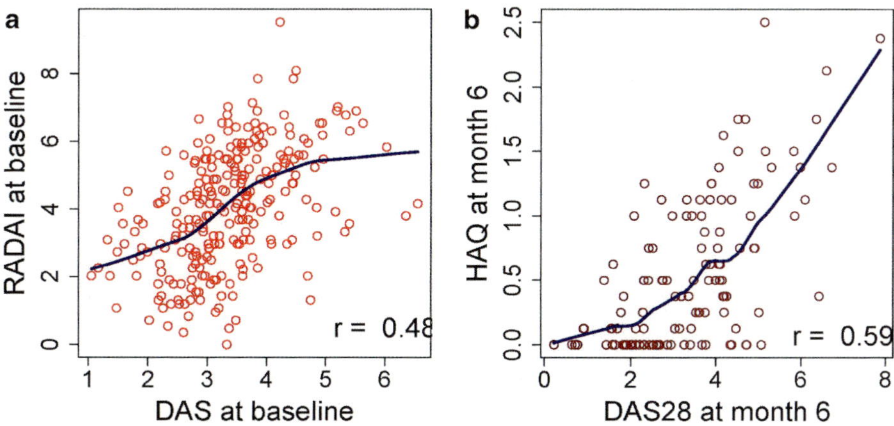

Fig. 5 (**a**) Scatterplot of DAS and RADAI at baseline (tREACH study), (**b**) scatterplot of DAS and HAQ at month 6 (RAPPORT study). In addition a smooth line representing the relationship is added (using *R* function lowess)

measurements show no association. In that case the scatterplot exhibits a circular figure (as a pizza) or in general a figure centered on the horizontal line. For a positive correlation, the two measurements evolve in the same direction, while for a negative correlation the opposite is true. The Pearson correlation between DAS and RADAI is equal to 0.48, which is appreciable but not particularly high. In absolute value, the maximal Pearson correlation is 1. The *coefficient* r_p is an estimate of the "true" correlation ρ which would be obtained if we relate all possible DAS and RADAI values obtained from the population from which the sample was taken. A significance test can then determine whether the true correlation is zero or not, i.e., whether H_0: $\rho = 0$. In addition a 95 % CI for ρ can be computed. For our example, $P < 0.001$, indicating that most likely the true correlation is not equal to zero, which is confirmed by the 95 % CI equal to [0.38, 0.57] since it does not include zero.

The Pearson correlation measures the linear relationship between two measurements. If the relationship has a "banana" shape, then the Pearson correlation does not estimate the (nonlinear) association properly. Furthermore, the significance test to evaluate H_0: $\rho = 0$ assumes that both measurements have a normal distribution. The smooth line (see section "Regression models") in the scatterplot shows an approximate straight line relationship. Thus, for the correct computation of the P-value associated with a Pearson correlation, both variables should have a normal distribution. In our example the distributions of DAS and RADAI appear to be normal. For non-normal distributions and/or a nonlinear relationship, the *Spearman rank correlation* r_s is preferred. To compute the Spearman correlation, the original data are first replaced by their ranks, and on these ranks the Pearson correlation is computed. Again, a P-value for $\rho = 0$ and a 95 % CI can be calculated. Typical for a nonparametric procedure, the Spearman correlation is robust against outlying values. The Spearman correlation between DAS28 and HAQ at month 6 in the RAPPORT study is $r_s = 0.59$ ($P < 0.001$). The scatterplot together with the smooth line in Fig. 5b suggests that there is a curvilinear relationship and a skewed distribution of HAQ. The Spearman correlation of DAS28 and HAQ at month 6 equals $r_s = 0.59$, which is lower than the Pearson correlation of 0.64.

We note that it often does not really make sense to evaluate a correlation with a P-value. Indeed, often a zero correlation is not expected (e.g., we do expect a nonzero correlation between DAS20 at baseline and DAS28 at month 12), but we rather wish to know the size of the correlation using a 95 % CI.

The Spearman correlation can also be used for ordinal data. For two binary outcomes, several measures have been suggested such as the *tetrachoric correlation*. An alternative measure is the *cross-ratio*, which is in fact equal to the odds ratio but now the two binary variables are interchangeable without harming the interpretation of the association (symmetric case). For the odds ratio one variable is often considered to represent the "cause" and the other the "result" (asymmetric case).

It often happens in an explorative study that many correlations are tested without a clear hypothesis to evaluate. This clearly inflates the Type I error rate tremendously and may lead to wild speculations of possible relations.

Agreement

Suppose that we want to measure how reproducible clinicians can score DAS28, both between occasions as well as between clinicians. That is, we wish to know the *intra-rater variability* (between occasions) and the *inter-rater variability* (between clinicians). Both measures of variability can be estimated by the *intra-class correlation* (*ICC*). We assume that there are either two clinicians who score DAS28 on RA patients, or that one clinician scores DAS28 twice on each patient. Let σ_B^2 represent the variance of the average of the 2 scores across the patients and σ_W^2 the variance of the scores within the same patient, then the population intra-class correlation is defined as

$$\mathrm{ICC} = \frac{\sigma_B^2}{\sigma_B^2 + \sigma_W^2}.$$

The above formula shows that ICC will always be positive, and must therefore be different from the classical (Pearson) correlation. In fact, ICC measures in a scatterplot the closeness of the points to the bisecting line, while the classical correlation measures the closeness of the points to the best straight line. The sample estimate of ICC, i.e., $\widehat{\mathrm{ICC}}$, is obtained by replacing in the above formula the true variances by their sample estimates, by s_B^2 and s_W^2. In Fig. 6 three fictive cases of two observers scoring the same patients are shown together with the intra-class correlations: (a) the scores were generated around the bisecting line whereby the within-patient variance of the scores remains constant with increasing values of the scores, (b) the same situation except that now the within-patient variance of the scores increases with increasing values of the scores, (c) the scores between the raters are closely related but are not located on the bisecting line. The corresponding Pearson correlations are equal to 0.78, 0.78 and 0.99, respectively, which illustrates that the two measures are different in nature. Again one can test whether ICC = 0, but we suggest to report the 95 % CI. As an example, the 95 % CI for ICC of Fig. 6a is equal to [0.71, 0.81].

Finally, to graphically represent whether the within-patient variability s_W^2 depends on the actual value, the *Bland-Altman plot* is used. The Bland-Altman plot is a scatterplot of the difference of the two values with their average.

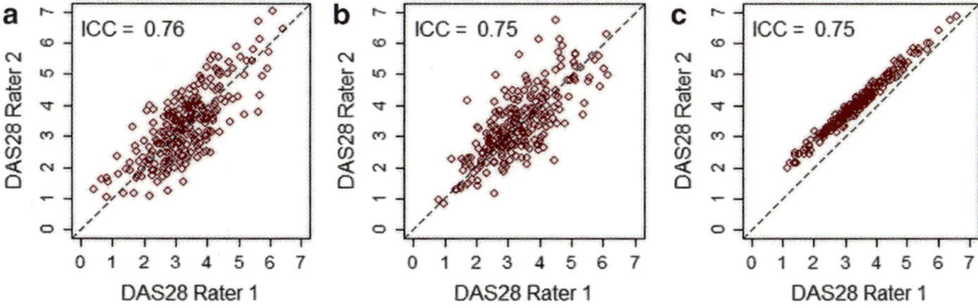

Fig. 6 Fictive data: three examples of two raters scoring DAS28. Panel (**a**) corresponds to ICC = 0.76, panel (**b**) corresponds to ICC = 0.75 and panel (**c**) corresponds to ICC = 0.75. Further information is given in the text

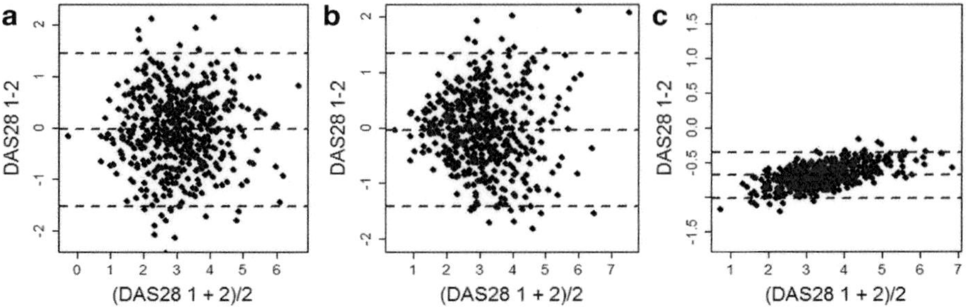

Fig. 7 Fictive data: three examples of a Bland–Altman plot corresponding to Fig. 6 (**a**), (**b**) and (**c**), respectively

In Fig. 7, the Bland-Altman plots corresponding to Fig. 6 are shown. In Fig. 6a s_W^2 remains constant across the different DAS28 values, while for Fig. 6b s_W^2 increases with DAS28 value. Clearly, Fig. 7a shows that the within-patient variability is constant, while for Fig. 7b the variability increases. Figure 7c shows that there is a problem with scoring.

Up to now, we have considered only the situation with two raters. The intra-class correlation, but also the agreement measures below can be extended to more than two observers. The actual expression of the agreement measure depends on whether the measure aims to estimate agreement between the selected observers in the study (study clinicians) or among all observers that belong to a particular population (all clinicians).

For binary, nominal or ordinal scores a popular measure of agreement is given by the *kappa coefficient* κ also called *Cohen's kappa*. For two binary scores, Cohen's kappa computes the relative degree of agreement, i.e., the agreement corrected for spontaneous agreement (also called agreement by chance). The theoretical formula for the true κ is given by

$$\kappa = \frac{\pi_o - \pi_e}{1 - \pi_e},$$

where π_o represents the (population) observed agreement and π_e the (population) agreement that happens by pure chance. In Table 4(a) π_o is estimated by $\hat{\pi}_o = \frac{82+324}{498} = 0.82$ whereas π_e is estimated by $\hat{\pi}_e = \frac{133}{498} \times \frac{124}{498} + \frac{368}{498} \times \frac{375}{498} = 0.62$. Then $\hat{\kappa} = 0.52$ is the estimated excess agreement above the agreement obtained by pure chance. For Table 4(b) and (c) we obtained $\hat{\kappa} = 0.60$ and $\hat{\kappa} = 0.25$, respectively. In addition one can compute a *P*-value for the null hypothesis. When kappa is zero, then the observed agreement is obtained by pure chance.

Agreement in ordinal data could be measured by *weighted kappas*. A greater weight is then assigned to cells that are further away from the diagonal in the table; popular are linear and quadratic weights. Note that there has been a lot of discussion in the statistical and epidemiological literature of the value of the kappa-statistic. For instance, it has been shown that it is difficult to compare kappa values obtained from different studies.

Table 4 Fictive study: three examples upon which Cohen's kappa is computed

	(a)			(b)			(c)		
	Rater 2			Rater 2			Rater 2		
Rater 1	82	51	133	97	33	130	21	98	119
	42	324	368	47	321	368	0	379	379
	124	375	498	134	364	498	21	477	498

The tables are obtained by binarizing the DAS28 scores with threshold 2.6, which represents the upper bound below which the disease activity is considered low

Regression Models

In this section we evaluate the strength of the relationship between two (or more) measurements. In addition, we now require also a mathematical expression that allows one measurement to "predict" from the other measurement(s). This entails an important class of statistical methods, called *regression methods*. First we treat linear regression models, where the response is continuous. Then binary and ordinal regression models are considered. We end with Cox regression, which is the most popular regression technique in survival analysis.

Linear Regression

Simple Linear Regression

In *simple linear regression* one variable, called the *response* or *outcome*, is predicted from another variable, called the *covariate*, *regressor* or *predictor*. In some textbooks the response is called the dependent variable and the covariate is referred to as the independent variable. However, this terminology may cause confusion in multiple linear regression introduced below and will therefore not be used here.

In Fig. 8 we show the regression line predicting DAS at month 12 in the tREACH study from the age (in years) of the patient. The straight line provides the "best" linear prediction of the response from the regressor, whereby "best" means that the squared deviations of the predicted response from the observed response are minimized with the regression line. The regression line is here given by the following formula: $\text{DAS} = 1.11 + 0.0086 \times \text{age}$. The coefficient 1.11 is called the (estimated) *intercept* and 0.0086 the (estimated) *slope*, they are also called the *regression coefficients*. The intercept represents the average DAS for $\text{age} = 0$, while the slope represents the increase of the average DAS when age is increased by one year. Clearly, the intercept has no physical meaning here. When the slope is zero, the regression line is horizontal and hence the response and regressor are not related. With a positive slope the response increases on average when the regressor increases, while for a negative slope the opposite is true. Note that the regression coefficients depend on the scale of the response and the regressor. For instance, when age is replaced by

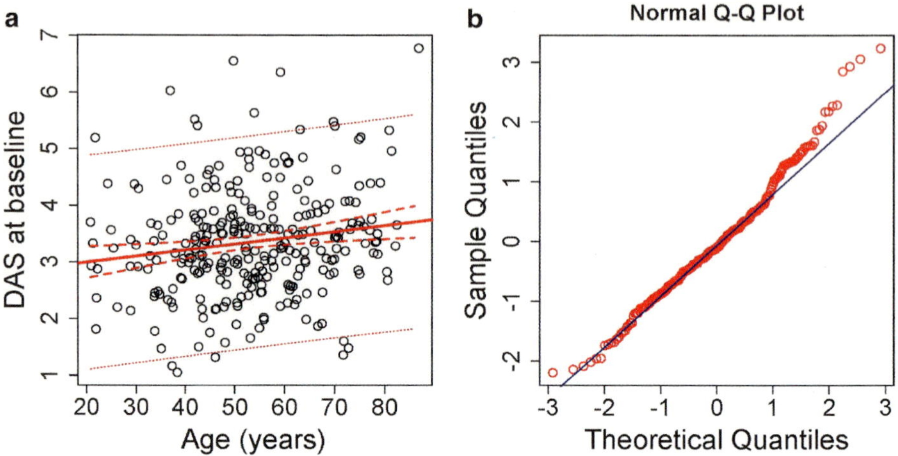

Fig. 8 tREACH study: (**a**) simple linear regression, regressing DAS at month 12 on age at baseline. The *solid straight line* is the estimated regression line, the *dashed lines* express the 95 % confidence bounds for the predicted values, and the *dotted lines* express the 95 % confidence bounds for the individual observations; (**b**) Q–Q plot to check normality of the residuals

age/10 the slope must be multiplied with 10. This dependence on the scale of the regressor, but also of the response, makes it difficult to compare the magnitude of the regression coefficients.

The regression coefficients 1.11 and 0.0086 estimate the true regression coefficients which relate the two variables in the population. The classical assumption of simple linear regression is that the response deviates in a Gaussian way around a straight line with a variance that remains constant across the values of the regressor. The true relationship of the response with the regressor is not known but assumed to be linear. Hence for the observed response for the *i*th subject, denoted here as y_i, it is assumed that

$$y_i = \beta_0 + \beta_1 x_i + \varepsilon_i,$$

with x_i the regressor value for the *i*th subject and ε_i the deviation of the response from the straight line, called the *i*th *residual*. It is assumed that this residual has a normal distribution. The true regression coefficients are estimated from the data. Here the estimates are: $\hat{\beta}_0 = 1.11,\quad \hat{\beta}_1 = 0.0086$. From these estimates the predicted response $\widehat{\mathrm{DAS}}_i = \hat{\beta}_0 + \hat{\beta}_1 \times \mathrm{age}_i$ can be determined for each subject. The above statistical assumptions (linear relationship, Gaussian distribution around the regression line with constant variance) allow to: (1) derive the standard errors of the estimates, (2) test the null hypotheses that the true regression coefficients are zero, i.e., $\beta_0 = 0, \beta_1 = 0$ and (3) provide (95 %) confidence bounds for the predicted values and the responses at the different regressor values.

In Table 5, a classical regression output is shown, with the regression estimates, their standard error, the computed *t*-value (estimate/SE) and the corresponding *P*-value. For both regression coefficients the null hypothesis is rejected, i.e., there is

Table 5 tREACH study: regression estimates for the regression model with response DAS at month 12 and age as regressor

Coefficient	Estimate	SE	*t*-value	*P*
Intercept	1.11	0.21	5.41	<0.001
Age (years)	0.0086	0.004	2.30	0.023

evidence that the true regression coefficients are not zero. However, we are only interested in verifying H_0: $\beta_1=0$. Since $P<0.05$, we believe that there is some relationship between DAS at month 12 and age. The strength of the relationship is classically expressed with the *coefficient of determination*, denoted as R^2. The coefficient of determination expresses the proportion of variability of the response that is explained by the regression model. The minimal value of R^2 is 0 when the regressor has no predictive ability. The maximal value of 1 is obtained when all points lie on a (non-horizontal) straight line. For our example, $R^2=0.021$ which is low and hence DAS is not well predicted from age. This example is an illustration that a significant relationship does not immediately result in good prediction. In addition, we can estimate the 95 % confidence boundaries for the predicted responses (dashed lines) and the future responses (dotted lines), they are both indicated in Fig. 8a. Finally, it can be verified that R^2 is equal to the square of the Pearson correlation, i.e. equal to r_p^2.

Each regression analysis should be accompanied by diagnostic plots that verify the statistical assumptions. Such an exercise is too often neglected in practice. Linearity of the relationship can be graphically inspected by comparing the linear regression line with a *smooth fit*. This is a curvilinear plot that expresses the relationship between response and regressor nonparametrically, i.e., without any restrictions. The assumption of normality can be checked with a *Q–Q plot* that plots the obtained residuals, here $\hat{r}_i = \text{DAS}_i - \widehat{\text{DAS}_i}$, on the *Y*-axis and their expected value (under normality) on the *X*-axis. If normality applies, a straight line is (approximately) obtained. Another possibility is to apply a *normality test*, which formally tests whether the distribution of residuals is Gaussian. For the model predicting DAS28, the Q–Q plot in Fig. 8b shows some deviation from normality for the distribution of the residuals. Fortunately, since linear regression is rather robust against non-normality of the residuals, there is no immediate reason to look for another model.

Multiple Linear Regression

In *multiple linear regression*, several regressors are involved in a linear relationship with the response. The computational procedure to determine the regression coefficients is similar as for simple linear regression. Also, the assumptions upon which the statistical tests are based are the same as for simple linear regression. Yet, finding the appropriate model and interpreting the regression coefficients is now far more complex than with simple linear regression. To better explain, let us suppose that in the tREACH study we wish to predict DAS at month 12 from DAS at baseline, age, gender, and the treatment (1) triple therapy + prednisone oral (A), (2) triple therapy + prednisone injection (B), or (3) MTX + prednisone oral (C). In Table 6 we

Table 6 tREACH study: regression model with response DAS at month 12 and DAS28 at baseline, age, gender, and treatment as regressors

Coefficient	Estimate	SE	*t*-value	*P*
Intercept	0.16	0.27	0.62	0.54
DAS baseline	0.13	0.051	2.45	0.015
Age (years)	0.010	0.003	2.86	0.0047
Gender (0 = male)	0.50	0.11	4.58	<0.001
Treatment B	0.11	0.12	0.86	0.39
Treatment C	0.19	0.12	1.55	0.12

show the estimates of the multiple regression model. From that table we conclude that only age and gender significantly influence DAS at month 12.

The regression model estimated in Table 6 can be written as

DAS month 12 = 0.16 + 0.13 × DAS baseline + 0.010 × age + 0.50 × gender + 0.11 × treatment B + 0.19 × treatment C.

The estimated regression coefficients tell us that (on average) DAS at month 12 is higher for females and for greater values of DAS at baseline and age. Treatment, on the other hand, appears not to have any significant effect. Thus, the interpretation of regression coefficients appears to be the same as with simple linear regression. However, there is an important difference, namely, the value and interpretation of the regression coefficient depends on which other regressors are in the model. To better understand this, let us look at the following fitted regression models to DAS (at month 12) for the tREACH data:

- Model 1: DAS = 1.11 + 0.0086 (0.023) × age
- Model 2: DAS = 0.59 + 0.012 (0.0015) × age + 0.53 (<0.001) × gender
- Model 3: DAS = 0.24 + 0.010 (0.0054) × age + 0.52 (<0.001) × gender + 0.13 (0.011) × DAS baseline
- Model 4: DAS = 0.85 + 0.0070 (0.24) × age + 0.13 (0.76) × gender + 0.0074 (0.32) × age × gender
- Model 5: DAS = 0.93 − 0.0025 (0.91) × age + 0.54 (<0.001) × gender + 0.00013 (0.52) × age^2

Each time, the *P*-value of the regression coefficient is given in parentheses. Model 1 is a simple linear regression model including only age. The model provides the *univariate effect* of age on the response, i.e., older age implies a higher DAS at month 12. The regression coefficient of age in Model 2 represents the effect of age when gender is kept constant, i.e., it represents the effect of age within males and females separately. It is said that the effect of age is *controlled for* gender and this significantly augments the effect of age here. This is called the *multivariate effect* of age when gender is included in the model. Note that the women are significantly younger in this study. Together with the fact that women have a higher DAS at month 12, it explains why this model shows a stronger effect of age. DAS at baseline value is included in Model 3, which has (as expected) a significant impact on the DAS value at the end. In Model 4, the product of age with gender, also called the *interaction between age and gender*, is added to the model. Now none of the age regression coefficients is significant anymore. This is an illustration of *multicollinearity* in the regressors. Multicollinearity is a common phenomenon when highly correlated regressors are included in the model causing unstable regression computations. Model 4 is a sign that one must be quite careful in building up the model and interpreting the regression coefficients. Model 5 illustrates that with linear regression nonlinear relationships can also be expressed. There is, however, again a multicollinearity problem since age is positively and highly (closely) linearly correlated with age^2. The linear relationship between age and age^2 can be removed by working with a centered age, namely, with *agec=age-mean* (*age*), and $agec^2$. For this model, the regression coefficients for gender and $agec^2$ remain the same but the regression coefficient of agec changes drastically and is now statistically significant ($P=0.0014$).

The above shows that building an appropriate multiple linear regression model may be not that easy. Below is a list of challenges that one may face in the model-building process:

- When a large number of regressors is available, it is not immediately clear which regressors to include in the model. It is popular to select regressors in an automated manner, using, e.g., *stepwise selection procedures*. However, it is known that these procedures do not necessarily result in a meaningful model. In addition, since such a procedure involves many decisions to include or exclude a regressor, the reported *P*-values therefore suffer severely from the multiple testing problem.
- In multiple linear regression, there is much more freedom to deviate from the model assumptions. In order to achieve an appropriate model, we might have to transform the regressors, add double products, and/or transform the response. Such transformations might also be needed to improve the normality of the residuals. When the variance of the response is not constant, the model needs to be further expanded and another computational procedure is needed.
- To find out whether the constructed model is appropriate, i.e., satisfies the statistical assumptions, a battery of diagnostic plots is needed. One example of such a plot, the Q–Q plot of the residuals, was seen for simple linear regression. However, many other residual plots are needed to check the multiple linear regression model. In addition, diagnostic procedures should be used that can highlight *influential observations*, i.e., observations that have an unduly large effect on the estimates of the regression coefficients.

Constructing the appropriate multiple linear regression model may therefore need considerable statistical background. All these efforts do not, however, guarantee that we find the true model, if such a thing exists. We can only hope for a useful one.

Logistic Regression

When the response is binary, linear regression is not appropriate anymore. Most popular is the *logistic regression model* whereby the probability of experiencing an event (scored as "1") is expressed as a function of the covariates using the logistic function. More specifically, let π_i be the probability of experiencing the event and x_i the regressor for the ith individual, then the simple linear logistic model is given by

$$\log\left(\frac{\pi_i}{1-\pi_i}\right) = \beta_0 + \beta_1 x_i,$$

whereby $\log\left(\frac{\pi_i}{1-\pi_i}\right)$ is also denoted as $\text{logit}(\pi_i)$. An equivalent way of specifying the model is

$$\pi_i = \text{expit}(\beta_0 + \beta_1 x_i) = \frac{\exp(\beta_0 + \beta_1 x_i)}{1+\exp(\beta_0 + \beta_1 x_i)},$$

where $\exp(a)=e^a$ and the function $\exp(a)/(1+\exp(a))$ is referred to in the literature as the *expit function*. The parameters β_0 and β_1 are again called the regression coefficients, with β_0 playing the role of an intercept and β_1 of a slope. In Fig. 9, four logistic models are shown in a fictive preclinical setting relating morbidity to the dose of an experimental drug. It is immediately seen that always $0 < \pi_i < 1$, whatever the values of β_0 and β_1 and of the regressor are. When $\beta_1 > 0$ ($\beta_1 < 0$), increasing (decreasing) the regressor will increase the probability of an event, while $\beta_1 = 0$ implies that the regressor has no impact on the response.

For a binary regressor, it can be shown that $\exp(\beta_1)$ expresses the odds ratio relating the binary response to the regressor. For a continuous regressor, $\exp(\beta_1)$ expresses the odds ratio of the response with the regressor when the regressor increases by one unit. In practice β_0 and β_1 are estimated from the data, resulting in $\hat{\beta}_0$ and $\hat{\beta}_1$. For each individual, the predicted response $\hat{\pi}_i$ can be computed by plugging in the estimates $\hat{\beta}_0$ and $\hat{\beta}_1$ in the expression for $\hat{\pi}_i$. Based on these estimates, one can test whether the true regression coefficients β_0 and β_1 are equal to zero. As for linear regression, we will be only interested in the test $\beta_1 = 0$. Again 95 % CIs for β_0 and β_1 can be computed.

As for linear regression, more than one regressor can be included in the logistic regression model. The interpretation of the regression coefficients then depends on which other regressors are included in the model. For instance, $\exp(\beta_1)$ then expresses the odds ratio of the regressor with the binary response but controlled for the other regressors.

The computational procedure to establish the estimates of the regression coefficients is iterative, i.e., the numerical algorithm needs several steps to end up in the estimates. This is in contrast to linear regression where analytical solutions are available for the regression coefficients. But, apart from the numerical procedure, the same challenges as in linear regression are to be dealt with in logistic regression.

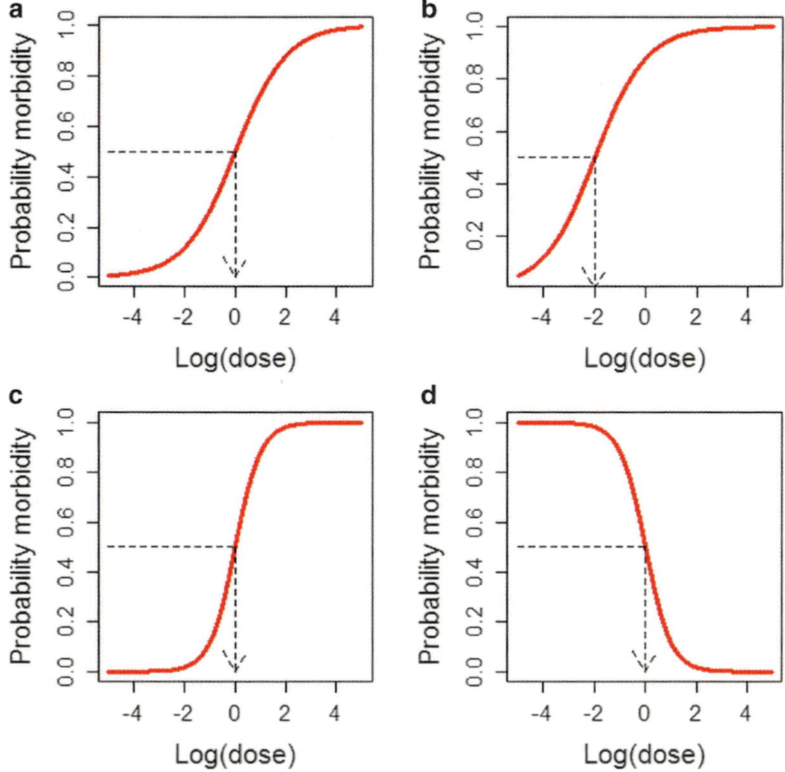

Fig. 9 Fictive preclinical study: four logistic models are shown relating $\pi_i = \exp(\beta_0 + \beta_1 x_i)/(1+\exp(\beta_0 + \beta_1 x_i))$ to x_i with: (**a**) $\beta_0=0, \beta_1=1$; (**b**) $\beta_0=2, \beta_1=1$; (**c**) $\beta_0=0, \beta_1=2$; and (**d**) $\beta_0=0, \beta_1=-1$. The solid line represents the logistic curve for different values of the log(dose). The dashed lines point to the log(dose) that corresponds to probability = 0.5

For instance, it is not immediately clear which regressors should be included in the model and whether they need to be transformed. Two measures of performance are popular: (1) an adapted R^2, called *Nagelkerke*'*s* R^2, such that its minimal value is 0 and maximal value is 1; and (2) a *concordance measure* (between 0.5 and 1), which measures the proportion of pairs of observations that have the same ordering in the observed (binary) responses as in the corresponding pair of predicted responses. For a non-predictive model, the concordance is equal to 0.5.

As an illustration, we explore in the tREACH study the relationship between a binary outcome bDAS (obtained from binarizing DAS at month 12 using threshold 2.4) and various regressors. Then, bDAS is 1 if there is low disease activity (<2.4), 0 otherwise. Three models express the probability of having low disease activity as a function of regressors. We obtain (within parentheses *P*-values):

- Model 1: logit (pDAS) = 2.53 − 1.23 (0.0078) × gender
- Model 2: logit (pDAS) = 4.02 − 1.39 (0.004) × gender – 0.025 (0.054) × age
- Model 3: logit (pDAS) = 4.62 − 1.38 (0.004) × gender – 0.023 (0.082) × age − 0.22 (0.23) × DAS baseline

In Model 1, only gender is included. According to the fitted logistic model, males in the tREACH study show a lower disease activity. The odds ratio for gender is equal to 0.29, with 95 % CI = [0.11, 0.72]; hence, female patients have a lower probability to have a low disease activity at the end of treatment. One can verify that these estimates are the same as those obtained from a 2×2 contingency table. In Model 2, age is added to the model. Now the regression coefficient of gender is controlled for age. The odds ratio is slightly decreased to 0.25 with 95 % CI = [0.098, 0.63]. In Model 3, the DAS value at baseline is added to the model, but surprisingly it appears to have no impact on the response. For the three models, Nagelkerke's R^2 is equal to 0.058, 0.083, and 0.092, respectively, while the concordance is for the three models 0.611, 0.663, and 0.674, respectively. We see some increase in predictive performance when age is added to the model, but none of the models does a satisfactory job in predicting low disease activity at the end of the study.

The logistic regression model is one of the most popular models in epidemiology to search for risk factors for a variety of diseases. Its popularity has much to do with the property that the odds ratio obtained from a logistic model obtained from a case–control study is equal to the odds ratio obtained from a logistic model applied to a corresponding cohort study (see chapter "Methodological issues relevant to observational studies, registries and administrative health databases in rheumatology").

Other models for binary outcomes in this class are the *probit* and *complementary log–log regression model*, for which the expit function is replaced by other S-shaped functions. An extended version of the logistic regression model has been suggested for an ordinal response, called the *ordinal logistic regression model.*

Finally, the logistic model belongs to a general and important class of statistical models, called *generalized linear models*. This class of models hosts many important models in statistics.

Cox Regression

A regression model for a survival response needs to take care of (right) censored observations. By far the most popular regression model for survival data is *Cox regression model* proposed by Sir D.R. Cox in 1972 [18]. Cox's approach is based on a fundamental assumption on the *hazard function*, which we first introduce. We recall that "survival" does not need to be interpreted literally, but rather "death" means the occurrence of an event, such as drug survival or the occurrence of arthritis in ACPA-positive arthralgia over time or cardiovascular events.

The Hazard Function

The hazard function expresses the instantaneous risk for "dying" as a function of time that applies to a subject. More formally, the hazard function $h(t)$ is defined as

$$h(t) = \frac{\text{Prob}\left(\text{death in}\left[t, t+\Delta t\right] \middle| \text{alive at } t\right)}{\Delta t},$$

for small Δt. The formula reads as follows: given that a subject is alive at time t, the hazard at time t is the probability of dying in an interval of size Δt immediately after time t, divided by Δt.

The survival function and the hazard function provide complementary information, with the former describing the cumulative process of dying. Further, for each (theoretical) survival function, there is a corresponding hazard function. In fact, when we know the survival function, we also know the hazard function and vice versa. It is illustrative to look at some common hazard functions in Fig. 10. The constant hazard is the hazard caused by a variety of causes that may happen during any time in the life of an individual, such as a fall, a car accident, etc. The hazard caused by surgery is typically high at the time of surgery and then decreases with time. The aging process causes people to die when they get older; hence, the hazard function increases with age. Finally, the bathtub hazard function is seen when the different risks jointly apply to a population.

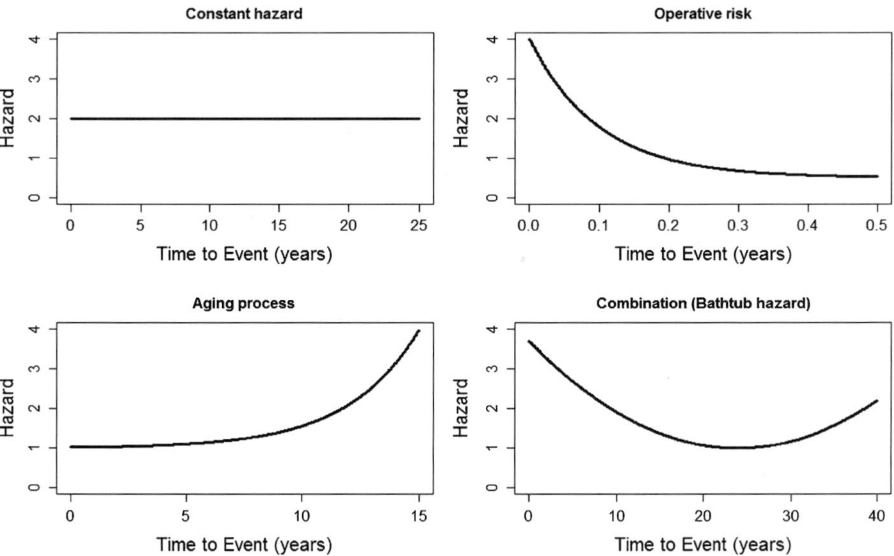

Fig. 10 Some examples of theoretical hazard functions

The hazard function can be easily computed when a parametric assumption of the survival distribution is made, such as a Weibull distribution. Without such an assumption, it is difficult to obtain a reliable estimate of the hazard function from the data. This was recognized by Cox in 1972, who proposed a method that allows estimating the effect of risk factors on survival without needing to estimate the hazard function.

The Proportional Hazards Assumption

The *proportional hazards assumption* (*PH assumption*) specifies that the impact of a regressor acts multiplicatively on the hazard function. In the case of a binary regressor, say gender, the PH assumption implies that the hazard function for males is proportional to that for females. When the hazard ratio is equal to 2, we have

$$\frac{h_{\text{Male}}(t)}{h_{\text{Female}}(t)} = 2.$$

This signifies that the instantaneous risk for men ($h_{\text{Male}}(t)$) is twice the risk for women ($h_{\text{Female}}(t)$). When the ratio is not constant, we say that the PH assumption is violated. The hazard ratio $h_{\text{Male}}(t)/h_{\text{Female}}(t) = c$ is equivalent with $h_{\text{Male}}(t) = h_0(t) \times \exp[\log(c)] = h_0(t) \times \exp[\beta_1 \times \text{gender}]$ with $\beta_1 = \log(c)$ and gender $= 0$ for a female and 1 otherwise. In the above re-expression, the hazard function of the female patients plays the role of a *baseline hazard*. When there are p regressors in the model, the PH assumption generalizes to

$$h_x(t) = h_0(t) \times \exp\left[\beta_1 x_1 + \beta_2 x_2 \cdots + \beta_p x_p\right].$$

Summarized, the PH assumption assumes that the regressors act multiplicative on the hazard function and their effect remains constant during the study. The regression coefficients represent, as for the other regression models, the strength of the regressors in the presence of the other regressors.

Cox Regression

In 1972, Cox proposed a method to estimate the regression coefficients under the PH assumption. His approach does not require estimating the hazard function and became the most important survival regression method.

For an illustration of Cox regression, we take a fictive example that compares the time in remission between men and women, see Figure 11. The tREACH data cannot be used as an example here since patients are examined when visiting their rheumatologist at regular time intervals, which implies that any event of interest (but not fatal) is interval censored. Cox regression was, though, proposed for right-censored survival times.

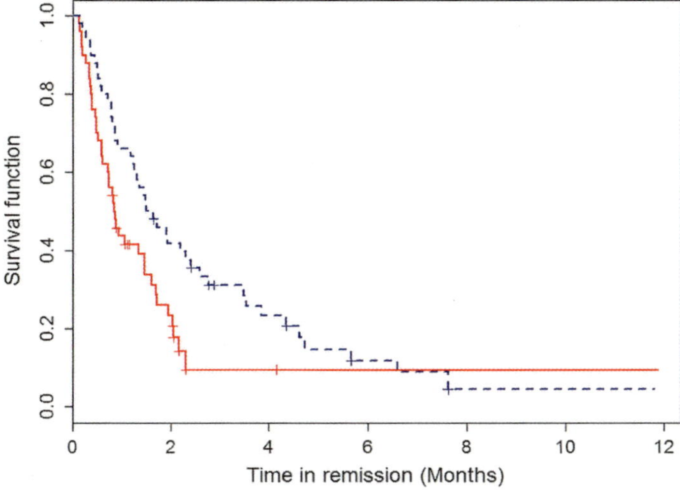

Fig. 11 Fictive study: Kaplan–Meier estimates of the survival functions for men (*dashed line*) and women (*solid line*)

As for logistic regression, an iterative procedure is needed to estimate the regression coefficients. In a Cox regression analysis, no intercept is estimated. This can be seen in the above expression of the general PH assumption. There is only one regressor x_1 equal to gender (female = 1). The estimate of β_1 is equal to 1.09, so that females go out of remission sooner than men. Now $\exp(\beta_1) = 2.97$ is an estimate of the hazard ratio, which is the coefficient c in section "The proportional hazards assumption." The 95 % CI for the hazard ratio, equal to [1.85, 4.77], does not include 1. We therefore conclude that females have a significantly higher risk to go out of remission than males ($P < 0.001$). An adapted R^2 and a concordance measure allow evaluating the predictive performance of the survival function. We obtained here $R^2 = 0.176$ and 0.636 for concordance.

As for the other regression models, several regressors can be included in a Cox regression model. The inclusion of other regressors will change the value and the meaning of the original regression coefficients. All issues that popped up with linear and logistic regression, such as which regressors to include and in what scale, also apply to Cox regression.

We note that the PH assumption is an assumption that needs to be verified. A sign of nonproportional hazards are crossing survival functions (if based on enough subjects) but also formal diagnostic procedures are available. When the effect of the regressors is not constant over time, one might extend the model by including interaction terms with time. It is also possible to assume some smooth dependence of the hazard ratio with time. Estimating the regression coefficients is then considerably more complex. It could also be that regressors change during the conduct of the study. They are called *time-dependent regressors* and can be incorporated in a classical Cox regression analysis. Recently another approach, based on *joint modeling* of a survival and a longitudinal process, has been proposed and looks quite promising [19].

Models for Longitudinal Studies

In a follow-up (FU) study, subjects are followed up in time. In the previous section, the time to an event was recorded in the FU study. Another example is when individuals are examined at several time points, which leads to a *longitudinal study*. Important examples of longitudinal studies are the randomized clinical trial (RCT) and the cohort study in epidemiology. To properly analyze longitudinal data, one needs to take into account the correlated nature of the repeated measures and one needs to address the fact that patients may miss examinations or drop out from the study. Many longitudinal studies in rheumatology are, however, analyzed inappropriately because of the unawareness of these two problems.

We first discuss the impact of missing data on the analysis of longitudinal studies, then give a brief review of some older, but still in use, statistical techniques possibly in combination with imputation techniques. We end with more modern techniques that incorporate flexibly the correlated nature of the data and allow for less restrictive missing data processes.

The Problem of Missing Data

Missing data can affect all kinds of studies, but with longitudinal studies, we have more tools to address the problems that missing data cause. The amount and the reason why data are missing dictate what statistical technique to use. First, note that subjects may miss a visit *intermittently* and then return afterward to the study or they may *drop out* completely from the study. The most serious problem is the latter situation upon which we will focus here. Leaving the study may happen for a variety of reasons. A classical taxonomy introduced by Little and Rubin [20] still dominates the missing data terminology. Here we discuss this terminology in the context of regression models, where we assume that the response may be missing, but not the regressors. One distinguishes:

- *Missing completely at random* (*MCAR*): A missing response occurs because of reasons completely unrelated to the response, i.e., by pure bad luck.
- *Missing at random* (*MAR*): The missing data mechanism is related to observed responses. For example, when in an RCT patients are removed from the study by the clinical investigator because their DAS28 is too high, the dropout process depends on the latest value of DAS28 recorded in the study.
- *Missing not at random* (*MNAR*): The missing data mechanism may not only be related to observed responses but also to unobserved responses. Take the previous example, but now assume that a visit to a rheumatology clinic outside the study reveals that the patient's DAS28 exceeds 5. The patient therefore decides to change medication and leaves unrecorded the study. Consequently, the dropout of the patient cannot be predicted within the study from the recorded past measurements.

Missing data may affect seriously the statistical analysis and the clinical conclusions. For instance, the descriptive statistics such as the mean, median, SD, etc. may be severely distorted with the MAR and MNAR missing data mechanisms, see, e.g., [21]. Most classical statistical techniques for the analysis of repeated measures are valid under MCAR (but their precision may be severely affected) but are likely to fail when the missing data processes are MAR or MNAR.

Classical Statistical Techniques

In clinical research, it is still common practice to compare two treatments in a longitudinal study by significance tests at each visit. Simplicity is the only advantage of this approach. Indeed, the *repeated significance testing approach* is flawed with various problems: (1) it suffers from the multiple testing problem, (2) this approach turns a longitudinal study into several cross-sectional studies and therefore neglects the correlation among the responses, (3) the approach can only be applied when the examination times are (roughly) regular, and finally, (4) with this approach, it is difficult to imagine what the results imply for future patients because at each visit the comparison of the treatments is done on a different set of patients, i.e., on only those patients that are present at the respective visits. It is an example of an *available case approach*, whereby only the patients available at the examination can be compared. Finally, it is only valid under the MCAR assumption.

To address the multiple testing issue, one could apply an ANOVA approach. There are two classical ANOVA techniques to analyze repeated measurements: *repeated measurements ANOVA* (*rANOVA*) and *multivariate ANOVA* (*MANOVA*). Both approaches were popular among statisticians about 50 years ago. However, these approaches are not suitable for contemporary studies in clinical research since they require the data to be balanced, i.e., all subjects should be measured at the same time points and the data are not plagued by missing values. For rANOVA and MANOVA, a subject will be removed from the analysis if he/she has missed only one measurement. In addition, rANOVA assumes that the correlation among all repeated measures is the same irrespective of the time lag between the measurements (*compound symmetry*). For MANOVA, the correlation matrix must be general (*unstructured*) and this might require too many variance and correlation parameters to estimate. For instance, when there are 6 visits, 21 correlations and variances need to be determined. This causes two problems: (1) estimating too many parameters for the given data reduces the power of the analysis considerably; (2) when there are relatively few subjects and many measurements per subject, the model parameters may be not estimable ruling out MANOVA as an option. The two ANOVA approaches are examples of the *complete-case approach*. They are only valid on the MCAR missing data mechanism. Despite the abovementioned drawbacks, the two ANOVA methods are still frequently used in the clinical literature.

Imputation Techniques

The above classical techniques may be combined with an approach that imputes reasonable values for the missing data. This may limit their efficiency loss in case of imbalance. A popular imputation approach in RCTs is the *last-observation-carried-forward (LOCF) approach*. This technique imputes for all the missing responses the last observed response value. Suppose that a patient dropped out at visit 3, then with the LOCF approach, the last recorded DAS28 value at visit 2 is repeatedly filled-in for all subsequent missing DAS28 values. There are, however, serious statistical as well as clinical problems with this approach. Indeed, it is now generally recognized that the LOCF procedure creates unrealistic profiles (both in terms of mean and variance). Further, the statistical properties of an analysis based on LOCF imputed data are unclear, see [21, 22].

An appropriate approach to impute missing data is the *multiple imputation (MI) approach*. The MI approach is based on a statistical model to impute the missing data stochastically. To reflect that filled-in data are subject to uncertainty, the imputation is done more than once (typically $M=3$ to 5 times) yielding M imputed data sets. The imputed data sets are then combined in a second step for the statistical analysis of the data. Any statistical model can be combined with MI approach. The MI approach can also be applied to impute missing regressor values.

More Recent Approaches to Analyze Longitudinal Data

We consider here two approaches: *mixed models* and *generalized estimating equation techniques*. We focus on continuous responses but mention also briefly the analysis of binary and ordinal responses.

Linear Mixed Models

A *linear mixed model* (LMM) assumes there exists an average profile for the population of patients from which the individual profiles deviate in a random manner by a subject-specific intercept, slope, quadratic term, etc. In Fig. 12, we give examples of LMMs whereby the evolution of the ith individual deviates from the overall downward linear trend in DAS28 by a subject-specific intercept b_{0i} (random intercept model) or additionally by a subject-specific slope b_{1i} (random intercept + slope model). The random intercept + slope model is given by

$$\text{DAS28}_{ij} = \beta_0 + \beta_1 \text{time}_{ij} + \cdots + b_{0i} + b_{1i}\text{time}_{ij} + \varepsilon_{ij},$$

with $\beta_0, \beta_1, \ldots$ called *fixed effects*. The sub index i pertains to the patient number; the sub index j (here 1 to 5) pertains to the visits with $j=1$ referring to the baseline visit and $j=5$ to the 5th monthly visit. The dots indicate that additional fixed effects can be included in the model. The solid thick line in Fig. 12 represents $\beta_0+\beta_1$ time$_{ij}$.

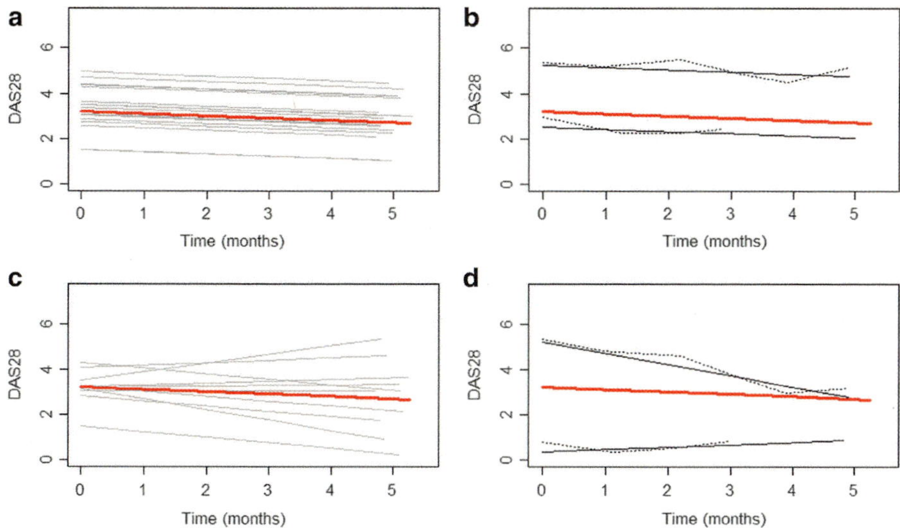

Fig. 12 Examples of mixed models. (**a**): random intercept model showing a sample of subject-specific linear trends and (**b**) two specific trends in the random intercept model together with observed profiles, (**c**) random intercept + slope model showing a sample of subject-specific linear trends, and (**d**) two specific trends in the random intercept + slope model together with observed profiles. In the different plots the solid thick line corresponds to the population average evolution. The thin solid lines correspond to the individual linear evolutions. The dotted lines in panels (**b**) and (**d**) represent the actual observed profiles

Note that here $\text{time}_{ij} = \text{time}_j$, which means that the time intervals between visits to were taken the same for all subjects. On the other hand, b_{0i}, b_{1i} represent the deviations of the subject-specific profiles from the population profile and are called *random effects*. Finally, ε_{ij} represents the measurement error, which is the fluctuation of the observed response around the subject-specific regression line ($\beta_0 + \beta_1 \text{time}_{ij} + \ldots + b_{0i} + b_{1i} \text{time}_{ij}$). The above model therefore reads as follows: the response (DAS28) at visit j of the ith patient is the sum of the overall trend seen in the population + the specific trend in patient i + the temporal fluctuation at visit j. As one can observe, the correlation among the repeated measurements is determined by the random intercept and slope, which ties together all observations from the same individual. For an LMM, no explicit imputation is involved, but there is still *implicit* imputation as can be seen in Fig. 12. In other words, for patients who drop out, it is assumed that their unobserved profile (after dropout) continues along their subject-specific profile.

The LMM allows for unequal time points. To estimate the model parameters (β_0, β_1, … and the variances of b_{0i}, b_{1i}, and ε_{ij}), distributional assumptions need to be made. Classically, it is assumed that b_{0i}, b_{1i}, and ε_{ij} have normal distributions with a zero mean and variances to be estimated by the data. The random effects are allowed to be correlated but should be independent from measurement error. Based on these assumptions, all parameters can be estimated. Given that the model is correctly specified, the parameters are well estimated for an MCAR or MAR dropout process,

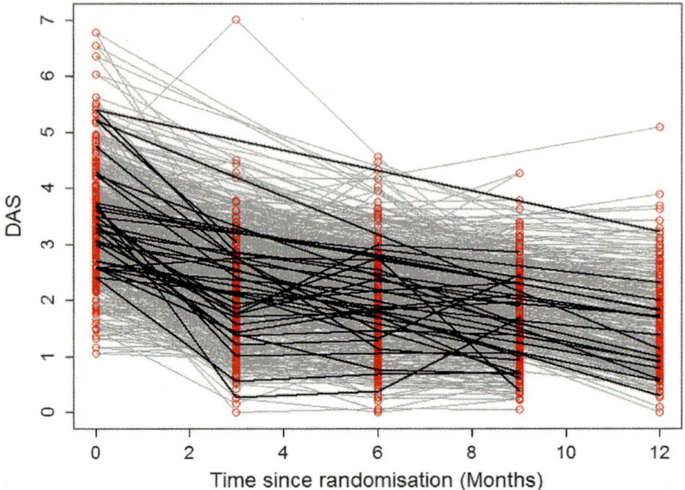

Fig. 13 tREACH study: spaghetti plot of observed longitudinal DAS profiles; for a random sample, the profile is printed in black; all others are printed in gray

but in principle not for an MNAR dropout process. We refer to [23] for the motivation of this result and further technical details.

As an illustration, we analyzed the longitudinal DAS responses from the tREACH study. It was planned that the RA patients were examined at baseline, 3, 6, 9, and 12 months. However, some of the patients missed visits and/or were dropouts. Of the 281 patients who were randomized to the three treatments (91 patients to treatment A, 93 to B, and 97 to C), 264 patients were still in the study at 3 months, 255 patients at 6 months, 250 patients at 9 months, and 248 patients at 12 months. Hence, only a relatively few patients dropped out. From experience, we know that most often the dropout mechanism is at least MAR, which motivates the use of the linear mixed model.

In Fig. 13 the individual profiles of all patients are plotted. We observe that overall there is a decrease in DAS but also that there is quite some variability. In Fig. 14, we show the mean ± SEM plots based on the observed data. For an MAR dropout process, we have seen above that these plots may be misleading but here the amount of dropouts is limited and hence the descriptive measures probably give a good picture of the true values.

The following LMM was fit to the DAS responses using the *R function lmer*:

$$\text{DAS}_{ij} = \beta_0 + \beta_1 \text{time}_{ij} + \beta_2 x_{1i} + \beta_3 x_{2i} + \beta_4 x_{3i} + \beta_5 x_{4i} + b_{0i} + b_{1i}\text{time}_{ij} + \varepsilon_{ij},$$

with

- Fixed effects, the regression coefficients of time (time_j), gender (x_{1i}), age at baseline (x_{2i}), treatment (x_{3i}), and duration of complaints (x_{4i}).
- Random effects: random intercept (b_{0i}) and slope (b_{1i}).

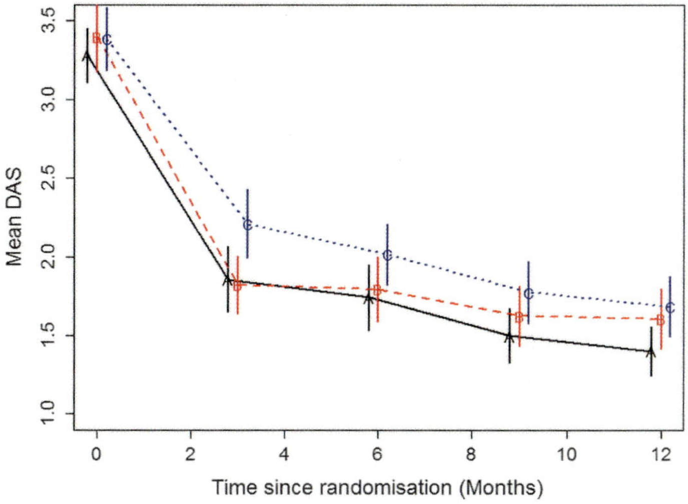

Fig. 14 tREACH study: mean ± SEM plots of DAS split up into the three treatment groups. The solid line corresponds to treatment arm A, the dashed line to treatment arm B and the dotted line to treatment C

Table 7 tREACH study: parameter estimates for the LMM with response: DAS and regressors: time since randomization, gender, age at baseline, treatment, and duration of complaints

Coefficient	Estimate	SE	*t*-value
Intercept	2.29	0.19	12.10
Time	–0.13	0.006	–22.93
Gender (0 = male)	0.39	0.086	4.57
Age (years)	0.011	0.003	3.91
Treatment B	0.03	0.098	0.34
Treatment C	0.19	0.097	1.97
Complaints	0.0004	0.00044	0.92

The results of this analysis are shown in Table 7. Note that the lmer function does not provide *P*-values. The reason is that the degrees of freedom of the *t*-distribution are quite hard to determine in the LMM. Nevertheless, we can deduce from Table 7 that except for treatment and duration of complaints all regressors have a significant impact on the response (*t*-values much larger than 2 in absolute value).

Also, the random intercept and slope of each patient can be estimated. Recall that b_{0i} expresses the subject-specific deviation of the intercept for the *i*th subject, while b_{1i} expresses the subject-specific deviation of the slope. In Fig. 15, the estimates of the random effects are shown. We notice that the histograms of the random effects show some mild deviation from normality. The scatterplot shows that compared to the overall trend, patients who start relatively low may have their DAS value increase or be roughly stable over time, while those who start relatively high have a tendency to decrease considerably.

The model in Table 7 is a starting point. We can then explore which other regressors should be included, whether polynomial terms in time or age are needed or

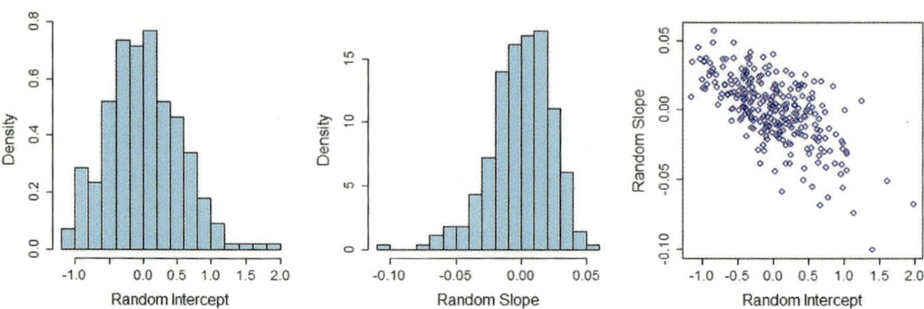

Fig. 15 tREACH study: histograms of the random intercept and slope and scatterplot of the random effects

double products, whether the random part should be made more complex by adding, say, a random quadratic term, etc. All of this can be done as in classical regression, and one can test which of the models is most appropriate.

We conclude that an LMM analysis provides a convenient way for analyzing contemporary follow-up studies, which are often hampered by many missing data. A condition is, however, that the LMM is (approximately) correctly specified and that the missing data process is at most MAR. However, one observes in simulations that the LMM often performs well in the case of MNAR especially if the repeated measurements are highly correlated. With regard to interpretation, a statistical analysis with a linear mixed model provides a treatment effect for the whole patient group if these patients were able to stay in the study until the end. This is different with the interpretation of a complete case analysis. Namely, a complete case analysis evaluates the treatment effect only for the patients still present at the end of the study and who never missed a visit. This is problematic since one cannot know in advance who will comply with the treatment during the whole of the study. On the other hand, with an LMM, none of the patients are excluded (provided they deliver at least one measurement), and all patients contribute to the estimated treatment effect.

Generalized Linear Mixed Models

A popular model to analyze longitudinal binary responses is the *logistic random effects model*. It is a generalization of the logistic model seen in section "Logistic regression" to include random effects. As an example, suppose that we are interested in the probability of remission in the tREACH study at each clinical examination. Let then π_{ij} be the probability that DAS < 1.6 at visit j and for patient *i*. A *logistic random intercept model* relating this probability to time and with the regressors of the previous section is given by the expression

$$\text{logit}\left(\pi_{ij}\right) = \beta_0 + \beta_1 time_{ij} + \beta_2 x_{1i} + \beta_3 x_{2i} + \beta_4 x_{3i} + \beta_5 x_{4i} + b_{0i}.$$

The random intercept b_{oi} is common to subject *i* and links all his repeated data. The fixed effects $\beta_0, \beta_1, \ldots, \beta_5$ have now a somewhat different interpretation than for a classical logistic regression model because of the inclusion of the random intercept into the model. Note that the above model does not have a measurement error. If needed, a random slope can be added to the model. The logistic random effects model has been further generalized to ordinal responses. We refer to [23, 24] for further technical details.

A special case of the logistic random intercept model is the *Rasch model*. This is a psychometric model for analyzing categorical data, such as answers to questions on a reading assessment or questionnaire responses. In [25], this model was used to determine whether the 14 questions (items) in the Completed Behçet's Disease Current Activity Forms form a hierarchical and unidimensional scale of disease activity. Specifically the authors used the model

$$\text{logit}\left(\pi_{ik}\right) = b_i - \beta_k,$$

with π_{ik} the probability that subject *i* will answer the item *k* correctly (or be able to do task *k*), b_i playing here the role of the disease activity of that subject, and β_k the item activity parameter. Hence, in this model, b_i is the random intercept that expresses the personal ability of a subject to answer the item correctly, while β_k is a fixed effect expressing the overall difficulty of answer item *k* correctly. This model is then fitted to each of the items.

Other repeated responses, such as counts, can be also analyzed with mixed effects models. A general class of such models is given by the *generalized linear mixed model*, extending the generalized linear models mentioned in section "Logistic regression" to include random effects. For all these mixed effects models, computations to determine the parameter estimates are considerably more involved (involving integral calculations) but are still feasible. Inference is again robust under an MCAR and MAR missing data process provided the model is (approximately) correctly specified.

Generalized Estimating Equations

The *generalized estimating equations* (*GEE*) approach is different in nature from the mixed model approach, where no complete model specification is required for the repeated measurements. The GEE approach can be applied to continuous and categorical outcomes. While for the mixed model approach, care should be taken that the mean structure and the correlation matrix should be correctly specified, with the GEE approach, only the mean structure needs to be specified correctly. For the correlation structure, just a rough guess is needed, called the *working correlation matrix*. While the GEE approach is a more robust approach to analyze longitudinal studies, it generally requires a larger sample size than the mixed model approach. Further, the basic version of GEE is only robust against an MCAR process. A *weighted GEE* or multiple imputation combined with GEE provides protection against an MAR process, at the expense of again a larger sample size.

Frailty Models

A generalization of Cox regression that includes random effects is called the *frailty model*. This approach consists of a variety of survival techniques to analyze clustered survival times occurring, e.g., when a patient suffers from several RA flares over time or RA patients cluster in groups because they have been treated in different hospitals, etc.

Approaches to Deal with MNAR Missingness

When the missing data or dropout process is of the MNAR type, in principle none of the approaches described above work. The problem of an MNAR process is that the probability of missing data/dropout depends on unobserved responses. Hence, there is no way to check what the specific missing data mechanism is. The only solution is to imagine different missing data processes and combine these with the primary analysis of the repeated measurements, i.e., to perform a *sensitivity analysis*. We refer to [23, 24, 26] for a further theoretical background and for practical guidelines.

Multivariate Methods

Up to now, we have considered only one response at a time. There is a whole class of statistical methods that allows exploring many responses at the same time; these are called *multivariate methods*. Note that multiple regression is often referred to in the literature as multivariate regression; this is however a wrong term because this statistical approach only involves one response.

Examples of multivariate techniques are *principal component analysis*, *factor analysis*, *biplot graphs*, etc. These approaches have in common that they aim to discover the intrinsic dimensionality of the multivariate response. For instance, in [27] 272 consecutive Turkish patients with Behçet's disease (BD) were examined for target organ associations. The authors extracted four factors using a factor analysis of the variables: oral and genital ulcers, erythema nodosum, papulopustular skin lesions, uveitis, superficial and deep vein thrombosis, and joint, arterial, neurological, and gastrointestinal involvement. These four factors explained 69 % of the information in the original measurements. We refer to the statistical literature for further details on this rich class of models.

The Bayesian Approach

There is a growing interest in an alternative approach for statistical inference. The basis for this approach goes back 250 years with Bayes' theorem, which was published in 1763. Two years after the death of reverent Thomas Bayes, his friend

Richard Price published the document "An Essay toward a Problem in the Doctrine of Chances," which is based on the writings of Bayes and which includes Bayes' theorem. Bayes' theorem expresses the uncertainty of the hypothesis of interest, after having collected experimental data and making use of what is known about this hypothesis. Formally, Bayes' theorem is given by

$$p(\text{hypothesis}|\text{data}) = \frac{p(\text{data}|\text{hypothesis})\, p(\text{hypothesis})}{p(\text{data})}.$$

The theorem reads: the hypothesis is strongly supported by the data ($p(\text{hypothesis}|\text{data})$ is high) when there is a relative strong prior belief in the hypothesis ($p(\text{hypothesis})$ is high) and/or the observed data fit well with the hypothesis ($p(\text{data}|\text{hypothesis})$ is high). The probability $p(\text{hypothesis}|\text{data})$ is called the *posterior probability*, $p(\text{data}|\text{hypothesis})$ is known as the *likelihood* of the data, and $p(\text{hypothesis})$ is the *prior probability* of the hypothesis.

A similar result can be formulated when we wish to know what the true value of a parameter θ is after having done an experiment. To explain this, suppose we wish to know the prevalence of RA in 2012 in Turkey. Browsing the Internet reveals that the RA prevalence around the globe varies from 0.2 to 1 % (excluding specific Indian tribes), but no value was found for Turkey. From these historical data, one could postulate that the prevalence for Turkey must be around 0.5 % but with uncertainty. This uncertainty can be expressed by a distribution, called the *prior distribution* shown in Fig. 16a. This distribution expresses that, with 95 % (prior) probability, we believe that the prevalence of RA lies between 0.25 and 0.89 %. Suppose now

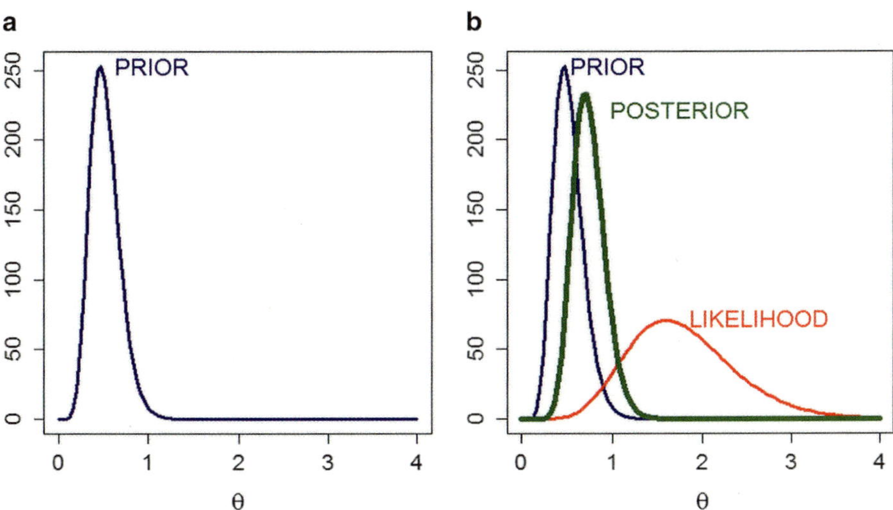

Fig. 16 Prevalence RA: (**a**) prior distribution of θ and (**b**) prior likelihood and posterior distribution of θ, with $\theta = \%\text{RA}$ in Turkey in 2012

that we have done a limited survey in 2012 examining 500 subjects in Turkey and found 8 subjects with RA. This gives an estimated prevalence of 1.6 % with a 95 % CI = [0.82 %, 3.12 %]. The likelihood function in Fig. 16b is based on the survey data and summarizes what we know of θ. This function is maximal for 1.6 % (hence, best supported prevalence value by the data), but also other not too different values for θ are relatively well supported (corresponding with a relatively high likelihood value). Bayes' theorem in this case is

$$p(\theta|\text{data}) = \frac{p(\text{data}|\theta)p(\theta)}{p(\text{data})}.$$

Hence, as before, the posterior probability is high for those values of θ that are well supported by the data, and the prior as can be inferred from Fig. 16b. The posterior distribution thus combines prior information with the information from the survey to arrive at a more precise statement on θ. The posterior uncertainty of the prevalence reduces to [0.44, 1.12 %]. The posterior distribution also delivers summary measures for θ characterizing its most likely value using the posterior mean, median, or mode and its (posterior) standard error. All can be computed from the posterior distribution.

There are three major aspects that distinguish the Bayesian approach from the classical frequentist approach:

- The Bayesian approach allows to include prior information into the analysis of data.
- In the Bayesian approach, the parameters have a distribution, which arises from the fact that we are always uncertain about the true value of that parameter.
- In the Bayesian approach we do not look at other possible samples as is done when computing the *P*-value. One says that the Bayesian approach is only based on the currently observed data; in other words, in the Bayesian approach, one conditions on the observed data.

While the classical frequentist approach is still most popular among clinicians, one might favor the Bayesian approach for the following reasons. After having done the experiment, the researcher invariably wishes to know how well his hypothesis is supported. As seen above, this is not given by the *P*-value, which only provides evidence against the observed results given the null hypothesis. In fact, $p(\text{hypothesis}|\text{data})$ is needed, but this can only be obtained from a Bayesian analysis. Further, the classical 95 % CI is interpreted as the interval that contains with 0.95 probability the true value. However, this is not the technical definition that applies in the frequentist approach (see section "Type I error, type II error and the power of a test") but has in fact a Bayesian flavor. Hence, the Bayesian approach may offer philosophical and conceptual advantages.

Nowadays, the Bayesian approach definitely offers to analyze more complex problems than the classical approach. However, it has taken more than 200 years before it was considered as a tool for the practical statistician, since for a long time, the approach could only be applied to (simple) textbook examples. Indeed, one must realize that in realistic examples the parameter θ quickly becomes a high-dimensional vector complicating the computation of the denominator $p(\text{data})$ in Bayes' theorem. Indeed, $p(\text{data}) = \int p(\text{data})p(\theta)\text{d}\theta$ involves the evaluation of an integral which can be quite complicated for high dimensions and often impossible to compute with classical numerical techniques. In that case, the posterior distribution cannot be determined and no inference is available. In other words, if the integral in the denominator cannot be computed, then the Bayesian approach cannot be applied.

A breakthrough was achieved by Gelfand and Smith [28] who suggested using a sampling technique to replace the integral calculations. The development of these *Markov chain Monte Carlo sampling techniques*, together with the development of the corresponding (Win)BUGS software [29], led to the great popularity of the Bayesian approach nowadays. The reason is that the sampling approach (together with WinBUGS and other recently developed Bayesian software) allows analyzing in principle any complex problem. We refer to the literature, especially the statistical literature (e.g., [30]), to appreciate the strength of the Bayesian approach, since space restrictions prevent us to illustrate its elegancy and power.

Despite its increasing popularity, the Bayesian approach is still criticized by many because it needs a prior distribution to make the computations happen. This prior distribution is inevitably (somewhat) subjective and therefore always a (small) subjective component creeps into a Bayesian analysis. The Bayesians argue that research is always somewhat subjective (and should be, otherwise it cannot be research). Secondly, they argue that (1) the prior distribution can be made so uninformative that it almost does not carry any prior information at all, (2) one can always vary the prior to evaluate its effect to see how much the posterior distribution is ruled by the prior information and how much by the data at hand, and (3) most often the information from the data dominates the prior information. What is important to realize is that the Bayesian approach offers a tool to combine prior knowledge with current data and hence mimics in this way how scientists organize their research and how humans in general go through life.

Statistical Guidelines

Motivated by the need to improve the standards of the methodology in clinical research, several guidelines to improve clinical research have been published in the literature. The earliest, and perhaps most well known, are the *CONSORT guidelines*. On the website http://www.consort-statement.org/, we can read that "CONSORT, which stands for Consolidated Standards of Reporting Trials, encompasses various initiatives developed by the CONSORT Group to alleviate the problems arising from inadequate reporting of randomized controlled trials (RCTs)." The main product of CONSORT is the *CONSORT statement*, which is an evidence-based, minimum set of recommendations for reporting RCTs. It offers a standard way for authors to prepare reports of trial findings, facilitating their complete and transparent reporting and aiding their critical appraisal and interpretation. The

CONSORT statement comprises a 25-item checklist and a flow diagram, along with some brief descriptive text. The checklist items focus on reporting how the trial was designed, analyzed, and interpreted; the flow diagram displays the progress of all participants through the trial.

The CONSORT guidelines constitute the start of a series of guidelines in different kinds of studies, such as *PRISMA* (guidelines for systematic reviews and meta-analyses), *STROBE* (guidelines for observational studies in epidemiology), etc. More guidelines can be found on the website of the *COCHRANE collaboration* (http://www.cochrane.org/). As we can read from the website: "The Cochrane collaboration is an international network to help healthcare practitioners, policy-makers, patients, their advocates and carers, make well-informed decisions about health care."

The above guidelines encompass more than just statistical guidelines; in fact, their purpose is to improve clinical research on the whole from the design to the reporting and interpretation stage. Various other guidelines can be found on the world wide web. And of course many statistical textbooks contain also guidelines; see, e.g., [4, 5].

Conclusions

This chapter had the intention to give a brief overview of the statistical methodology used to analyze clinical studies, with examples from two rheumatologic studies. It was only possible to discuss the topics briefly, and we had to refer to the reader to the literature where for each topic a multitude of books has been written. In addition, the statistical discipline has seen an explosion in the last five decades and especially in the last two decades due to the enormous evolution in computing power. Therefore, many topics were not addressed at all or could only touched upon briefly, such as with the large class of multivariate statistical techniques, the exploratory Bayesian approaches, etc. The explosion in the development of new statistical approaches will not and cannot stop, since the medical society is collecting increasingly more data and more complex data. And statistics is by excellence the science that aims to make sense out of these data.

References

1. R Development Core Team. R: a language and environment for statistical computing [computer software]. Vienna: R Foundation for Statistical Computing; 2010.
2. SAS® version 9.3 Cary, NC, USA, SAS Institute Inc. 2012.
3. IBM Corp. Released 2012. IBM SPSS statistics for windows, version 21.0. Armonk: IBM Corp.
4. Bland M. An introduction to medical statistics. 3rd ed. Oxford: Oxford University Press; 2002.
5. Petrie A, Sabin C. Medical statistics at a glance. 3rd ed. Chichester: Wiley; 2009.

6. Walter MJM, Mohd Din SH, Hazes JMW, Lesaffre E, Barendregt PJ, Luime JJ. Is tight controlled disease activity with online patient reported outcomes possible? J Rheumatol. 2014;41:640–7.
7. Van der Heijde D, Jacobs J. The original "DAS" and the "DAS28" are not interchangeable: comment on the articles by Prevoo et al. Arthritis Rheum. 1998;41:942–50.
8. Van der Heijde D, Van't Hof M, Van Riel R, et al. Judging disease activity in clinical practice in rheumatoid arthritis: first step in the development of a disease activity score. Ann Rheum Dis. 1990;49:916–20.
9. Bruce B, Fries J. The health assessment questionnaire (HAQ). Clin Exp Rheumatol. 2005;23: S14–8.
10. Fransen J, Langenegger T, Michel B, Stucki G. Feasibility and validity of the RADAI, a self-administered rheumatoid arthritis disease activity index. Br Soc Rheumatol. 2000;39:321–7.
11. Wolfe F. Fatigue assessments in rheumatoid arthritis: comparative performance of visual analog scales and longer fatigue questionnaires in 7760 patients. J Rheumatol. 2004;31: 1896–902.
12. Claessen SJ, Hazes JM, Huisman MA, van Zeben D, Luime JJ, Weel AE. Use of risk stratification to target therapies in patients with recent onset arthritis; design of a prospective randomized multicenter controlled trial. BMC Musculoskelet Disord. 2009;18(10):71.
13. de Jong PH, Hazes JM, Barendregt PJ, et al. Induction therapy with a combination of DMARDs is better than methotrexate monotherapy: first results of the tREACH trial. Ann Rheum Dis. 2013;72(1):72–8.
14. Visser H, le Cessie S, Vos K, Breedveld FC, Hazes JM. How to diagnose rheumatoid arthritis early: a prediction model for persistent (erosive) arthritis. Arthritis Rheum. 2002;46(2):357–65.
15. Aletaha D, Neogi T, Silman AJ, et al. Rheumatoid arthritis classification criteria: an American College of Rheumatology/European League Against Rheumatism collaborative initiative. Arthritis Rheum. 2010;62(9):2569–681.
16. Royall R. Statistical evidence. A likelihood paradigm. London: Chapman and Hall; 1997.
17. Svejgaard A, Ryder LP. HLA and disease associations: detecting the strongest association. Tissue Antigens. 1994;43:18–27.
18. Cox DR. Regression models and life-tables (with discussion). J R Stat Soc B. 1972;34: 187–220.
19. Rizopoulos D. Joint models for longitudinal and time-to-event data: with applications in R. Boca Raton: Chapman and Hall/CRC; 2012.
20. Little RJA, Rubin DB. Statistical analysis with missing data. 2nd ed. New York: Wiley; 2002.
21. Lesaffre E. Longitudinal studies in rheumatology: some guidance for analysis. Bull NYU Hosp Jt Dis. 2012;70(2):65–72.
22. Panel on Handling Missing Data in Clinical Trials; National Research Council. The prevention and treatment of missing data in clinical trials. Washington, DC: The National Academic Press; 2010.
23. Verbeke G, Molenberghs G. Linear mixed models for longitudinal data. New York: Springer; 2000.
24. Molenberghs G, Verbeke G. Linear models for discrete longitudinal data. New York: Springer; 2005.
25. Lawton G, Bhakta BB, Chamberlain MA, Tennant A. The Behçet's disease activity index. Rheumatology. 2004;43:73–8.
26. Molenberghs G, Kenward M. Missing data in clinical studies. West Sussex: Wiley; 2007.
27. Tunc R, Keyman E, Melikoglu M, Fresko I, Yazici H. Target organ associations in Turkish patients with Behçet's disease: a cross sectional study by exploratory factor analysis. J Rheumatol. 2002;29(11):2393–6.
28. Gelfand AE, Smith AE. Sampling-based approaches to calculating marginal densities. J Am Stat Assoc. 1990;85:398–409.
29. Lunn DJ, Thomas A, Best N, Spiegelhalter D. WinBUGS – a Bayesian modelling framework: concepts, structure, and extensibility. Statistics Comput. 2000;10:325–37.
30. Lesaffre E, Lawson A. Bayesian biostatistics (statistics in practice). New York: Wiley; 2012.

Disease Classification/Diagnosis Criteria

Hasan Yazici and Yusuf Yazici

The science and practice of rheumatology rely heavy on criteria. This is true for both clinical practice and research. This chapter will focus on disease classification and diagnostic criteria only. Outcome and remission criteria are handled in chapter "Outcome measures in rheumatoid arthritis".

The prevailing view is that we should have separate criteria sets for research and diagnosis, the former requiring *classification* and the latter *diagnostic* criteria. We propose this is not only unnecessary but unfounded. The main aim of this chapter is to discuss why we indeed have to put heavy emphasis on disease criteria in rheumatology and how we should we go about it and why it is wrong to have separate classification and diagnostic criteria for any one disease. In doing this we will resort to specific examples from the recent attempts in criteria making for rheumatoid arthritis (RA) and vasculitides, especially Behçet's syndrome (BS).

H. Yazici, MD (✉)
Division of Rheumatology, Department of Medicine, Cerrahpasa Medical Faculty, Cerrahpasa Hospital, University of Istanbul, Cerrah PaÅŸa Mh No 53, Istanbul 34098, Turkey
e-mail: hasan@yazici.net

Y. Yazici, MD
Division of Rheumatology, Department of Medicine, Seligman Center for Advanced, Therapeutics and Behcet's Syndrome Center, NYU Hospital for Joint Diseases, New York University School of Medicine, New York University, 333 East 38th Street, New York, NY 10016, USA
e-mail: yusuf.yazici@nyumc.org

H. Yazici et al. (eds.), *Understanding Evidence-Based Rheumatology*,
DOI 10.1007/978-3-319-08374-2_3

A Brief History of Disease Criteria in Rheumatology

Generations of physicians around the globe have been and still are taught the Jones criteria to diagnose rheumatic fever [1]. These criteria were developed by Dr. Jones in 1944 by a strictly ad hoc and eminence based approach and we are afraid this legacy continued in several later updates. The last attempt to better these criteria was a consensus conference in 1992 [2]. In this last conference the issue of potential geographical differences in the utility of these criteria were brought up, as if this was something unique to rheumatic fever. As we will bring up once more below, the utility of *any* diagnostic criteria is strictly dependent in the setting in which the criteria are applied. It is no surprise then that more recent formal surveys keep on showing that the sensitivity of the Jones criteria for diagnosing rheumatic fever is only around 30 % in endemic areas like India [3].

In 1974 Dr. Desmond O'Duffy proposed his Behcet's Disease criteria [4]. The more senior author of this chapter (HY) was in the audience as a young fellow when this set of criteria was presented in a rheumatology meeting. At the end of the presentation he got up and had the courage to ask the presenter " How successfully do your criteria tell Behcet's from ingrown toe nails, particularly since I saw no attempts to prospectively test these criteria in a real setting nor a control group in your exercise?" There was little discussion and few heated exchanges, but this outburst was probably the initial stimulus for the latter work related to the formulation of the International Study Group Criteria for Behcet's Disease (ISGC) [5] currently in use.

Perhaps a new era began in criteria making when American College of Rheumatology (ACR) began publishing criteria for many of the vasculitides [6]. These criteria were no longer ad hoc. A survey was conducted seeking formal sensitivity and specificity for many of the common primary vasculitides. Granted they were based on retrospective analyses and lacked prospective testing, they were an important step away from sheer eminence.

Then came the realization that these ACR vasculitis criteria were not useful for diagnostic purposes [7]. In a formal sensitivity and specificity study it was shown that these criteria had limited (17 % to 29 %) positive predictive values when applied to 198 patients with various vasculitides and connective tissue diseases. Two years later, a further study showed that Chapel Hill Consensus Conference (CHC) criteria, another widely recognized vasculitis criteria set mainly based on the size of the vessel involved, correctly identified only 8 of 27 patients with Wegener's granulomatosis and 4 of 12 patients with microscopic polyangiitis [8]. The response to this issue was that these two sets of criteria were not intended for diagnostic use but were strictly classification criteria for research and educational purposes [9]. This contention sounded very reasonable when first heard and over the years it became the standard to call all disease criteria classification criteria. This was followed by a new desire and the promise to prepare diagnostic criteria in addition to classification criteria for our diseases, an exercise, which we are afraid, might be likened to constructing a perpetual motion machine.

Why do we Need Disease Criteria?

As with other major and hotly debated issues the "why" of an exercise is often a neglected caveat. Apart from preparing for boards and other such evils there are some very good reasons for having disease criteria. These include:

1. To diagnose diseases to help our patients. This encompasses both managing and explaining to the patient the nature of his/her illness.
2. To conduct valid clinical or basic research about these conditions.
3. To explain to the public, health authorities, third party payers, research supporters and financial source allocators the nature of our patients' illnesses.

The presence of separate reasons, at first sight, might be taken to indicate that we might actually need separate classification criteria for research and diagnostic criteria for our patients but perhaps other sets of criteria for still other purposes and even perhaps one for Brussels and another for Washington, as well. We, however, propose that one set of criteria should be good enough for diagnosis, research and public awareness as long we explain, first to ourselves, then to our patients and rest of the public what we intend to with these criteria openly, frankly admitting we cannot diagnose every ill we see. This explanation should obviously continue with the explanation that we can manage some of these ills rather effectively even when we do not know what the exact diagnosis is.

Rheumatologic Diseases as Constructs

As we emphasized in the previous chapter, many rheumatologic diseases do not have specific clinical, histologic, laboratory or radiologic features. Hence we have to come up with constructs to specify what we mean by a "disease". For example if we have a shoulder which is swollen in the shape of a shoulder pad and when we biopsy it we find amyloidosis, we do not have to come up with a construct to tell us and the patient that he/she has amyloidosis. The same is true for a painful, hot and swollen knee from which you isolate staphylococci. On the other hand, in a patient with chronic mouth ulcers, attacks of diarrhea and episodes of uveitis you have to build up a construct to identify Behçet's syndrome and another to identify Crohn's. Still yet, you have to build up a construct to tell one from the other. Why do you have to resort to constructs? Simply because neither Behçet's nor Crohn's can be identified by a specific appearance, histology or a laboratory finding. So you need to build up a concept composed of specific features, in other words *a construct*. Surely the need for such constructs in rheumatology is not as extensive as in psychiatry with their voluminous standard reference manual, DSM (Diagnostic and Statistical Manual of Mental Disorders) of the American Psychiatric Association which includes definitions of over 400 different mental disorders [10] but we still need them. A set of criteria in turn is nothing more or less than the declaration of the components of a construct with some hierarchy (more commonly called weighing) of these components. It is to be underlined that elements which we decide to exclude from this construct make up the exclusions of our criteria. We propose that the first step in understanding disease criteria is to realize that they are constructs put together for specific purposes to explain and convey departures from the normal. In addition such constructs are needed not only for diseases of unknown origin. Sometimes we resort to constructs in handling diseases we know in depth the etiology and/or the pathogenesis of. For example in a tuberculosis endemic area we can justifiably begin treating a patient with a cough for so many weeks and a chest radiograph according to a well built up construct for diagnosis of tuberculosis or admit a patient with a chest pain for a suspected myocardial infarction if he/she fulfills the Cook County criteria for chest pain [11]. The main message then is that in the science and practice of medicine a diagnosis is needed mainly after we consider what we do with it.

The Basic Elements of Criteria Making

We have emphasized that we need disease criteria especially when our disease is a construct. The 3 basic elements of criteria making all have to do with concepts in probability. They are sensitivity, specificity and the pretest probability.

Sensitivity: Sensitivity is an easy concept. It is simply the percentage of true positives. If 95 % of patients with systemic lupus erythematosus (SLE) are positive for antinuclear antibodies (ANA) then the sensitivity of ANA for SLE is 95 %. Alternatively if 85 % percent of patients fulfilling a particular set of disease criteria for SLE then it is said that this set of criteria is 85 % sensitive in detecting SLE.

Specificity: Specificity is a more difficult concept. It is the percentage of true negatives. Following the example we gave in defining sensitivity, if 80 % of all people *not* having SLE are *not* positive for ANA, then the specificity of ANA for SLE is 80 %. Similarly if a particular set of criteria is negative in 85 % among a group of individuals without SLE then we say that this set of criteria is 85 % specific in detecting SLE. Why is specificity more difficult [12]? We propose two reasons. First, before defining either the sensitivity or the specificity of any finding or a set of criteria for any disease, we have to first define what we mean by individuals with and without the disease. This is intuitively easier in sensitivity where our job is to only define what we mean by the disease we are interested in. If we are trying to assess the sensitivity of laboratory finding we are only concerned with one disease, SLE. We can surely also specifically want to assess the sensitivity among a subset of SLE patients like early, mild or severe disease. Whichever is the case, when at the end we say that "The sensitivity of the test A is 75 % in SLE we say practically all that needs to be said. With specificity, however the situation is more involved. When we declare that "The test A is 70 % specific for SLE." the information we convey is incomplete. What we need to define here is not SLE but *what is not SLE*. On the one hand, we can make our test very specific if we test it among healthy people only or we can make it noticeably less specific for SLE if we test it among patients with a particular disease with a known propensity for having a positive test A. In brief, the definition of specificity of any finding for any disease is incomplete unless we also clearly define the population without having the disease of our concern. What needs to be said is "The test A is 70 % specific for SLE when tested among x number of healthy individuals, y number of patients with disease B and z number of patients with disease C".

The second reason we propose for what makes specificity more difficult to grasp than sensitivity is the way we verbalize either concept. When we say "Among 100 patients with SLE 95 patients were ANA positive. Therefore the sensitivity of having a positive ANA test is 95 % sensitive for SLE.", three positive bits of information follow each other. On the other hand, when we declare "Among 100 patients without SLE, 70 were negative for ANA. Therefore the specificity of having a positive ANA is 70 % specific for SLE." we again verbalize three consecutive bits of fact however, now, the first two of these are negative while the 3rd is a positive bit of information. We propose that this mental incongruity is the second reason why specificity is a relatively more difficult concept to remember.

Confidence Intervals Around Sensitivity and Specificity

As we will repeatedly see in this book some of the evidence behind evidence-based medicine is surprisingly new. Recall that when we defined sensitivity above, we only gave a percentage. It does not require a great insight to realize that the quality of information coming from 700/1000=70 % and 7/10=70 % differ substantially.

It is also sobering to note that confidence intervals are still not popular with criteria makers of our day. On the other hand this should not be surprising in that it was as late as 1995 that the science of medicine was introduced to confidence intervals around sensitivity and specificity [13].

The Inverse Relation Between the Sensitivity and Specificity – The ROC

A further important point to be discussed about sensitivity and specificity is their inverse relationship. The graphic description of this relationship is the so-called ROC (receiver operating characteristics) curve. The term comes from signal detection used by engineers for military purposes during World War II [14]. A graph is constructed by plotting the sensitivity (the so called true-positives) against 1- specificity (the so – called false negatives) for a series of hypothetical criteria to diagnose a disease. The criteria set A with a 90 % sensitivity and 85 % specificity will correctly pick up 90 % of the patients with the disease while it will also falsely designate 15 % of the individuals without the disease as having the disease. On the other hand the criteria set B with 95 % sensitivity but this time with 75 % specificity will identify 95 % of all the patients with the disease, however this time a considerably more portion, 25 %, of the individuals without the disease will be incorrectly labeled.

It can be said that a substantial portion of medical decision making is, or more realistically should be, based on constantly working with mostly conceptual ROCs. For example, when confronted with a patient with chest pain you want have criteria as sensitive as possible to put him in a coronary care unit for observation. You can afford to be not very specific for diagnosing him/her as having a myocardial infarction. A short time later when you are debating whether to put a coronary stent in you have to be more specific with a trade off in sensitivity. The decision for a coronary bypass is again another point on the curve, etc. In brief, the relation between what you want to do and where you are on the ROC is all important and without the appreciation of its importance all exercise related to criteria making is in vain.

Importance of Pretest Probabilities and Likelihood Ratios in Making Criteria

It is intuitive that more frequent a disease is, more likely it will be diagnosed and vice versa. Bayes' theorem (BT) expresses this numerically. The importance of disease frequency (pretest probability in Bayesian terms) in making a diagnosis is not well appreciated in that the usefulness of any disease criteria ultimately depends on this theorem. BT states that given a set of disease criteria is positive in an individual, the probability of that individual having the sought disease is the product of the positive likelihood ratio (LR^+) multiplied by the pretest probability (PrP) of that disease in the setting where the patient is seen [15]. Briefly A (the probability of disease being present if the criteria are positive) = B (the PrP) X C (the LR^+ as defined by the disease criteria at hand). The formula is usually given in odds but it works with probabilities as well. Since physicians are more used to probabilities we suggest they use these, remembering that a probability is the likelihood of an event happening against the sum of the probabilities of its happening *and* not happening and thus always expressed as a fraction of unity. The odds, on the other hand, is the ratio of the number of times an event can happen versus the number of times it cannot happen. For example if an event has a 80 % probability of happening then the odds of that event happening versus not happening would be 4:1.

A different type of LR, LR^- also helps us in decision making. While a LR^+ is expressed is sensitivity/1-specificity or more simply the ratio of the %'s of true positives to false positives while a LR^- is expressed as 1-sensitivity/specificity or more simply the ratio of false negatives to the true negatives.

To give an example, we know that the sensitivity of the most popular criteria for Behcet's syndrome (BS), ISGC criteria [5] is 93 % while its specificity is 97 %.

With these specifications it means that the LR^+ of the ICBD criteria is = 31 while its LR^- is = 0.07. So if we apply the ISGC set to 100 consecutive patients in an outpatient clinic and the pretest probability of having BS in this clinic is 1.0 %, then the probability that any one patient fulfilling the ISBD criteria would have BS in this clinic would be 23.7 %. Conversely the probability of any one patient not fulfilling these criteria to have BS in this clinic would be 0.07 %. In this example it is clear that ISGC were considerably more useful in ruling out than ruling in BS in this clinic. One also sees from this example how important the pretest probability is to judge the usefulness of any criteria set.

It should be intuitively apparent to the reader from the above discussion that the diagnostic usefulness of both the LR^+ and the LR^- of criteria set depends very much on the PrP of the presence and the absence of the disease in the setting the disease is being sought. There are two additional arithmetic indices that help us here. The first is the "positive predictive value" which is the ratio of true positives to all (true + false) positives and the second is the "negative predictive value" which is the ratio of true negatives to all (true + false) negatives. The arithmetic formula for the first is:

Positive predictive value = sensitivity X PrPd/sensitivity X PrP + (1-specificity) X (1-PrP)

and for the second is:

Negative predictive value = specificity X PrPnd/specificity X PrPnd + (sensitivity) X (PrPnd)

where PrPd represents the prevalence of the disease in the population we are concerned with and the PrPnd stands for the prevalence of nondiseased (including those individuals with diseases other than the one we are trying to diagnose) in the same population.

Going back to the LRs two more important uses should be underlined. They are used to devise disease criteria themselves and they can also be used to find the inherent prevalence of the disease (PrP) we are seeking to diagnose in the setting we practice or for comparing prevalence between different settings in many situations where we do not know the differing inherent frequencies.

In either instance the basic method is the same. What needs to be done is to collect a large group of patients and suitable controls from diseases which come into the differential diagnosis. We then numerically compare the frequency of the individual clinical and laboratory findings of the diseases that come into the differential diagnosis. This process is commonly known as making "a clinical prediction" rule. The usual arithmetic involved is a step down logistic regression to identify which clinical and/or laboratory findings independently contributed to a diagnosis already established.

For example in order to prepare the ISGC set already alluded to a group of BS patients already diagnosed as such were taken [5, 16]. The frequencies of a group of selected clinical findings (since this syndrome has no specific laboratory or histologic findings) of the BS group were compared to the frequencies of the same clinical findings among, again, an already diagnosed patients' diseases that usually come into the differential diagnosis of BS. Thus for each clinical feature a sensitivity and a specificity were calculated. These made up the LR^+ and the LR^- for that symptom. Following this a step down logistic regression was made, to see which clinical features weighed the most in the differential diagnosis. In a hierarchical scheme from high to low only those features that added up to an increased ability to differentiate BS from the control group made up the disease criteria. Once made, this set of criteria had its own sensitivity, specificity and LRs to tell BS from other conditions. So, in brief, a diagnostic criteria set is nothing more or less than a LR, which has positive and negative components.

As said the LRs can also be used to estimate the disease prevalence (the PrP) in a practice setting. An excellent example for this is how cardiologists used it in the past to determine the PrP of coronary artery disease (CAD) in 2 cardiology and 2 general medicine settings [17]. They wanted to know this to better judge whether a patient presenting with chest pain had a higher, different chance of having CAD when he/she presented to a cardiology clinic versus a general medicine facility. In this exercise they used how various clinical and laboratory features at the time of presentation, through the LRs similarly calculated told, whether they were eventually diagnosed or not as having CAD. In short the clinical decision rule thus prepared from a list of separate LR's was the LR or C in the Bayes' formula as given above. The A was the probability of CAD as observed and the B was the prevalence eventually estimated in the 4 different settings. It indeed turned out that the two general medicine settings had lower PrPs than the two cardiology settings.

One final word before we leave the discussion about LRs is the rather confusing statements in many expert sources is that LRs do not depend on disease prevalence [18]. The issue is that they do not depend on any frequency once the disease criteria or a clinical prediction rule is formulated but they are very much dependent on disease or a disease feature frequency when they are initially formulated and this directly takes us to the next item to be discussed about disease criteria.

Circularity in Criteria Making

A master of quantitation in rheumatology James Fries had once said [19]: *Presence of disease "criteria" affirms our ignorance of the essence of disease. If we understand a disease, we can ascribe the elements that are necessary and sufficient for its diagnosis. One can so define gouty arthritis, in which joint fluid crystals serve as a "gold standard" against which to measure the usefulness of other observations. No other major rheumatic disease, including SLE, has such a standard. Thus, criteria must be constructed in a circular manner, by testing variables against a diagnosis based on intuition. The 'best' criteria therefore only describe the current conventional wisdom in an efficient manner.*

We believe, especially for the practicing rheumatologist, rather lengthy discussion in the previous section about the Bayes' theorem and the LRs were helpful regarding how circular indeed is all criteria making.

However, here we have to make a distinction between a *circular manner* and a *circular reasoning*. When Humpty Dumpty used a word it meant exactly what he chose it to mean "neither more nor less". This is rather similar to the exercise of making criteria to identify a disease X . Once we make it, when the next patient presents with this construct we say this patient has that disease. This identification has surely been made in a *circular manner* as it was ought to be. Now let us assume we had included in our disease criteria the positivity of the laboratory findings y or z as a prerequisite for a diagnosis and tabulate our experience in time the characteristics of the patients we had seen with this disease. If we then say "We saw 100 patients within the last 3 months with the disease X and very noticeably all of them were y or z positive . This is *circular logic* par excellence. While our readers will find many definitions of circular logic in sources starting from ancient Greece, a quite workable definition of circular logic is "coming to a conclusion *unaware* (italics added) that the conclusion reached was inescapable" [20].

Disease Criteria: Classification Versus Diagnostic Criteria

Many of the current disease criteria we use include a sentence to the effect *this set of criteria are useful after other disease are excluded* [5, 21] which indeed deserves the naughty reply, *If so why do I need these criteria to start with?* Another common statement is "*These are classification criteria and we hope to follow up with diagnostic criteria soon.*" As recently admitted in an otherwise excellent review [22] the authors acknowledged there were no diagnostic criteria at hand for vasculitis. We agree, however , the authors continued to give the old promise of diagnostic criteria to come. We are afraid that this urge to prepare universal diagnostic criteria for many of our diseases is rather like the ancient hopes of the alchemists or the zealots of perpetual motion machines.

Why is this so? There are several possible explanations:

First, as brought up in the first chapter and reiterated here many of our diseases are constructs without any specific causes and known pathogenic mechanisms. As such their definition is almost solely dependent on how we define them. Even slight differences in these constructs can make their subsequent identification rather difficult. We will return to this more in the next section on the new ACR/EULAR criteria for rheumatoid arthritis. Second, physicians [23] and their patients are not well trained in probabilities. The all-important Bayesian approach with its pivotal PrP is still not widely appreciated. LR is not a frequently heard term in everyday medical parlance. The Bayesian probabilities dictate that when the PrP of a disease is small even with diagnostic criteria with high $^{+}$LRs the chances of false positive diagnoses too high to be useful in the individual patient. Third, as we have noted in the previous 2 sections the LRs of a diagnostic criteria set are very much dependent on the setting in which the criteria was made. So the true validation of any criteria set should be made in the real clinical setting and this is seldom available.

Next, the well intentioned truism that to classify is somewhat different from to diagnose has compounded the problem. To diagnose is nothing more or less than to classify in the individual patient [12]. The cerebral process between the two is virtually the same. It is also self-deceiving to say, as is frequently done, "We classify when we do research and diagnose when we treat a patient." Of note is the not much appreciated hidden implication of this statement. How can we convince ourselves that we can be more objective and more scientific when we do research and be less scientific and less objective when we try to manage an illness? Such a contention may not even be ethical. Lastly, the patients, the health authorities including the third party payers and most importantly us physicians almost always expect a formal and tangible diagnosis rather than a mere classification from physicians. It is important to note that the historically much older word to "diagnose" goes back to ancient Greece and means to discern including "*knowing the nature of*". The word "classify", however, is 17th century and simply means allocating to different classes. Thus a mere classification implies less precision and even less of an attempt "to better comprehend the nature of" [20]. When confronted with a patient, we prefer to diagnose and when we do research, we like to classify. However, in many instances we do not openly admit we cannot make a specific diagnosis in many of our patients. There are also many instances, while we do not exactly know what a patient has, we do much better in recognizing what he/she does not have. This consideration is particularly relevant in situations where we are confronted with a patient with a hitherto undefined disease. It is indeed puzzling why, as physicians, we do not more frequently admit that most of what we diagnose are based on probability, rather than certainty. Perhaps as the proverbial healer we do want to play down our image.

What was Wrong with the 2010 ACR/EULAR Criteria for Early RA?

We chose to give a special place to the 2010 ACR/EULAR criteria for early RA [24–26] in this chapter for the main reason that some of the shortcomings in the design, execution and interpretation of this major effort were rather representative of how the rheumatology discipline, we suggest, inadequately addressed the whole issue of criteria making

The main drive behind the creation of such a criteria set was that within the preceding two decades rheumatologists understood that earlier we treated RA the better the patient outcomes were. It was clear that methotrexate (MTX) was the anchor drug in managing RA but the new biologic agents were also quite promising. Nevertheless, this needed to be officially announced not only to all the rheumatologists but also to the public where the patients and the third party payers came from. In Fries' words about all criteria quoted above [19] the aim was to *describe the current conventional wisdom in an efficient manner.* Finally, the criteria then at hand to classify RA [27] did this in an inefficient way because it identified the disease late in the game, mainly among patients with already serious morbidities.

However the definition of "early RA" was difficult in that in any setting there were (and are) differing views about what constituted early RA. So a construct was needed to define this. The authors decided to select a group of patients from 9 different early arthritis cohorts from either side of the Atlantic. The main 2 main inclusion criteria were that patients had to have inflammatory arthritis (synovitis/swelling) at least in 1 joint and they had to be prescribed MTX at most within a year of their initial presentation. On the other hand the main exclusion criterium was that patients who had an apparent diagnosis, other than RA.

The authors chose MTX initiation within a year of arthritis as the golden inclusion rule for this exercise. They reasoned that a good rheumatologist invariably prescribed MTX to those patients whom he/she thought was developing or have already developed within a certain time, the erosive, deforming bad disease (construct) which we call classic RA today. They did not want to consider fulfilling the older criteria as the golden rule since, they reasoned, this would cause circularity as this set of criteria particularly identified patients with advanced disease, the outcome they wanted to particularly avoid with the use of the new data set. They emphasized it was important to avoid circularity [24, 26].

The exercise had 3 phases. First, the data driven phase, where chiefly by a factor analysis the main elements that prompted a rheumatologist to start MTX therapy in a patient with early inflammatory arthritis were determined. The second phase was a *consensus-based, decision science–informed approach* with the purpose of deriving a clinician based judgement as to which clinical, laboratory, radiographic clues were determinants of eventually developing bad disease in RA. These clinicians not only used their expertise but were also "informed" of the results of Phase 1 in this undertaking. Finally, the third phase was integration of the information from Phases 1 and 2 with a final validation of the criteria set among 3 of the 9 cohorts not analyzed in Phases 1 and 2.

So what are the outstanding problems with this exercise?

A. There was no intention at formulating specificity of these criteria. It followed that there were no control groups with other diseases that come in the differential diagnosis of RA.
B. The authors reiterated that they wanted to avoid circularity by their design. However as highlighted above, circularity is an essential component of criteria making. We find it hard to understand why the authors did not decide to delinieate which factors were more important to recognize in a patient with early arthritis to cause severe disease later on. In such a scheme the control groups for the eventual LRs would naturally be those patients who would not eventually develop the disease construct as defined by the older 1987 criteria. An additional end point would have been to add a construct of a milder RA at, say, one year, i.e. increasing number of joints involved, more seropositivity etc.
C. They said that "One limitation of the new criteria is that they are based on current knowledge." [24] This statement is superflous. *All* criteria are based on current knowledge.

D. After their exercise the authors made the default promise of diagnostic criteria to come [24].
E. The whole exercise was about what prompts a rheumatologist to start MTX in early undifferentiated arthritis. It is unfortunate that the authors did not call the exercise just this.
F. Finally, it was indeed curious why the authors chose to give the gender distribution of the rheumatologists involved. Are there gender differences in decision making in rheumatology, particularly as related to RA?

Since there were no comperator groups with any other diseases at any phase of development of these criteria, many such studies about these criteria followed. These showed in brief that 18 % of patients with early arthritis filfulling these criteria in Leiden had a different diagnosis at the end of one year. Of the 198 patients who were classified differently, 46 developed psoriatic arthritis while 6 turned out to have arthritis associated with cancer [28]. In another cross sectional study among patients receiving routine clinical care in an university outpatient clinic in New York, the sensitivity and specificity of the 2010 criteria were 97 vs 55 % respectively while the corresponding values for the 1987 criteria were 93 vs 73 %. More specifically 67 % of patients with SLE and 50 % of patients with osteoarthritis could be classified as having RA by the 2010 criteria [29]. A recent systemic literature review of publications assessing the preformance of the 2010 criteria came up with similar figures for sensitivity and specificity [30]. It was also interesting to note that the authors of this systemic review concluded that the 2010 criteria was more for classification rather than diagnosis.

What to do?

We must first reconcile ourselves that unless the specific cause/ pathogenesis/ histology of a condition is known a fool proof diagnosis is almost impossible. We always have to deal with probabilities especially when we have to manage diseases we recognize only as constructs. Then we have to teach both our patients and the health authorities what we first have convince ourselves. The patient has to know that the basis of most of our medical interventions are based on probabilities. Similarly, and especially, the health authorities and the third party payers should come to grips with the same.

Finally, after first admitting that diagnostic and classification criteria are one and the same, we must begin formulating how we can make a classification scheme more useful for diagnosis. We propose several approaches:

1. To popularize the understanding that many of our existing disease criteria are much more useful to exclude diseases as we gave the example for BS. Devising criteria specific for excluding diseases can be a novel approach.
2. Tailoring disease criteria to a practice setting is another approach. These, if you will, setting-specific criteria will have the potential to be much more useful in

that the PrP will remarkably increase, and the number of conditions that come into the differential diagnosis will decrease, increasing the specificity of the criteria set. To give an example [12] we recognize that the prevalence of BS is may be 1000 fold greater in Japan [31], as compared to North America [32]. On the other hand, if you go to a dedicated uveitis clinic in either country, you will find that the proportion of BS patients that seen in either setting differs only by several fold, 2.5 % in North America and 6.2 % in Japan. This certainly increases the PrP of BS in North America, while the number of conditions to be differentiated from BS as far as eye involvement is considered will be comparatively few. Similarly, a simple disease criteria set to differentiate BS from inflammatory bowel disease for the gastroenterologist would be most useful.

3. Including family history of the disease being sought, surely very important in making a diagnosis, is for some reason, frequently omitted from disease criteria [33]. This needs to change.
4. The scientific journals might consider always requesting confidence intervals around the LRs whenever we devise new criteria. Similarly a systematic effort can be made to add confidence intervals to criteria commonly used. It is disconcerting to note that confidence intervals are not provided in the final criteria set in any of the classification criteria sets published by the ACR.

References

1. Jones TD. The diagnosis of rheumatic fever. JAMA. 1944;126:481–4.
2. Ferrieri P. Jones Criteria Working Group. Proceedings of the Jones Criteria workshop. Circulation. 2002;106:2521–3.
3. Pereira BA, da Silva NA, Andrade LE, et al.Jones criteria and underdiagnosis of rheumatic fever. Indian J Pediatr. 2007;74(2):117–21
4. O'Duffy JD. Suggested criteria for diagnosis of Behçet's disease. J Rheumatol. 1974;1 suppl 1:18 (abstr).
5. International Study Group for Behçet's Disease. Criteria for diagnosis of Behçet's disease. Lancet. 1990;335:1070–80.
6. Hunder GG, Arend WP, Bloch DA, et al. The American College of Rheumatology 1990 criteria for the classification of vasculitis: introduction. Arthritis Rheum. 1990;33:1065–7.
7. Rao JK, Allen NB, Pincus T. Limitations of the 1990 American College of Cardiology classification criteria in the diagnosis of vasculitis. Ann Intern Med. 1998;129:345–52.
8. Sorensen SF, Slot O, Tvede N, Petersen J. A prospective study of vasculitis patients collected in a five year period: evaluation of the Chapel Hill nomenclature. Ann Rheum Dis. 2000;59:478–82.
9. Hunder GG. The use and misuse of classification and diagnostic criteria for complex diseases. Ann Intern Med. 1998;129:417–8.
10. American Psychiatric Association. Diagnostic and statistical manual of mental disorders. 5th ed. Arlington: American Psychiatric Publishing; 2013.
11. Reilly BM, Evans AT, Schaider JJ, et al. Impact of a clinical decision rule on hospital triage of patients with suspected acute cardiac ischemia in the emergency department. JAMA. 2002;288(3):342–50.
12. Yazici H. Diagnostic versus classification criteria – a continuum. Bull NYU Hosp Jt Dis. 2009;67:206–8.

13. Reid MC, Lachs MS, Feinstein AR. Use of methodological standards in diagnostic test research. Getting better but still not good. JAMA. 1995;274(8):645–51.
14. Fan J, Upadhye S, Worster A. Understanding receiver operating characteristic (ROC) curves. CJEM. 2006;8(1):19–20.
15. Max MB, Lynn J (editors). Symptom research: methods and opportunities. Bethesda: National Institutes of Health, Department of Health and Human Services. Available at: http://symptomresearch.nih.gov/tablecontents.htm. Accessed 4 Apr 2009.
16. International Study Group for Behçet's Disease. Evaluation of diagnostic ('Classification') criteria in Behçet's disease. Br J Rheumatol. 1992;31:299–308.
17. Sox HC, Hickam DH, Marton KI, et al. Am J Med . 1990; 89:7-14.
18. Greenberg RS, Flanders WD, W, Eley JW, Boring, III, JR. Diagnostic testing *in* Medical Epidemiology, 4th Edition; Lange Medical Books 2004, p.9.
19. Fries JF. Disease criteria for systemic lupus erythematosus. Arch Intern Med. 1984;144: 252–3.
20. Yazici H. A critical look at diagnostic criteria: time for a change? Bull NYU Hosp Jt Dis. 2011;69:101–3.
21. Dasgupta B, Cimmino MA, Kremers HM, et al.. Provisional classification criteria for polymyalgia rheumatica: a European League Against Rheumatism/American College of Rheumatology collaborative initiative. Arthritis Rheum. 2012;64(4):943–54.
22. Waller R, Ahmed A, Patel I, Luqmani R. Update on the classification of vasculitis. Best Pract Res Clin Rheumatol. 2013;27(1):3–17.
23. Cahan A, Gilon D, Manor O, Paltiel O. Probabilistic reasoning and clinical decision-making: do doctors overestimate diagnostic probabilities? QJM. 2003;96(10):763–9.
24. Aletaha D, Neogi T, Silman AJ, et al. 2010 rheumatoid arthritis classification criteria: an American College of Rheumatology/European League Against Rheumatism collaborative initiative. Ann Rheum Dis. 2010;69(9):1580–8.
25. Funovits J, Aletaha D, Bykerk V, et al. The 2010 American College of Rheumatology/ European League Against Rheumatism classification criteria for rheumatoid arthritis: methodological report phase I. Ann Rheum Dis. 2010;69:1589–95.
26. Neogi T, Aletaha D, Silman AJ, et al. The 2010 American College of Rheumatology/European League Against Rheumatism Classification Criteria for Rheumatoid Arthritis: phase 2 methodological report. Arthritis Rheum. 2010;62:2582–91.
27. Arnett FC, Edworthy SM, Bloch DA, et al. The American Rheumatism Association 1987 revised criteria for the classification of rheumatoid arthritis. Arthritis Rheum. 1988;31: 315–24.
28. van der Linden MM, Knevel R, Huizinga TWJ, van der Helm-van Mil AHM. Classification of rheumatoid arthritis. Comparison of the 1987 America College of Rheumatology criteria and the 2010 American College of Rheumatology/American League Against Rheumatism criteria. Arthritis Rheum. 2011;63:37–42.
29. Kennish L, Labitigan M, Budoff S, et al. Utility of the new rheumatoid arthritis 2010 ACR/ EULAR classification criteria in routine clinical care. BMJ Open. 2012;2(5):pii: e001117.
30. Sakellariou G, Scirè CA, Zambon A, Roberto Caporali R, Montecucco C. Performance of the 2010 Classification Criteria for Rheumatoid Arthritis: a systematic literature review and a meta-analysis. PLoS One. 2013;8:e56528.
31. Rodriguez A, Calonge M, Pedroza-Seres M, et al. Referral patterns of uveitis in a tertiary eye care center. Arch Ophthalmol. 1996;114:593–9.
32. Goto H, Mochizuki M, Yamaki K, et al. Epidemiological survey of intraocular inflammation in Japan. Jpn J Ophthalmol. 2007;51:41–4.
33. Yazici H, Yazici Y. Criteria for Behçet's disease with reflections on all disease criteria. J Aotoimmun. 20014; 48-40: 104-7.

Biomarkers, Genetic Association, and Genomic Studies

Mehmet Tevfik Dorak and Yusuf Yazici

Abbreviations

ABCC3	ATP-binding cassette, subfamily C member 3
ACPA	Antibodies to citrullinated protein antigen
ACR	American College of Rheumatology
ACYP1	Acylphosphatase 1, erythrocyte
AFP	Alpha-fetoprotein
AIF1	Allograft inflammatory factor 1
ANA	Antinuclear antibody
anti-CarP	Anti-carbamylated protein
anti-CCP	Anti-cyclic citrullinated protein
anti-TNF	Anti-tumor necrosis factor
ARHGEF16	Rho guanine exchange factor 16
AUC	Area under "ROC" curve
BF	Factor B
BMI	Body mass index
BRAF	v-raf murine sarcoma viral oncogene homologue B1

M.T. Dorak, MD, PhD
School of Health Sciences, Liverpool Hope University,
Hope Park, HCA-EW 208, Liverpool L16 9JD, UK
e-mail: dorakm@hope.ac.uk; mdorak@fiu.edu; mtd3053@gmail.com

Y. Yazici, MD (✉)
Division of Rheumatology, Department of Medicine, Seligman Center for Advanced Therapeutics and Behcet's Syndrome Center, NYU Hospital for Joint Diseases, New York University School of Medicine, New York University,
333 East 38th Street, New York, NY 10016, USA
e-mail: yusuf.yazici@nyumc.org

H. Yazici et al. (eds.), *Understanding Evidence-Based Rheumatology*,
DOI 10.1007/978-3-319-08374-2_4

CACNB2	Calcium channel, voltage-dependent, beta 2 subunit
CDAI	Clinical disease activity index
CEA	Carcinoembryonic antigen
cfNRI	Category-free NRI
COL4A1	Collagen, type IV, alpha 1
COMP	Cartilage oligomeric matrix protein
CRP	C-reactive protein
CTX-I	Collagen cross-linked C-telopeptide
CXCL13	C-X-C motif chemokine 13
DAS	Disease activity score
DMARDs	Disease-modifying antirheumatic drugs
EGF	Epidermal growth factor
EHD1	EH domain-containing 1
EIF3S9	Eukaryotic translation initiation factor 3, subunit 9 eta
ESR	Erythrocyte sedimentation rate
EULAR	European League Against Rheumatism
F2RL1	Coagulation factor II receptor-like 1
FHL3	Four and a half LIM domains 3
FLS	Fibroblast-like synoviocytes
FVT1	Follicular lymphoma variant translocation 1
GADD45A	Growth arrest and DNA-damage-inducible, alpha
GAS	Global arthritis score
GWAS	Genome-wide association studies
HSPA1A	Heat shock 70 kDa protein 1A
IDI	Integrated discrimination improvement
IL-15	Interleukin-15
IL-6	Interleukin-6
LTBR	Lymphotoxin-beta receptor
MALDI-TOF-MS	Matrix-assisted laser desorption/ionization time-of-flight mass spectrometry
MBDA	Multi-biomarker disease activity
MDHAQ	Multidimensional health assessment questionnaire
mHAQ	Modified health assessment questionnaire
MIF	Migration inhibitory factor
MLL	Myeloid/lymphoid or mixed-lineage leukemia
MMP-1	Matrix metalloproteinase-1
MMP-3	Matrix metalloproteinase-3
NPV	Negative predictive value
NRI	Net reclassification improvement
OMERACT	Outcome Measures in Rheumatology
OPG	Osteoprotegerin
OR	Odds ratio
PAD4	Peptidyl arginine deiminase type 4
pain VAS	Pain visual analogue scale
PGA	Patient global assessment

PhGA	Physician global assessment
PPP1R12B	Protein phosphatase 1, regulatory subunit 12B
PPV	Positive predictive value
PRMT2	Protein arginine methyltransferase 2
PSA	Prostate-specific antigen
PSMB8	Proteasome subunit, beta type, 8
PTPN22	Protein tyrosine phosphatase non-receptor 22 gene
RA	Rheumatoid arthritis
RANKL	Nuclear factor kappa-B ligand
RAPID-3	Routine assessment of patient index data-3
RF	Rheumatoid factor
ROC	Receiver operating characteristics
RPIA	Ribose 5-phosphate isomerase A
SAA	Serum amyloid A protein
SDAI	Simplified disease activity index
sICAM-1	Soluble intercellular adhesion molecule-1
sIL-2Ralpha	Soluble interleukin-2 receptor alpha
SJC	Swollen joint count index
SKIL	SKI-like oncogene
SLE	Systemic lupus erythematosus
SPRY2	Sprouty homologue 2 (*Drosophila*)
STNFRII	Soluble tumor necrosis factor receptor II
STNFRs	Soluble tumor necrosis factor receptors
sVCAM-1	Soluble vascular cell adhesion molecule-1
TCR	T-cell receptor
TFCP2	Transcription factor CP2
TJC	Tender joint count
TLR	Toll-like receptor
TNFAIP3	Tumor necrosis factor-alpha-induced protein 3
U-CTX-I/II	Urine C-telopeptide of types I and II
VEGF-A	Vascular endothelial growth factor-A
YKL-40	Cartilage glycoprotein-39

The group of tests commonly collected under the name "biomarkers" have been touted for their promise of helping in the diagnosis, treatment, and ultimately prognosis of many conditions. Rheumatoid arthritis (RA), the most common autoimmune inflammatory joint disease, with its clinical heterogeneity, availability of multiple treatment options, and quite variable individual patient responses is a good model to discuss the making and implementing biomarkers in rheumatic diseases in general. Being aware of room for improvement in both diagnosis and management of RA mainly using biomarkers, the European League Against Rheumatism (EULAR) and American College of Rheumatology (ACR) are jointly in the process of producing improved clinical criteria for diagnosis and classification of RA. Validated biomarkers have already had an impact in the treatment of other conditions such as multiple sclerosis [1], Alzheimer disease [2], Parkinson disease [3], and cancer [4]. There are also advances in biomarker development for diagnosis of RA and its subtypes, prognostic assessment and personalized treatment choice, and treatment monitoring [5–10]. In this chapter, the controversy regarding what constitutes a robust biomarker and how to rigorously investigate biomarkers will be discussed, and recent progress in the field of biomarkers as well as genetic associations will be presented.

What Is a Biomarker?

Biomarkers are often thought of as serologic, perhaps because currently the most commonly used biomarkers relate to oncology like prostate-specific antigen (PSA), carcinoembryonic antigen (CEA), or alpha-fetoprotein (AFP) whose levels are measured in the serum. A biomarker, however, can be clinical (disease activity score), histologic (synovial pathology), functional (glomerular filtration rate), an imaging parameter (macrophage positron emission tomography), or a molecular one (autoantibodies, genotypes, gene expression signatures, proteins, metabolites). From available definitions of a biomarker [11], a biomarker for the purposes of this chapter is "a characteristic that is objectively measured and evaluated, and may influence, explain or predict the incidence or outcome of a disease, or individual response to a treatment." Molecular biomarkers may be serologic, genomic, metabolomic, or proteomic. Any biomarker may be a proxy for changes early in the disease development (descriptive biomarker), may be involved in disease pathogenesis (mechanistic biomarker), or appears in response to treatment (dynamic biomarker). Genomic biomarkers for *BCR-ABL* translocation in chronic myeloid leukemia, *HER2* and *BRAF* mutations (in breast cancer and melanoma, respectively) have recently been used for treatment choices with great success, and expectations are high for any other disease to benefit from progress in genomics and other omics [12]. Besides cancer-specific mutations, gene expression signatures have proven very useful, in particular, in defining a subset of a disease for the most optimal treatment or for prognostic stratification. One such genetic expression signature test, MammaPrint, incorporating expression levels of 70 genes, has been FDA approved for prognostic classification of breast cancer cases [13, 14]. Individual markers may be good indicators of disease risk or prognosis at the population level, but their value for individual assessment is limited as will be discussed below [15, 16]. The most successful biomarkers have been a panel of biomarkers with increased sensitivity and specificity [7, 8, 10, 17, 18].

Biomarkers Can Have Multiple Uses

In routine care, biomarkers may be used (1) to identify genetically predisposed individuals for active surveillance; (2) for early diagnosis to start therapeutic intervention; (3) to assess, predict, or monitor disease severity; (4) to select the most

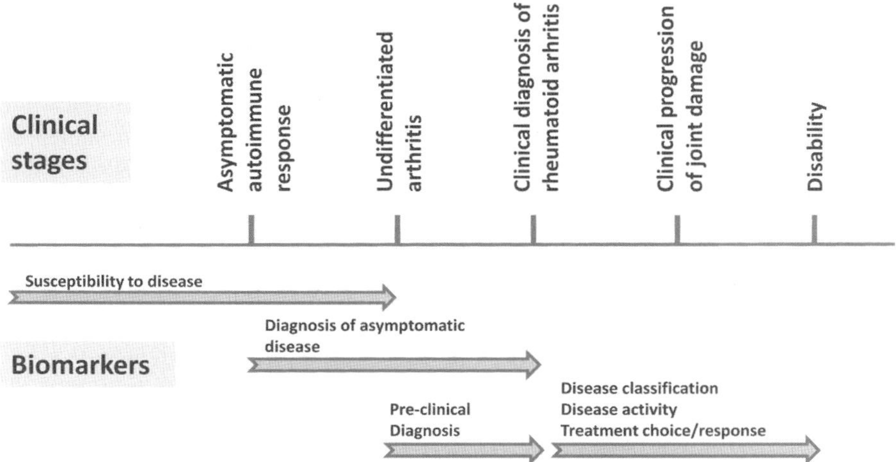

Fig. 1 Types of biomarkers that can be used at different stages of rheumatoid arthritis

optimal treatment for each individual; and (5) to monitor response to treatment (Fig. 1). RA has a high degree of heterogeneity in clinical presentation, progress, and response to treatment, which makes it possibly a good condition for biomarker development with beneficial use in practice.

The majority of biomarkers in RA are also molecular like autoantibodies, cytokines, and acute-phase reactants. Genetic markers have long been recognized as markers of susceptibility, clinical classification, and prognostic classification, but none has yet achieved a biomarker status. Recent genome-wide association studies (GWAS) have identified strong markers for susceptibility, disease classification, drug response, and prognosis, but their development into biomarkers will pose difficulties as will be explained below. This is an important issue for RA is one of the diseases with a high heritability [19–22]. The markers identified to date, however, do not account for the large portion of this genetic risk. It is expected that with the expansion of search for genetic markers for predisposition to epigenetic markers [23–25], the "missing heritability" may be uncovered.

Risk Markers Are Not Necessarily Biomarkers

A common misconception is that any marker that shows an association with any aspects of a disease, i.e., a risk factor, can be used as a biomarker. In practice, however, it is not that straightforward [15, 16, 26, 27]. Even a risk factor whose association with a trait yields a relative risk or odds ratio (OR) of 5.0, which is a high value for any epidemiologic association, is unlikely to be an informative biomarker at the individual level. For a risk factor to have a detection rate of 80 % for a false-positive rate of 5 %, the OR should reach more than 2,000, which corresponds to almost exclusive presence in the group of interest. This is exactly the problem with most risk factors, in particular, for genetic markers in that a lot of healthy people will also carry the marker without any sign of the disease. By using the copresence of multiple markers, a threshold may be obtained that the combination of markers would only be present in patients and absent in healthy subjects. Although achievable, this situation will only apply to a minority of patients and a minority of controls resulting in low specificity and sensitivity for the marker as a biomarker.

It may appear paradoxical that a strong risk marker yielding a very high relative risk with a very strong statistical result is not as useful for biomarker development as expected. First of all, a statistical result only shows that the marker is a classifier – in the sense that it classifies a subject as a case or control – and this is less likely to be due to chance. As will be discussed, a likelihood ratio (which incorporates specificity and sensitivity), area under the receiver operating characteristic (ROC) curve analysis, and reclassification statistics are better indicators of the value of a test as a biomarker. The ultimate aim is to have a marker able to classify a subject as diseased or healthy, rather than estimating the risk of disease, i.e., how many folds increased risk a subject has. An ideal biomarker is present in all diseased subjects (100 % sensitivity), and it is totally absent in non-diseased (healthy or those patients with other diseases) subjects (100 % specificity) yielding a likelihood ratio of infinity. As an example, the FDA-approved 70-gene signature in breast cancer for overall survival [28] corresponds to $P<0.001$ and a hazard ratio of >2.0, but a sensitivity of 90 % and a specificity of 40 %, with the resulting AUC value of around 0.65 for survival. These figures correspond to a poor-to-modest classifier: to identify correctly 90 of the 100 patients with poor prognosis (and missing 10 of them), 60 of 100 patients with good prognosis are also identified as candidates for poor prognosis [27].

Biomarker Development

The initial discovery phase is just a start in a rather involved process of biomarker development. This process involves (1) discovery and replication, (2) analytic validation, (3) clinical validation, (4) determination of clinical utility, and (5) clinical use following regulatory approvals (Fig. 2). Taking a simple association study to a clinically useful biomarker is a process as detailed and elaborate as drug development [29, 30]. Such a successful translation requires work in basic, translational, and regulatory science and a comprehensive collaboration among laboratory scientists, technology developers, clinicians, statisticians, and bioinformaticians. Several guidelines have been published for different aspects of biomarker development studies: molecular epidemiology (STROBE-ME) [11], early clinical trials of novel agents [31], tumor marker prognostic studies (REMARK) [32], genomic applications (EGAPP) [33], genetic risk prediction (GRIPS) [34], and biospecimen-based studies (BRISQ) [35]. These and other [36–38] guidelines aim to prevent the use of biomarkers in the absence of high levels of evidence supporting their clinical utility

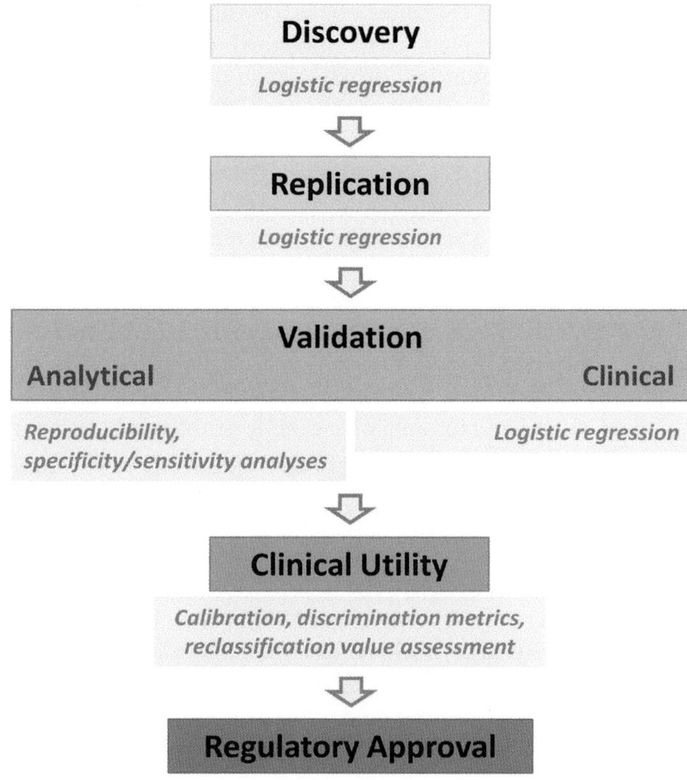

Fig. 2 Steps to be taken to convert an experimental finding into a clinical biomarker

and help the investigators to design biomarkers that can lead to true personalized care with high confidence.

It is important to appreciate that the discovery phase is just the beginning, but still strict guidelines of study design should be followed [30, 39, 40].

The discovery phase studies tend to be retrospective and small in size and suffer from well-recognized problems such as cross-validation for replication and extensive subgroup analysis. Instead, emphasis should be given to statistically adequately powered, prospective studies. This can be achieved using stored biospecimens of ongoing or completed cohort studies or randomized clinical trials as long as samples from placebo arm or standard treatment are used [30], bearing in mind the caveats of inclusion criteria for clinical trials. Since the rest of the development program will be based on these initial results, extreme care at this stage will pay off later.

Once the initial results are obtained in the discovery phase, the validation phase begins with examination of analytical validity as the next step. This is a technical checklist of the analysis methods used in the measurement of the biomarker candidate. The specific assay test for the biomarker is examined for its accuracy and precision. For a genetic variant, this step makes sure that the genotyping assays perform well with acceptable concordance rates by different operators, in different laboratories using different platforms. Analytical validity is measured in the laboratory by calculating the test sensitivity, which provides the probability that a positive test is truly positive (e.g., will yield is a positive results when the marker is in fact present), and test specificity, which provides the probability that the test will not detect the marker when it is not present. This calculation is performed by testing the analysis method against a gold standard or by using samples known to be positive and negative for the presence of the marker. Ideally, both parameters should be 100 %.

In the clinical validity step, the power of the biomarker candidate to show statistical correlation with the phenotype of interest or intended clinical endpoint is reexamined and confirmed. It is in this step that potential confounders (age, sex, race/ethnicity, die, medications) are also examined. Measures of sensitivity and specificity are evaluated in a representative sample of the population for whom the test is intended using appropriate epidemiologic study designs ideally including an independent replication study. These studies also establish the positive predictive value, which reflects the probability that a person with a positive test result has or will have the phenotype for which the marker is believed to be a predictor. Confirmed clinical validity does not necessarily mean that a biomarker can immediately be used in patient care. This is achieved in the next clinical utility step. Only biomarker candidates with confirmed analytical and clinical validity are submitted to the formal assessment of clinical utility. In this step, large, independent, and well-designed studies evaluate the biomarker's expected utility using formal statistical tools. It is this stage that is usually underappreciated in discussions of the value of a marker as a biomarker. Only after passing this step, a marker attains a biomarker status with clinical utility meaning that it provides information that is useful in the clinic in making decisions about disease susceptibility, disease classification, prognostic stratification, or response to a given treatment. Once evidence of utility in real clinical settings is generated, the regulatory process begins for introduction of the biomarker for use in routine clinical care (Fig. 2).

Evaluation of a Biomarker for Clinical Utility

A biomarker is a classifier that classifies a group of people into separate groups like susceptible and non-susceptible individuals, one subgroup of a disease and another, or a subgroup with good prognosis and another without. The clinical utility of a biomarker is assessed in a different manner from the way a case–control study evaluates an association. Here the focus is on whether by using a biomarker subjects can be reclassified in a class different from where they would be classified using existing evidence. An ideal biomarker, say, for disease susceptibility, with its high specificity and sensitivity (positive in every predisposed subject and negative in every subject that will remain disease-free, thus, yielding a high likelihood ratio), is well calibrated (the predicted risk for developing the disease corresponds to real risk and not over- or underestimated) and therefore would classify every subject as predisposed or not. Once this ideal stage is reached, the positive and negative predictive values for the marker will also be ideal demonstrating the benefits and risks from both positive and negative results. Such an imaginary biomarker would have a value of 100 % for each of sensitivity, specificity, and area under "ROC" curve (AUC). This scenario is only true for some monogenic Mendelian disorders where the genetic effect is not modified by the environment.

In the ultimate stage of biomarker development preceding the regulatory approval, statistical evaluation is most rigorous. Logistic regression and its output of effect size, the OR, are not good indicators of the clinical utility of the biomarker candidate. The OR is not an estimate of individual-level risk nor a diagnostic test or classifier; and the OR should not be used in a predictive study as the effect size [41]. A high OR (or relative risk) associated with a marker even after adjusting for established risk factors does not necessarily translate into better risk prediction. The statistical considerations differ between etiologic risk studies and studies on biomarkers that are going to be used to classify subjects. Studies that use the OR as the effect size use multiple markers with small effect sizes simultaneously to increase the effect size. This approach certainly increases the effect size, but the multimarker set is still not a good classifier. In a simulation study of 40 independent genetic risk markers each yielding an odds ratio of 1.2–2.0 and a sample size of one million, the best results in discriminative accuracy quantified as the AUC were obtained when the risk genotypes were all common (≥30 %) and odds ratios were closer to 2.0. Even with this unrealistic scenario, the AUC was 0.93 [42]. This example shows that even simultaneous use of most common and strong risk markers may still not have a large discriminatory value between disease and healthy states.

The ROC curve analysis is a commonly used measure of performance of a predictive test. An ideal marker has an AUC of 1 representing perfect discrimination between the diseased and nondiseased subjects; in other words, all subjects are correctly classified by the test. The baseline value for an AUC is 0.5 which represents no discrimination at all; in other words subjects are classified no more correctly than can be attributed to by chance. AUC plots the sensitivity of the marker against (1 – specificity) for all possible cutoff values. In the case of a binary marker, this is just a single point. The c-index is numerically equivalent to the AUC. A serious issue with the AUC is that it does not measure the ability of a new marker to add value to a preexisting prediction model. Thus, a new marker may have a good performance, but whether adding the new marker to existing markers will improve the performance needs to be known. This is usually done by generating two ROC curves, one with and one without the new marker using information on existing markers, and observing whether there is a difference between them. The difference can be formally assessed by the c-statistics if the change in AUC appears to be substantial enough.

However, useful ROC curves may be for classification; evaluation of predictive models cannot rely solely on the ROC curve, but should assess discrimination and calibration using new metrics (Table 1). Jakobsdottir et al. looked at this formally [16]. They compared the utility of genetic markers of a number of complex disorders

Table 1 Comparison of models for risk prediction

Association	Logistic regression
Global model fit	Likelihood ratio test; Bayes information criterion
Discrimination	ROC; concordance (or c)-statistics
Calibration	Hosmer–Lemeshow statistic for goodness of fit
Risk reclassification	Integrated discrimination improvement (IDI); net reclassification improvement (NRI); category-free NRI (cfNRI); decision curve analysis

From Refs. [43–47]

identified by GWAS using ROC curve analysis against conventional risk markers already known and concluded that small *P* values, high ORs, and AUCs do not guarantee good prediction of actual risk. The AUC should be considered as a first step in evaluating a model or in comparing two models against each other. The AUC value is, however, insufficient on its own to show that a model would improve decision-making. One criticism aimed at the AUC analysis in clinical utility determination is that it gives equal weight to specificity and sensitivity, hence to false positives and false negatives, which may not be the case in a real clinical situation [43]. Published estimates of disease prevalence and heritability or sibling recurrence risk for 17 complex genetic diseases have been used to calculate the proportion of genetic variance that a test must explain to achieve an AUC = 0.75, which is a modest value. For 17 diseases, the proportion of genetic variance that have to be explained by genetic markers for the predictive model to attain an AUC value of 0.75 varied from 0.10 to 0.74. In other words, depending on disease prevalence and heritability, genetic markers can explain as little as 0.10 or as high as 0.74 of the heritability to yield an AUC value of 0.75, the threshold regarded as making a diagnostic classifier clinically useful when applied to a sample considered to be at increased risk [42]. On the other hand, a threshold AUC value is 0.99 for a predictive test to be a classifier when applied to the general population. Given the prevalence and heritability of RA, the maximum value for genetic markers in RA for prediction of disease susceptibility can get close (0.98) but not quite reach this threshold [48].

For clinical utility assessment, additional statistical methods including discrimination metrics (c-statistics), measures of calibration (addressing how close the predicted risks are to the actual observed risks), and reclassification (addressing whether the model including the novel biomarker changes a person's risk sufficiently to move them to a different risk category) are needed (Table 1) [44–46, 49, 50]. Calibration is essential for good decision-making. A model is well calibrated when the predicted risk is equal to the observed risk. Calibration takes into account the average risk in a population. Although essential in biomarker development, calibration is *not* sufficient for clinical utility. What is most crucial for determination of clinical utility in biomarker development is reclassification, which aims to do at the individual level what AUC analysis does at the group level. In reclassification analysis, each individual's data is considered to see whether the new marker changes their risk classification. This is achieved by reclassification tables that show changes in individual risk classifications with the addition of the new marker to the prediction model. It has been pointed out that a marker which has only modest or no effect by AUC analysis may still improve risk classification at the individual level [44, 45].

Past Mistakes in Biomarker Development

It is important to learn from past mistakes for current efforts in biomarker development to be more productive. It is well known that most claims of classification performance are overly optimistic, lacking verification by replication with questionable generalizability. Ioannidis reviewed the most common causes of biomarker failures [51]. He has pointed out that despite the introduction of so many biomarkers into clinical practice, the health impacts have not been favorable in general. Four types of failures have been recognized as summarized in Table 2. The most dramatic of these failures concerns the PSA. Initially introduced in the 1980s for monitoring treatment response, PSA testing has found a place as a biomarker for screening and early diagnosis of prostate cancer [52]. The AUC for PSA in ROC curve analysis is 0.68 for cancer versus no cancer. Given that a test that performs no better than chance yields an AUC of 0.5, this value does not suggest a high clinical utility in classifying subjects as having prostate cancer or not. PSA is believed to have done more harm and good, by drastically increasing overdiagnosis and overtreatment of prostate cancer [53]. The problem with PSA was that it was not subject to a robust assessment before being used for screening and actual clinical use disappointed. A search for biomarkers is still ongoing. The PSA example illustrates the importance of following the steps shown in Fig. 2 before introducing a biomarker to clinical use.

Table 2 Types of biomarker failures

	Type A	Type B	Type C	Type D
Problem	A biomarker makes it to the clinics, but does not fulfill the promise	A biomarker is reported to have strong features, but cannot be validated by following studies	A biomarker is found in one study, but clinical optimization is lacking	A biomarker is promoted despite lack of promising evidence
Example	Prostate-specific antigen (PSA)	Proteomic markers of ovarian cancer	Gene expression signatures in cancer	Direct-to-consumer genetic risk determination
Solution	Satisfactory assessment of clinical utility before introducing it into practice	Verification of analytical validity before proceeding with the development	Use of robust statistical methods at the development phase and follow-up toward clinical implementation	Better assessment of incremental benefit of using these markers over existing risk markers

Adapted from Ioannidis [51]

An ideal biomarker for clinical use should have three major characteristics: (1) It should be safe and easy to measure preferably noninvasively and with good reproducibility; (2) it should have a high sensitivity, high specificity, and high positive and negative predictive values (PPV and NPV, respectively) for its intended outcome; and (3) it should improve decision-making abilities in line with clinicopathological parameters. Any attempt to introduce a single marker to routine care as a biomarker will probably suffer one of the types of failure listed in Table 2. If a single biomarker cannot fulfill all the expectations, which is usually the case, a panel of multiple biomarkers if performing better than any single biomarker may be used. Indeed, most common biomarkers used in RA to assess disease activity (multi-biomarker disease activity or MBDA) are of this type.

Validity of Existing Biomarkers for Rheumatoid Arthritis

In RA, associations of markers, especially those that are genetic, have been widely reported as valid for a number of outcomes, but the development of biomarkers based on those findings has been either unsuccessful or slow. As discussed above, a high OR is no indication of success for a biomarker, and the strongest HLA region association in RA has an OR of 5–10. Even the strongest HLA association in any disease with an OR of around 100 as in ankylosing spondylitis may not turn out to be a good biomarker. This highlights the difficulty with converting even the strongest risk markers to biomarkers.

As discussed below, there are a number of biomarkers used for RA diagnosis, disease activity, assessment, or prognosis. A survey analyzed the validity of biomarkers as reported in 170 articles [40]. Most common biomarkers were gene expression profiles. Flaws were identified in most reports. Less than half of the studies incorporated study-design features important for valid clinical associations: age and sex-matched groups and controlling for medications used. These issues concerned mainly the discovery stage studies. Even at that stage, which forms the foundation of a long process, no more than half of the studies were satisfactory by simple epidemiologic criteria. This is not a promising start to the process of biomarker development if biomarkers with genuine clinical utility are the aim.

To avoid future mistakes in biomarker development and to aid with valid ones, an independent initiative called OMERACT (Outcome Measures in Rheumatology) consisting of international health professionals interested in outcome measures in rheumatology was formed in 1992. OMERACT has played a critical role in the development and validation of clinical and radiographic outcome measures in RA and other rheumatic diseases. A special interest group developed validation criteria for soluble biomarkers of structural joint damage [36]. These criteria have been further developed and put to test for existing biomarkers [54–57]. Neither a baseline C-reactive protein (CRP) test nor later tests on five more soluble biomarkers receptor activator of nuclear factor kappa-B ligand (RANKL; TNFSF11), osteoprotegerin (OPG), matrix metalloprotease (MMP-3), and urine C-telopeptide of types I and II collagen (U-CTX-I and U CTX-II) produced strong evidence that these biomarkers could substitute for radiographic endpoints in RA. The OMERACT validation criteria are based on three domains: *truth* (is the measure truthful, does it measure what it intends to measure? Is the result unbiased and relevant?), *discrimination* (does the measure discriminate between situations that are of interest?), and *feasibility* (can the measure be applied easily, given constraints of time, money, and interpretability?) This initiative together with other published guidelines for various aspects of biomarker development studies are expected to result in the development of reliable biomarkers with enhanced validity and clinical utility.

Biomarkers in RA

Earliest Biomarkers in RA

Like many other complex disorders, RA is a heterogeneous disease. Traditionally, RA has been classified as rheumatoid factor (RF) positive and RF negative, but more recently, antibodies to citrullinated protein antigen (ACPA), also referred to as anti-CCP (Anti-cyclic citrullinated protein), are used in the classification of RA. Of the two, ACPA is more specific to RA as RF is more likely than ACPA to be positive in other rheumatic disorders [58]. These autoantibodies were therefore the earliest biomarkers for RA diagnosis and classification (Table 3). It is very important to take this heterogeneity into account in any study, but especially in studies of primary susceptibility. Thus, biomarkers should be developed for these subtypes separately. ACPA has different fine specificities, but they do not seem to provide additional information regarding the clinical phenotype at present. Isotype usage in ACPA

Table 3 Disease classification by ACPA antibody status

Characteristic	ACPA positive	ACPA negative
Heritability	~60 %	~60 %
Disease course	Severe	Milder
Drug-free remission probability	Lower	Greater
HLA (shared epitope) association	Yes (*HLA-DRB1**01; *04)	No
Other HLA associations	*HLA-DRB1**15	*HLA-DRB1**03; *13
PTPN22 association	Yes	No
Other genetic associations	*CTLA4*, *STAT4*, *PADI4*, *CTLA4*, *TNFAIP3-OLIG3*, *TRAF1/C5*, *FCGR*, *IL2RA*, *IL2RB*, *CD40*, *CTL21*, *CCR6*, and others	*IRF5*, *STAT4*
Smoking association	Yes and only in HLA shared epitope-positive subjects	No

response increases to include more diverse antibodies (IgM, IgA, all IgG subclasses, and IgE) together with the titer of ACPA before the development of full-blown disease [59]. In contrast, isotype usage does not change once RA settles as the full-blown disease.

More recently, another antibody specificity has been identified in RA. Anti-carbamylated protein (anti-CarP) antibodies are formed against homocitrullinated proteins with little or no cross-reactivity to ACPA [59]. Similar to ACPA positivity, anti-CarP antibodies have been proposed to predict the development of RA in patients with undifferentiated arthritis or arthralgia and predict joint damage [10, 59–61]. Anti-CarP antibodies may be detected in both ACPA-positive and ACPA-negative RA patients, and the unfavorable effect on the clinical course is more prominent in ACPA-negative patients [60]. More specific and sophisticated versions of the earliest autoantibodies are now available especially for early diagnosis of RA in patients who present with arthritis and will be discussed below.

Biomarkers for Disease Susceptibility

Genetic Markers for Disease Susceptibility

To examine genetic markers for disease susceptibility, it should be first established that the disease has genetic background. In the case of RA, this is well established. Both early candidate gene studies [62] and a major GWAS [63] have provided strong evidence for genetic susceptibility to RA (reviewed in [64]) (Table 4). Stronger evidence comes from classical twin studies which have estimated that heritability of RA exceeds 50 % [19–21]. The concordance rate for RA among monozygotic twins is higher in all studies (12–15 %) than among dizygotic twins (4 %) [19, 20] although heritability estimates based on familial resemblance are a little lower [22]. In twin studies, heritability estimates between ACPA-positive and ACPA-negative RA do not differ much: 68 % vs. 66 % [20]. Genetic contribution in similar magnitude has also been documented for the progression of joint damage in RA [79]. While it is clear that there is sizeable genetic contribution, environmental contribution is probably equally large. In another study of 13 monozygotic twin pairs discordant for RA and smoking, in 12 of 13 pairs, the smoking twin member was also the proband [80]. This example shows the importance of considering genetic and environmental factors in any study investigating susceptibility to RA. Besides smoking, alcohol consumption is an important risk modifier for RA. On the other hand when it comes to disease progression, countries where smoking is more prevalent, i.e., Turkey, severity of disease seems less.

Alcohol reduces the risk for RA as well as joint damage measured by X-ray [81].

As ACPA-positive disease makes up around 70 % of all RA cases, most genetic association studies and almost all major GWAS have been conducted in ACPA-positive cases. The largest study ever conducted in ACPA-negative cases only examined known risk markers for ACPA-positive disease at the time of the study [82].

Table 4 Genetic modifiers of RA susceptibility identified in GWAS and meta-analysis of multiple GWAS currently listed in GWAS catalog

Chromosome region	Chromosome position	Gene	SNP	*P* value	Odds ratio (95 % CI)	Population	Features	Reference
6p21.1	44232920	*NFKBIE*	*rs2233434*	1E–15	1.20 (1.15–1.26)	Japanese	Double hit[a]	[65]
10q21.2	63958112	*RTKN2*	rs3125734	5E–9	1.20 (1.13–1.27)	Japanese		[65]
2p15	62452661	*B3GNT2*	rs11900673	1E–8	1.11 (1.07–1.15)	Japanese		[66]
4q21.21	79513215	*ANXA3*	rs2867461	1E–12	1.13 (1.09–1.17)	Japanese		[66]
5q31.1	131430118	*CSF2*	rs657075	3E–10	1.12 (1.08–1.15)	Japanese		[66]
6p23	14096658	*CD83*	rs12529514	2E–8	1.14 (1.09–1.19)	Japanese		[66]
6p21.1	44232920	*NFKBIE*	*rs2233434*	6E–19	1.19 (1.15–1.24)	Japanese	Double hit[a]	[66]
10q21.2	63785089	*ARID5B*	rs10821944	6E–18	1.16 (1.12–1.20)	Japanese		[66]
11q13.4	72373496	*PDE2A, ARAP1*	rs3781913	6E–10	1.12 (1.08–1.16)	Japanese		[66]
14q32.33	105391005	*PLD4*	rs2841277	2E–14	1.15 (1.11–1.19)	Japanese		[66]
18p11.21	12797694	*PTPN2*	rs2847297	2E–8	1.10 (1.07–1.14)	Japanese		[66]
11q24.3	128492739	*ETS1, FLI1*	rs4937362	8E–7	1.09 (1.06–1.13)	Japanese		[66]
14q22.2	55348118	*GCH1*	rs3783637	2E–6	1.10 (1.06–1.14)	Japanese		[66]
14q23.1	61908332	*PRKCH*	rs1957895	4E–7	1.09 (1.05–1.13)	Japanese		[66]
15q26.1	90893668	*ZNF774*	rs6496667	1E–6	1.09 (1.05–1.13)	Japanese		[66]
16p12.2	23888840	*PRKCB1*	rs7404928	4E–6	1.08 (1.05–1.12)	Japanese		[66]
16q24.1	86018633	*IRF8*	rs2280381	2E–6	1.12 (1.07–1.17)	Japanese		[66]
6p21.33	31622606	*APOM*	rs805297	3E–10	1.56 (1.36–1.80)	Korean	HLA region	[67]
6p21.32	32429643	*HLA-DRA*	rs9268853	5E–109	2.40 (2.20–2.60)	European	HLA region	[68]
6p21.32	32602269	*HLA-DQA1*	rs9272219	1E–45	1.92 (1.75–2.08)	European	HLA region	[68]
6p21.33	31379931	*MICA*	rs1063635	1E–17	1.35 (1.27–1.45)	European	HLA region	[68]
6p22.1	29789171	*HLA-G*	rs1610677	4E–15	1.32 (1.79–1.41)	European	HLA region	[68]
22q12.3	37551607	*IL2RB*	rs743777	2E–6	1.19 (1.10–1.30)	European		[68]

(continued)

Table 4 (continued)

Chromosome region	Chromosome position	Gene	SNP	*P* value	Odds ratio (95 % CI)	Population	Features	Reference
21q22.3	45709153	*AIRE, PFKL*	rs2075876	4E–9	1.18 (1.11–1.24)	Japanese		[69]
6p21.32	32218989	*NOTCH4*	rs9296015	2E–38	NR	Japanese	HLA region	[69]
1p36.13	17674537	*PADI4*	*rs2240335*	2E–8	NR	Japanese	Only observed in Asians; double hit[a]	[69]
8p23.1	11359638	*BLK*	rs1600249	5E–6	1.30 (1.16–1.45)	Korean		[70]
12q21.1	72724034	*TRHDE*	rs12831974	6E–6	1.27 (1.14–1.40)	Korean		[70]
3p14.3	56966246	*ARHGEF3*	rs2062583	2E–6	1.59 (1.30–1.92)	Korean		[70]
6p21.32	32680928	*HLA-DRB1*	rs7765379	5E–23	2.51 (NR)	Korean	HLA region	[70]
1p36.13	17674537	*PADI4*	*rs2240335*	2E–8	1.50 (NR)	Korean	Only observed in Asians; double hit[a]	[70]
6q27	167532793	*CCR6*	rs3093024	8E–19	1.19 (1.15–1.24)	Japanese		[71]
6p21.32	32671103	*HLA-DRB1*	rs13192471	2E–58	1.97 (1.82–2.14)	Japanese	HLA region	[71]
2q32.3	191964633	*STAT4*	*rs7574865*	2E–6	1.17 (1.10–1.25)	Japanese	ACPA-positive and ACPA-negative disease; double hit[a]	[71]
6q23.3	138196066	*OLIG3,TNFAIP3*	rs2230926	2E–6	1.31 (1.17–1.46)	Japanese	ACPA-positive and ACPA-negative disease	[71]
2p14	65595586	*SPRED2*	rs934734	5E–10	1.13 (NR)	European		[72]
5q11.2	55438580	*ANKRD55,IL6ST*	rs6859219	1E–11	1.28 (NR)	European		[72]

5q21.1	102596720	*C5orf30*	rs26232	4E–8	1.14 (NR)	European	ACPA-positive and ACPA-negative disease	[72]
3p14.3	58556841	*PXK*	rs13315591	5E–8	1.29 (NR)	European		[72]
4p15.2	26108197	*RBPJ*	rs874040	1E–16	1.14 (NR)	European		[72]
6q27	167534290	*CCR6*	rs3093023	2E–11	1.13 (NR)	European		[72]
7q32.1	128594183	*IRF5*	rs10488631	4E–11	1.19 (NR)	European	Stronger in ACPA-negative disease	[72]
2q11.2	100806940	*AFF3*	rs11676922	1E–14	1.12 (NR)	European		[72]
9p13.3	34743681	*CCL21*	rs951005	4E–10	1.19 (NR)	European		[72]
10p15.1	6098949	*IL2RA*	rs706778	1E–11	1.14 (NR)	European		[72]
1q24.2	167408670	*CD247*	rs840016	2E–6	1.11 (NR)	European		[72]
4q27	123218313	*IL2,IL21*	rs13119723	7E–7	1.12 (NR)	European		[72]
12q24.12	111884608	*SH2B3*	rs3184504	6E–6	1.08 (NR)	European		[72]
14q24.3	75960536	*BATF*	rs7155603	1E–7	1.16 (NR)	European		[72]
17q12	38040763	*IKZF3*	rs2872507	9E–7	1.10 (NR)	European		[72]
21q22.3	43836186	*UBASH3A*	rs11203203	4E–6	1.11 (NR)	European		[72]
1p36.32	2553624	*TNFRSF14*	rs3890745	4E–6	1.12 (1.06–1.18)	European		[72]
1p13.2	114377568	*PTPN22*	*rs2476601*	9E–74	1.94 (1.81–2.08)	European	Strongest non-HLA risk marker; double hit[a]	[72]
2p16.1	61136129	*REL*	rs13031237	8E–7	1.13 (1.07–1.18)	European		[72]
2q11.2	100835734	*AFF3*	rs10865035	2E–6	1.12 (1.07–1.17)	European		[72]

(continued)

Table 4 (continued)

Chromosome region	Chromosome position	Gene	SNP	*P* value	Odds ratio (95 % CI)	Population	Features	Reference
2q32.3	191964633	*STAT4*	*rs7574865*	3E–7	1.16 (1.10–1.23)	European	ACPA-positive and ACPA-negative disease; double hit[a]	[72]
2q33.2	204738919	*CTLA4*	rs3087243	1E–8	1.15 (1.10–1.20)	European		[72]
6q23.3	138006504	*TNFAIP3*	rs6920220	9E–13	1.22 (1.16–1.29)	European		[72]
9q33.2	123690239	*TRAF1,C5*	*rs3761847*	2E–7	1.13 (1.08–1.18)	European	Double hit[a]	[72]
10p15.1	6393260	*PRKCQ*	*rs4750316*	2E–6	1.15 (1.09–1.22)	European	Double hit[a]	[72]
20q13.12	44747947	*CD40*	rs4810485	3E–9	1.18 (1.11–1.25)	European		[72]
1p34.3	38624129	*POU3F1*	rs12131057	4E–7	1.16 (NR)	European		[72]
15q23	69995344	*KIF3*	rs17374222	2E–6	1.13 (NR)	European		[72]
6p21.32	32282854	*HLA-DRB1*	rs6910071	1E–299	2.88 (2.73–3.03)	European	HLA region	[72]
2p16.1	61164331	*REL*	rs13017599	2E–12	1.21 (1.15–1.28)	European		[73]
2q33.2	204693876	*CTLA4*	rs231735	6E–9	1.17 (1.11–1.23)	European		[73]
8p23.1	11343973	*BLK*	rs2736340	6E–9	1.19 (1.13–1.27)	European		[73]
1p13.2	114377568	*PTPN22*	*rs2476601*	2E–21	NR	European	Strongest non-HLA risk marker; double hit[a]	[73]
9q33.2	123652898	*TRAF1, C5*	rs881375	4E–8	NR	European		[73]
1p36.32	2553624	*MMEL1,TNFRSF14*	rs3890745	1E–7	1.12 (NR)	European		[74]
7q21.2	92246744	*CDK6*	rs42041	4E–6	1.11 (NR)	European		[74]
9p13.3	34710260	*CCL21*	rs2812378	3E–8	1.12 (NR)	European		[74]
12q13.3	57968715	*KIF5A,PIP4K2C*	rs1678542	9E–8	1.12 (NR)	European		[74]
20q13.12	44747947	*CD40*	rs4810485	8E–9	1.15 (NR)	European		[74]

10p15.1	6393260	*PRKCQ*	*rs4750316*	4E–6	1.14 (NR)	European	Double hit[a]	[74]
1p13.2	114303808	*PTPN22*	*rs6679677*	6E–42	1.79 (1.65–1.94)	European	Double hit[a]	[74]
6p21.32	32663999	*HLA-DRB1*	rs6457620	4E–186	2.55 (2.40–2.71)	European	HLA region	[74]
6q23.3	138006504	*OLIG3, TNFIP3*	rs6920220	2E–9	1.24 (1.16–1.32)	European		[74]
18q23	76409597	*SALL3*	rs2002842	6E–6	1.61 (NR)	Spanish		[75]
6p21.32	32663851	*HLA-DQA1, HLA-DQA2*	rs6457617	1E–9	NR	Spanish	HLA region	[75]
6q23.3	138002637	*TNFAIP3, OLIG3*	rs10499194	1E–9	1.33 (1.15–1.52)	European		[76]
6q23.3	138006504	*TNFAIP3, OLIG3*	rs6920220	1E–7	1.22 (NR)	European		[76]
9q33.2	123690239	*TRAF1-C5*	*rs3761847*	4E–14	1.32 (1.23–1.42)	European	Double hit[a]	[77]
1p13.2	114377568	*PTPN22*	*rs2476601*	2E–11	1.72 (NR)	European	Strongest non-HLA risk marker; double hit[a]	[77]
6p21.32	32577380	*HLA-DRB1*	rs660895	1E–108	3.62 (NR)	European	HLA region	[77]
7q32.3	131370039	*Intergenic*	rs11761231	4E–7	1.32 (NR) (women)	European		[78]
22q12.3	37551607	*NR*	rs743777	1E–6	1.09 (0.97–1.24)	European		[78]
21q22.2	42511918	*NR*	rs2837960	2E–6	1.05 (0.93–1.20)	European		[78]
4p15.2	25417244	*NR*	rs3816587	9E–6	1.09 (0.96–1.25)	European		[78]
6p21.32	32574171	*HLA-DRB1*	rs615672	8E–27	NR	European	HLA region	[78]
1p13.2	114303808	*PTPN22*	*rs6679677*	6E–25	1.98 (1.72–2.27)	European	Double hit[a]	[78]
6p21.32	32663851	*HLA-DQB1*	rs6457617	5E–75	2.36 (1.97–2.84)	European	HLA region	[78]

NR not reported

[a]Double hit: GWAS hit in more than one study in this table

Thus, there is still need to examine risk markers exclusive to ACPA-negative disease. In fact, this approach is likely to be fruitful since heritability estimates for ACPA-positive and ACPA-negative RA are similar at least in twin studies, but the contribution of HLA complex to these estimates is much higher in ACPA-positive RA [20]. Thus, ACPA-negative RA is expected to have non-HLA markers stronger than those observed in ACPA-positive RA. The recently identified subtype characterized by anti-CarP antibodies has yet to be examined for genetic associations.

Although there have been a large number of candidate gene studies and have shown associations with RA susceptibility, RA is one of those diseases that have been most extensively studied by GWAS. Genome-wide association studies conducted in large discovery and replication samples have identified more than 45 confirmed associations (Table 4). After the first-generation GWAS, cumulative results have been subjected to meta-analyses [66, 72, 83, 84] and finally the Immunochip custom SNP array analysis [85]. Overall GWAS results indicate that heritability of RA is more than 50 %, of which HLA explains 36 % [21, 85]. This estimate of the contribution of HLA to RA heritability is considerably higher than a previous estimate based on a twin study in which the presence of the HLA shared alleles explained 18 % of the genetic variance of ACPA-positive RA but only 2.4 % of the genetic variance of ACPA-negative RA [20]. Anti-CCP development has also been examined for its genetic associations [86]. The strongest associations map to the HLA region to the class III and class II region border. The statistically most significant result was achieved by rs1980493 ($P=6\times10^{-5}$). This association was still strong after adjustment for the presence of the shared epitope. This SNP is in an intergenic region between *BTNL2* and *HLA-DRA*. Bioinformatic analysis shows its involvement in transcriptional and splicing regulation (functionality score = 0.50; range = 0–1).

The original HLA association was with HLA-Dw4 corresponding to HLA-DR4 [62]. It was refined to be the shared epitope (QR*RAA*, RR*RAA*, and QK*RAA*) encoded by the amino acids in positions 70–74 of HLA-DRβ1 molecule [87]. Further exploration of the "shared epitope" revealed that the association of the *RAA* sequence occupying positions 72–74 is modulated by the amino acids at positions 71 and 72. At position 71, K confers the highest risk, R an intermediate risk, A and E a lower risk; and at position 70, Q or R confers a higher risk than D [88]. The shared epitope predisposes an individual to ACPA production and in interaction with smoking [89, 90]. The association of HLA-DR shared epitope with the disease itself, and its clinical development is secondary to its association to anti-CCP [89]. In ACPA-negative cases, HLA shared epitope shows no association, but instead *HLA-DRB1**03 is a risk factor [91]. Besides the shared epitope association in ACPA positive with risk of RA mediated by ACPA production, *HLA-DRB1**1301 is also associated with RA but with protection [92].

In the most recent study of RA associations with individual amino acids positions in 5,014 ACPA-positive cases and almost 15,000 controls, three positions (11, 71, and 74) in HLA-DRβ1 and two in other HLA proteins (position 9 in HLA-B and position 9 in HLA-DPβ1) appeared to explain the risk conferred by the HLA complex [93]. All these positions are located in the peptide-binding grooves and suggest that

HLA associations are causally related to peptide presentation function of HLA molecules although shared epitope is implicated in signal transduction too [94]. The most significant association within the HLA region is with the imputed SNP rs17878703 (allele A), a quadrallelic SNP in the second nucleotide of *DRB1* codon 11 (OR = 3.7, $P<10^{-526}$) [93]. As this SNP is in one of the most polymorphic regions in the genome and quadrallelic (i.e., all four nucleotides are alleles of this SNP), it is not included in current genotyping platforms for GWAS due to technical difficulties and has to be imputed.

In the largest meta-analysis of more than 2.5 million SNPs in 5,539 RA cases and 20,169 controls of European descent, the top five ranking candidate causal SNP associations were all from the HLA complex (rs1063478, rs375256, rs365066, rs2581, and rs1059510) [84]. These results were subjected to pathway analysis to learn more about disease biology. HLA region associations contributed to the most strongly associated pathway. The *HLA-DMA* SNP rs1063478 is a missense variant (V166I) and alters the role of HLA-DM protein in antigen processing and presentation. Together with the peptide-binding groove polymorphisms, overall results in the HLA region implicate the antigen processing and presentation as the major biological pathway in the pathogenesis of RA. The *HLA-DRB1* association is not only the strongest for RA susceptibility but is also associated with systemic forms of RA [95, 96] and with radiologic damage [97].

Among the non-HLA region associations, that of protein tyrosine phosphatase non-receptor 22 gene (*PTPN22*) is outstanding [98]. The SNP rs2476601 (R620W) alters the role of the PTPN22 protein in the context of immune response-activation cell surface receptor signaling pathway. The *PTPN22* association is exclusive to European populations as the risk allele is either absent or very rare in Asians and Africans. Interestingly, these populations respond to the same treatments for RA, and phenotypically the disease is indistinguishable. Other noteworthy associations are with *CD40, STAT4, PRM1, PADI4, TRAF1/C5, and TNFAIP3* variants (Table 4). The tumor necrosis factor-alpha-induced protein 3 (*TNFAIP3*) SNP rs2230926 (F127C) alters the role of TNFAIP3 in the context of the CD40L signaling pathway [84, 99]. The *PADI4* association is strongest in Asian populations [100]. *PADI4* encodes the type 4 peptidylarginine deiminase enzyme, which posttranslationally converts peptidylarginine to citrulline, generating citrullinated proteins. Its association with RA risk is, therefore, biologically plausible. Of the genetic associations, *IRF5* association is exclusive to anti-CCP-negative subset of RA [101]. It has been, however, proven difficult to unravel genetic associations exclusive to ACPA-negative subset either by a case–control or a case-only design [82, 102]. The case-only design which compared ACPA-positive with ACPA-negative cases noted that the largest difference between the two subtypes lies within the HLA complex [102].

Pathway analyses have been used by a number of investigators to make better use of GWAS data. Including the antigen processing and presentation and CD40 ligand pathways [84], most pathways suggested by the GWAS data to be involved in disease susceptibility are also related to immune functions [103]. However, many other pathways have shown statistically significant associations, one of the strongest ones being "neuroendocrine defects," specifically in the secretion of macrophage migration inhibitory factor (MIF) in the development of RA [103]. A review of pathway analysis in RA identified multiple specific pathways as both predicted by computational methods and verified experimentally [104]. These include MAPK, JAK/STAT, Toll-like receptor (TLR), and T-cell receptor (TCR) signaling pathways and leukocyte transendothelial migration pathway. Other experimentally verified pathways include neurotrophin and chemokine signaling and cancer pathways [104]. An epigenomic study also found DNA methylation changes in multiple pathways related to cell migration, including focal adhesion, cell adhesion, transendothelial migration, and extracellular matrix interactions [105]. This backdrop may help future studies to shift the focus from hypothesis-free studies to studies with a prior hypothesis.

Although a lot of non-HLA genetic associations have been described for RA susceptibility, most effect sizes measured as OR are around 1.1–1.2 in comparison to the HLA shared epitope association which yields an OR of greater than 5.0. The non-HLA association with the highest OR is between 1.5 and 2.0 and is conferred by *PTPN22* rs2476601 [83]. As in other diseases, GWAS results in RA have delineated useful biological information [103, 106]. Most of the strongest genetic association concerns genes that are involved in a pathophysiologic pathway for RA development (such as *PTPN22* and TCR signaling; *STAT4* and T-helper type 1 response; *CD40* and signaling in B cells, monocytes, and dendritic cells). The power of the genetic risk markers identified in GWAS as predictive markers is, however, questionable. This issue has been addressed in other complex disorders with disappointing results [16], and at present, there is no reason for optimism that the situation is any different for RA.

Epigenetic Markers for Disease Susceptibility

GWAS have been very useful in the discovery of variants that participate in the disease process, and this information has been used to learn about disease biology, but a large proportion of heritability remains to be discovered even after multiple GWAS have been done in complex disorders [107]. Part of the missing heritability may be due to the lack of consideration of "epigenetic" variation [108, 109]. In RA, the twin concordance rate of only around 15 % despite high (>50 %) heritability suggests a possible role for epigenetics in susceptibility.

Heritability is an important parameter which allows a comparison of relative importance of genetic and nongenetic contributions to a phenotype but is subject to misinterpretation [110]. It is a population- and environment-specific parameter measured at a specific point in time. Heritability indicates the proportion of phenotypic variance that is caused by additive genetic effects in a given population in a specific environment at a specific point in time. Assortative matings in human populations, presence of major genes in disease pathogenesis, and environmental variation are sources of error in heritability estimates. Gene and environment covariation or gene and environment interaction are usually ignored (due to them not being estimated) in heritability calculations. If they exist, either genetic or environmental variance estimates will be inflated, respectively, resulting in biased heritability estimates. Since epigenetic changes are mainly caused by environmental exposures and transmissible, their contribution, if any, to current heritability estimates may be missing [111].

Epigenetic changes are either biochemical changes in the DNA or histones which do not result in the nucleotide sequence, but still influence the gene function or involve the noncoding RNA machinery. Biochemical changes are usually methylation of the cytosine nucleotide (C>Cm) or methylation or acetylation of histone molecules. Both modifications activate or, more commonly, silence gene transcription. MicroRNAs are small noncoding RNA molecules that regulate gene expression levels post-transcriptionally. MicroRNAs play an important role in immunity and inflammation. Their own increased or reduced expression levels make a difference on the translation of gene products.

The effect of epigenetics on gene function has been demonstrated in twin studies: among healthy twins, epigenetic profiles are indistinguishable during the early years of life, but older monozygotic twins exhibit differences in their overall content and genomic distribution of DNA methylation and histone acetylation, affecting gene expressions [112]. Monozygotic twins are near identical in their DNA sequence, despite that there are cases of phenotypic discordance, which provides an opportunity to explore epigenetic factors for phenotypic differences. In systemic lupus erythematosus (SLE), epigenetic differences that are mainly found in genes with immune-related functions go with discordance among monozygotic twins [113]. However, a similar study in multiple sclerosis has failed to implicate epigenetics in this line [114]. No similar twin study has been performed in RA yet, but strong evidence has been presented for the involvement of epigenetics in RA susceptibility and disease progression [115–117] (for reviews, see [23, 24, 118–122]).

Epigenetic changes on DNA or histones are induced by environmental exposures. All common lifestyle factors have been shown to change epigenetic profile in peripheral blood cells [123–125]. Specifically, smoking is a strong modifier of DNA methylation [126–129]. Since smoking is the strongest environmental risk factor for ACPA-positive RA, its mode of action may include epigenetic modifications, but this issue has not yet been formally addressed. In two independent epigenomic studies not designed to examine RA associations, a region in 6p21.33 (chr6: 30720080) near the HLA complex consistently showed one of the strongest methylation differences in smokers [129, 130]. Although the hypomethylated site is intergenic in the HLA class I region, the SNP rs1140809 (chr6: 30719655) nearest to the site which is strongly hypomethylated is a replicated risk marker for RA [73, 77]. No link is known between rs1140809 and methylation, but given that DNA sequence variants may correlate with methylation levels, it may be worthwhile for future studies examining an interaction between rs1140809 and smoking for RA association.

Gene-specific methylation changes (generally hypomethylation) are also associated with serum CRP level increases [131]. Genome-wide methylation changes associated with CRP levels concern the genes involved in immune system process, immune response, defense response, response to stimulus, and response to stress, which are all linked to the functions of leukocytes. Identification of the origin and inducers of such changes in epigenetic profile of people with high CRP levels may help understanding the pathogenesis of RA and the discovery of useful biomarkers.

A critical issue in epigenetics studies is the importance of studying a single cell type as each cell lineage inherently has a unique methylation profile. Thus, the methodology in genotype analyses where any nucleated cell type can be studied is different from epigenetic research. Another difference is the ambiguity of the cause–effect relationship of disease-associated epigenetic markers. While germline DNA sequence variants are always present before the disease occurrence, with epigenetic markers, it is not clear whether they have caused the disease or the disease caused the epigenetic changes. Case–control studies useful in genetic association studies are not useful in epigenetic studies, which require prospective studies using single cell types. Since RA is a disease of the synovium, it is ideal to examine the epigenetic changes in the synovium, especially in fibroblast like synoviocytes (FLS), the effector cells of cartilage and bone destruction. Several studies have analyzed methylation status of FLS in RA (Table 5). In one of those studies, the methylome profile in FLS included changes in genes most consistently from the KEGG "rheumatoid arthritis" pathway [115].

Another important clue to suggest that epigenetics may indeed explain the missing heritability in the post-GWAS era has come from another methylome study which used the peripheral blood cells but controlled for the cellular heterogeneity [143].

Epigenetic changes also concern histones and microRNA as other components of the epigenetic machinery. Studies on animal models of RA have suggested the involvement of epigenetic modifications of histones in inflammatory arthritis pathogenesis (reviewed in [119, 122, 142, 144]). Histone modification studies in humans have focused on acetylation as a post-translational histone modification, which tends to be increased in RA [25]. Likewise, increased or reduced expression of selected microRNAs (such as miR-155, miR-203, miR-146, miR124a, and miR34a) in RA has been reported [119, 145, 146]. Epigenetics has been recently added to the mix in RA, and the initial observations are promising. These developments will potentially lead to stronger markers for susceptibility and disease progression, which may then be converted to biomarkers.

Biomarkers for Diagnosis

Biomarkers are not only useful for clinical diagnosis of RA or differential diagnosis in patients presented with arthritis but also for early detection of disease even when it is still asymptomatic. This, in turn, can help the clinician to decide starting disease-modifying interventions for prevention of serious disease and its complications. The importance of early diagnosis stems from the expectations that early initiation of treatment specific for RA in subjects with signs of undifferentiated arthritis combat disease progression [147, 148]. Since biologic and nonbiologic therapeutic options are expanding, it maybe felt that it is crucial to reach an unambiguous diagnosis as early as possible to start treatment. However, in many cases

Table 5 DNA methylation changes reported in RA

Study design	Cell type	Finding	Reference
Quantitative PCR	Peripheral blood T cells	Global genomic hypomethylation	[132]
Bisulfite sequencing, quantitative PCR, and flow cytometry	Peripheral blood T cells	Hypomethylation of *CD40L* in females with subsequent increased *CD40L* mRNA expression	[133]
Bisulfite sequencing	Peripheral blood cells	Hypomethylation of -1099C position in relation to the *IL6* gene.	[134]
ELISA	Peripheral blood mononuclear cells	Global genomic hypomethylation in ACPA-positive subset	[135]
Quantitative PCR	Synovial pellet	Retrotransposable L1 elements are associated with genomic DNA hypomethylation	[136]
Bisulfite sequencing and methylation-specific PCR	Synovial cells	Hypermethylation of the DR3 gene promoter and subsequent downregulation of its expression in synovial cells leading to resistance to apoptosis	[137]
Immunohistochemistry and flow cytometry	Fibroblast-like synoviocytes	Global genomic hypomethylation and subsequent upregulation of relevant genes	[138]
Bisulfite sequencing and McrBC assay	Fibroblast-like synoviocytes	DNA hypomethylation in *CXCL12* promoter leading to endogenous activation of synoviocytes	[139]
Illumina microarray	Fibroblast-like synoviocytes	Hypomethylation (*CHI3L1*, *CASP1*, *STAT3*, *MAP3K5*, *MEFV*, and *WISP3*) and hypermethylation (*TGFBR2* and *FOXO1*) in key genes. Hypomethylation in pathways related to cell migration, focal adhesion, cell adhesion, transendothelial migration, and extracellular matrix interactions	[105]
Quantitative PCR and Western blotting to assess DNA methyltransferase expression	Fibroblast-like synoviocytes	Exposure to proinflammatory mediators alters DNA methylation by decreasing DNA methyltransferase expression and function	[140]
Flow cytometry, ELISA, fluorometry	Fibroblast-like synoviocytes	Recycling of polyamines contributes to methylation changes in synoviocytes	[141]
Illumina microarray and bisulfite sequencing for validation	Fibroblast-like synoviocytes	Hypomethylation (*CAPN8*, *SERPINA5*, *FCGBP*) and hypermethylation (*HOXC4*, *SPTBN1*, *BCL6*) in key genes	[142]

this is not possible and treatment still needs to be initiated; for this purpose, it may not be possible to rely on clinical criteria solely, and biomarkers may be expected to be more useful.

Conventional clinical criteria have been assessed for their usefulness in predicting RA in patients with undifferentiated arthritis. Older age, male gender, longer symptom duration at first visit, involvement of lower extremities, high acute-phase reactants, and presence of IgM-RF, anti-CCP2 antibodies, anti-modified citrullinated vimentin antibodies, and *HLA-DRB1* shared epitope alleles have been reported to be risk markers, whereas a high BMI was associated with a lower rate of joint destruction in a European study [149]. In Canadian patients, the number of tender and swollen joints, RF positivity, ACPA positivity, poor functional status, and high disease activity are associated with development of RA [150]. The strongest genetic risk markers for RA susceptibility, namely, *HLA-DRB1* shared epitope alleles and *PTPN22* rs2476601, also increase the relative risk for disease development mainly by contributing to development of ACPA [151]. Gadolinium-diethylenetriamine-enhanced MRI of wrists and finger joints has also been evaluated, and detection of symmetric synovitis and bone edema and/or bone erosions was found to be predictive of future RA development [152].

As an autoimmune disorder, RA has been traditionally diagnosed in part by detection of autoantibodies. Initially, this was RF with moderate sensitivity and low specificity due to positivity in disorders other than RA. The specificity of the more recently used ACPA is higher (>97 %) for RA, but its sensitivity is less than ideal at 68 %; in other words, it is only detectable in 68 % of RA cases. In different series, 50–80 % of cases are positive for RF, ACPA, or both. Newer-generation ACPA assays which are based on artificial optimized peptides to detect ACPA provide high specificity, and when combined with RF, the sensitivity is also increased [58]. Some of the more sophisticated versions of cyclic citrullinated peptide and carbamylated peptide autoantibodies (including those against peptidylarginine deiminase type 4 (PAD4) to BRAF (v-raf murine sarcoma viral oncogene homologue B1)) appear to detect up to 40 % of ACPA-negative patients. Multimarker combinations of these novel biomarkers (UH.RA 11 plex and UH.RA 14 plex) have the potential to detect up to 70 % of ACPA-negative RA patients, but clinical utility studies have not yet been performed [17]. The presence of ACPA is associated with a specific disease course and unique genetic associations [153] (Table 3). Anti-CarP antibodies have also been examined for their predictive role in undifferentiated arthritis. These antibodies are present in about 40 % of patients with arthralgia, and their presence predicts the development of RA in the entire group of cases and more strongly in anti-CCP2 antibody-positive subgroup [61].

A number of observations suggest that changes in autoantibody and cytokine levels are present years before symptomatic disease is diagnosed. Appearance of autoantibodies and changes in serum cytokine levels can identify asymptomatic subjects destined to develop RA years later [154–156]. It was found that ACPA specificity and the number of ACPA isotypes (IgG and IgA anti-CCP2) increase before diagnosis. The autoantibodies target innate immune ligands such as citrullinated histones, fibrinogen, and biglycan at the earliest timepoints. The ACPA response is followed by elevations in many inflammatory cytokines including TNF-alpha, IL-6, IL-12p70, and IFN-gamma [155, 156]. In some people, autoantibodies are detectable up to 10 years before the diagnosis [155]. A proxy for TNF-alpha levels (soluble tumor necrosis factor receptor II or sTNFRII), which is a biomarker associated with active RA, is detectable among female patients up to 12 years before diagnosis [157], yet without further studies, this line of research and related results may be too optimistic.

Other autoantibodies have also been used to diagnose of RA. These include anti-keratin antibodies, without a high sensitivity and specificity [158], and the antinuclear antibody (ANA), which has low sensitivity and specificity for RA (64 and 41 %, respectively) as opposed to the latter's very high sensitivity (95 %) but still low specificity (57 %) in SLE. Thus, traditional laboratory diagnostic methods are not perfect, and the search for new biomarkers with high specificity and sensitivity to improve the diagnosis of RA continues. Proteomic techniques, such as matrix-assisted laser desorption/ionization time-of-flight mass spectrometry (MALDI-TOF-MS), currently have the highest potential to identify new biomarkers, and research is moving toward that direction for unbiased characterization of potential biomarkers.

Gene expression signatures have been frequently used as biomarkers in various diseases and have shown some potential usefulness despite notable failures. One of the earliest studies in RA had aimed to subclassify RA according to gene expression signatures in rheumatoid synovium [159]. Two main groups of gene expression signatures were identified. In the first group, 121 genes were expressed at higher levels, and it was a different set of 39 genes that were overexpressed in the other group. In the first group, a cluster of overexpressed genes were from the HLA complex (HSPA1A/heat shock 70 kDa protein 1A, BF/factor B, HLA-DRB1, P5-1/MHC class I region ORF T58146, HLA-DPA, TPA1, AIF1/allograft inflammatory factor 1, PSMB8/proteasome subunit, beta type, 8, and GABBR1/GABA B receptor 1 with fold changes in expression from 1.5 to 7.3). This finding again pointed out the HLA region and the adaptive immunity pathway as a major player in RA pathogenesis. The analysis of the gene expression signature in the other group suggested the involvement of the fibroblast dedifferentiation pathway. These results are, however, related to the already established disease process and may reflect more the effect of the disease rather than the cause. An important conclusion was the confirmation of the heterogeneous nature of RA and the still unsatisfied need to subclassify patients for optimum treatment [159].

Biomarkers for Disease Activity, Treatment Response, and Outcome

The clinical course of RA is highly variable with the outcome ranging from self-limiting disease to uncontrollable progressive deterioration. Although a systemic disease, RA mainly affects joints, and joints are the primary focus of disease activity assessment. The first index of disease activity and the one that predicted the development of RA in patients with undifferentiated arthritis was the Swollen Joint Count (SJC) index [160]. Tender joint count (TJC), disease activity score (DAS), simplified disease activity index (SDAI), clinical disease activity index (CDAI), global arthritis score (GAS), patient global assessment (PGA), physician global assessment (PhGA), pain visual analogue scale (pain VAS), modified health assessment questionnaire (mHAQ), and multidimensional health assessment questionnaire (MDHAQ) are the other indices in use and rely on inflamed joint counts, patient self-assessment, and laboratory tests such as erythrocyte sedimentation rate (ESR) and CRP measurements (except CDAI). The Routine Assessment of Patient Index Data-3 (RAPID-3) is, on the other hand, based solely on patient-reported outcomes. Most RA patients are currently assessed for disease activity by ACR/EULAR 2010 criteria which include assessment of joints, disease duration as well as autoantibody status and ESR/CRP levels [161]. These indices are subject to intra- and inter-assessor variability and confounding by comorbidities or accumulated joint damage resulting from long-standing disease. Besides ESR and CRP, many other proteins also correlate with disease activity [7]. Among the conventional risk factors, alcohol consumption reduces the severity of RA [81].

Since the disease primarily affects synovia, emphasis has been on the detection of changes in synovial cells, especially FLS, or changes correlating with synovial pathology that ultimately lead to joint damage. Since the rate of joint destruction is quite variable, biomarkers would be most useful to predict who is at high risk for progressive joint damage. The factors contributing to disease progression are, however, incompletely understood. It has been observed that rapid progression of joint damage is associated with pain score, total radiologic score, an elevated acute-phase response (such as ESR, CRP), the presence of *HLA-DRB1* shared epitope, autoantibodies (IgM-RF, ACPA), and inversely with body mass index (BMI) [162–165]. However, since genetics in determining RA severity is documented and the heritability of joint destruction has been estimated to be between 45 and 58 % [79], emphasis has been on genetic associations [166] (Table 6). Genetic markers also have a number of advantages over conventional markers. Genotypes are stable from birth to death, measurable at disease onset (does not have to be measured before disease onset to avoid reverse causation), remain unchanged by treatment, and can be measured by high-throughput assays using DNA that can be stored for a long time. None of the genetic markers have been, however, validated as biomarkers, and replication success rate is low [166]. Curiously, unlike the HLA antigens, the *PTPN22* susceptibility risk allele is not associated with the rate of joint destruction in ACPA-positive RA [179].

Gene expression profiling has also been used to predict disease activity in RA. Combinations of the expression levels of 19 "predictor genes" in peripheral blood correlate with follow-up disease severity scores [180]. The predictor genes are divided into two groups based on under- or overexpression patterns. *FVT1* (follicular lymphoma variant translocation 1), *EHD1* (EH domain-containing 1), *COL4A1* (collagen, type IV, alpha 1), *PRMT2* (protein arginine methyltransferase 2), and *TFCP2* (transcription factor CP2) are *underexpressed* in the severe patient group compared to the mild patient group. *FHL3* (four and a half LIM domains 3),

Table 6 Genetic markers for disease activity in RA

Gene(s)	SNP or marker	Remarks	Reference
HLA-DRB1	Amino acids K-R-A-A in positions 71–74	Also a susceptibility marker; only in ACPA-positive RA	[97]
TRAF1/C5	rs3761847		[77]
C5orf30	rs26232		[167]
CD40	rs4810485	In ACPA-positive RA	[168]
FCRL3	rs7528684	Correlates with 10-year radiographic progression	[169]
IL2RA	rs2104286	Associated with slower progression of joint destruction as well as lower circulating levels of soluble interleukin-2 receptor alpha (sIL-2Ralpha), which itself correlates with a lower rate of joint destruction	[170]
IL4	rs2070874	Correlates with severe disability as assessed by HAQ	[171]
IL4R	rs1805011, rs1119132		[172]
IL15	rs7667746, rs7665842, rs4371699, rs6821171	(IL15 levels are increased in the serum, synovium, and bone marrow of RA cases)	[173]
TGFB; *IL6*	rs1800470, rs1800795	Progression of bone-erosive damage detected by ultrasound	[174]
DKK1	rs1896368, rs1896367, rs1528873	Cases with RA who are positive for risk alleles of *DKK1* have higher serum levels of DKK1 and more progressive joint destruction	[175]
GZMB	rs8192916	Also correlated with *GZMB* expression	[176]
MMP9	rs11908352	Also correlated with MMP-9 serum levels	[177]
SPAG16	rs7607479	Influences MMP-3 regulation and protects against joint destruction in ACPA-positive RA	[178]

SKIL (SKI-like oncogene), *RPIA* (ribose 5-phosphate isomerase A), *SPRY2* (sprouty homologue 2 (*Drosophila*)), *F2RL1* (coagulation factor II receptor-like 1), *PPP1R12B* (protein phosphatase 1, regulatory subunit 12B), *LTBR* (lymphotoxin beta receptor), *GADD45A* (growth arrest and DNA-damage-inducible, alpha), *ARHGEF16* (Rho guanine exchange factor 16), *MLL* (myeloid/lymphoid or mixed-lineage leukemia), *ACYP1* (acylphosphatase 1, erythrocyte), *EIF3S9* (eukaryotic translation initiation factor 3, subunit 9 eta), *CACNB2* (calcium channel, voltage-dependent, beta 2 subunit), and *ABCC3* (ATP-binding cassette, subfamily C member 3) are *overexpressed* in the future severe patient group compared to the future mild patient group [180]. The promising aspect of this observation is that peripheral blood cells can be used for prediction, but whether these changes reclassify the patients for future disease characteristics needs to be further assessed. In a study of FLS, *CD147* overexpression was found to be potentially responsible for the enhanced MMP secretion and activation and for the invasiveness of the synoviocytes [181]. Again, none of these markers has been evaluated for their properties as biomarkers.

Most conventional markers of disease activity are biochemical like CRP. In addition to the DKK1 and MMP-9 serum level correlations with respective SNPs and clinical course, other notable biochemical markers of disease activity are listed in Table 7.

The inverse correlation of BMI with radiographic progression in RA is curious [165]. The mechanism of this association is thought to be mediated by the soluble mediators (adipokines) secreted by adipose tissue. Indeed, tumor necrosis factor-α (TNF-α), interleukin-6 (IL-6), leptin, resistin, and visfatin are proinflammatory adipokines, but adiponectin may be anti- or proinflammatory depending on its molecular form. The serum level of IL-6 is high in patients with RA and correlates with inflammation markers (ESR, CRP) and disease activity scores. It was recently reported that serum IL-6, visfatin, and adiponectin levels in patients with RA were associated with radiographic joint damage in cross-sectional studies (reviewed in [165]). In a prospective study, levels of IL-6, TNF-alpha, visfatin, and adiponectin were also positively correlated with radiographic progression over 4 years independent of BMI, but only the adiponectin association retained statistical significance after adjustment for the presence of ACPA [196].

Multi-biomarkers for Disease Activity

In a complex disease, an individual marker is unlikely to earn a biomarker status with a high sensitivity and specificity. Recent efforts have focused on the development of multimarker combinations with better properties. One such biomarker is the MBDA score for the assessment of RA disease activity [18, 200]. This effort began with selection of 130 candidate serum protein biomarkers from extensive literature screens, bioinformatics databases, and available mRNA expression and protein microarray data. Each candidate biomarker was assessed for correlations to the currently used metric for RA activity (e.g., DAS28-CRP). After a stepwise approach, 12 serum-based biomarkers (SAA, IL-6, TNFRI, VEGF-A, MMP-1, YKL-40, MMP-3, EGF, VCAM-1, leptin, resistin, and CRP) were selected to generate an MBDA score between 1 and 100 as a measure of RA disease activity. This significantly correlated with DAS28-CRP and discriminated patients with low vs. moderate/high clinical disease activity. The MBDA outperformed any other individual biomarker, correlated with DAS28-CRP, and traced it during follow-up. There was also good agreement with ultrasonography and radiography-measured joint damage. The MBDA score seems to perform equally well in seropositive and seronegative RA patients [201].

Table 7 Nongenetic markers assessed for disease activity in RA

Protein	Remarks	Reference
Cartilage oligomeric matrix protein (COMP, thrombospondin 5)	Associated with joint damage progression over the first 5 years in patients with RA	[182]
Collagen cross-linked C-telopeptide (CTX-I)	Baseline levels were higher in progressors and correlated with 10-year change in radiographic damage score, but not a stronger classifier than ACPA	[183]
Matrix metalloproteinase-1 (MMP-1)	Serum levels decline with treatment in parallel with other markers of inflammation	[184]
Matrix metalloproteinase-3 (MMP-3)	Predicts radiographic progression at 8.2-years	[185]
Soluble intercellular adhesion molecule-1 (sICAM-1); vascular cell adhesion molecule-1 (sVCAM-1); E-selectin (sE-selectin); and vascular endothelial growth factor-A (VEGF-A)	Correlate with disease activity	[186]
C-X-C motif chemokine 13 (CXCL13)	Correlates with disease activity	[187]
Epidermal growth factor (EGF)-like growth factors	Amphiregulin (AREG) shows the highest correlation with disease activity; inhibition of EGF receptor ameliorates a mouse model of RA	[188, 189]
Serum amyloid A protein (SAA)	More sensitive than CRP in monitoring disease activity	[190]
Cartilage glycoprotein-39 (YKL-40)	Correlates with progression in Larsen score and disease activity	[191, 192]
Anti-CarP antibodies	Predicts a more severe disease course in ACPA-negative patients as measured by radiological progression	[60]
Interleukin-6 (IL-6)	Serum levels correlate with development of bone erosions or disease activity scores	[192, 193]
Interleukin-15 (IL-15)	High baseline levels predict a more severe disease and more intensive treatment	[194]
Soluble tumor necrosis factor receptors (sTNFRs)	Serum levels correlate with clinical improvement	[195]
Adiponectin; leptin; resistin	Adiponectin is associated with radiographic progression (independent of BMI); leptin shows an inverse association with disease activity; resistin correlates with disease activity markers	[196–199]

The MBDA score is made up of various components of the Swollen Joint Count (SJC28), tender joint count (TJC28), patient global assessment (PGA) equations as well as CRP [8]. Quantification of 12 biomarkers is performed with multiplexed sandwich electrochemiluminescence immunoassays in three panels [18]. In the analytical validity step, each biomarker was assessed for parallelism, dynamic range, cross-reactivity, and precision as well as the interference by serum proteins, heterophilic antibodies, and common RA therapies. The median coefficient of variation of the MBDA score was <2 % across the score range. Although the MBDA score performs very well, there is still room for improvement as the algorithm currently uses serum biomarkers that were measurable in RA patient serum with commercially available assays, and not cytokines and mediators that are likely to be highly expressed within the joint. One predicts that such an improvement would be most useful also for prediction of clinical RA in people with undifferentiated arthritis.

The MBDA algorithm has been evaluated and validated in multiple independent cohorts from different populations [201–203]. Further studies are ongoing for analysis of clinical validity and the relationship between the MBDA score and other measures of disease activity, and most importantly, the ability of the MBDA score to indicate the risk of joint damage progression. The MBDA score has not yet attained a biomarker status. For this, clinical utility studies in the form of prospective studies incorporating the MBDA score to assess calibration and reclassification properties are still required [200].

While a large number of risk markers for RA have been identified thanks to the work of large international consortia, the speed of translating these results into biological knowledge has been slower. The latest approach to this problem is a very large crowdsourcing project that will use large-scale genetics and omics data to identify predictors of response to immunosuppressive therapy in RA [204].

Recent Developments in Biomarkers for Assessing Treatment Response and Outcome

Disease-modifying antirheumatic drugs (DMARDs) and biological treatments such as Anti-tumor necrosis factor (anti-TNF) agents are the mainstay of treatment in RA. However, considerable variability, in both efficacy and toxicity, is observed. GWAS may have failed in uncovering missing heritability for disease susceptibility, but in pharmacogenetics it has been most successful and provided results most of which have already been translated into clinical medicine in conditions other than RA [205, 206]. Examples include HLA typing before initiation of treatment with abacavir (HLA-B*57:01), carbamazepine (-B*15:02), and allopurinol (HLA-B*58:01) to avoid potentially fatal drug hypersensitivity reactions. It is possible that genetic component may also influence drug treatment outcome in patients with RA [207]. Notable progress has been made in determination of the predictors of response to drug treatment in RA in recent years, which has made the talk of "personalized medicine" more promising for RA patients [207–210].

Pharmacogenetic studies in RA have also been useful in the development of matrices for the assessment of the effect of the initial treatment in each patient. These matrices use basic criteria at the baseline. Besides CRP serum levels, the autoantibody status (ACPA and RA), SJC28, and erosion score were used to evaluate the efficacy of treatment options using rapid radiological progression or RRP as the outcome measure. RRP is defined as damage progression in joints according to the Sharp–van der Heijde method with an increase of five points or more during the first year. The most popular matrices for this purpose are BeST, ASPIRE, and ESPOIR, some of which also use SJC28 in assessment (reviewed in [208]). Existing data suggest that there are probably other variables to predict RRP in established RA and these models need some refinement, perhaps by addition of more sensitive biomarkers.

Methotrexate was one of the first DMARDs used to treat RA and is still in use. Toxicity, side effect, and nonresponse are important issues. Associations of genetic markers with clinical response and high remission rate as well as overall toxicity, including variants affecting transport (in *MDR1*, *RFC1*) and intracellular metabolism (in *MTHFR*, *TYMS*, *ATIC*) of methotrexate, have been reported (reviewed in [207, 210]). Unfortunately, most of these associations either have not been replicated yet, or replication attempts have failed. A meta-analysis concluded that *MTHFR* rs1801133 (677 C>T) shows a dominant model association (CT/TT) with increased methotrexate toxicity [211]. This conclusion is based on four independent reports showing an association and an additional four showing no association, and the effect size is modest (OR = 1.7). Thus, the clinical value of this association is questionable.

Other DMARDs such as leflunomide and sulfasalazine are also used in treating RA. Pharmacogenetic studies to determine markers of adverse effects and efficacy of these agents have also been conducted (reviewed in [210]). Notable findings in terms of effects sizes are the CYP1A2*1F (rs762551) association with overall leflunomide-induced toxicity (OR = 9.7 for the CC genotype in comparison to CA/AA genotypes) [212] and NAT2*4 association (a multiSNP haplotype lacking wild-type alleles) with severe adverse events by sulfasalazine (OR = 24.6) [213]. It is this magnitude of effect sizes rather than the *P* values that will determine which association may have the potential to become a biomarker with clinical utility in the future.

The first biologics to be introduced in the treatment of RA were the TNF blockers (infliximab, etanercept, adalimumab). These biologics are usually the first choice in high-risk patients or if synthetic DMARD therapy fails in other patients. Not all patients respond to this treatment, and 30–40 % of patients have little or no response. Given the obvious benefit of TNF blocker treatment, it has been a very active area of research to find out markers to predict TNF blocker response. Already known nongenetic markers of good response include not smoking, good functional ability, being male, younger age, concomitant use of DMARDs and NSAIDs, and need for concomitant use of corticosteroids, but these studies have not necessarily yielded consistent results. Around 60–70 % of patients respond well to this treatment, and a large number of genetic markers have been identified to predict a good response [207, 208]. These studies ranged from examining the known RA susceptibility markers for their associations with anti-TNF treatment, candidate gene studies examining inflammation-related genes, and also totally agnostic or hypothesis-free GWAS. Although individual studies reported promising associations, most of them need validation in cohort studies before being considered for biomarker development (reviewed in [207, 208]) (Table 4).

One marker that has shown consistent associations in two large (>1,000 patients) studies is between *PTPRC* (CD45) rs10919563 and improved treatment response, with a meta-analysis showing a strong statistical significance ($P=5\times10^{-5}$) [214, 215]. Of particular interest is the polymorphism within the TNF gene itself as predictors of response to anti-TNF therapy. A meta-analysis of nine studies showed that the common TNF-alpha promoter polymorphism rs1800629 (–308 G>A) is associated with poor response to anti-TNF treatment with an OR of just above 2.0 ($P=0.0002$) [216].

Because of the stringency in quality control steps, statistical data analysis, sample size requirements, and the built-in replication arm, GWAS results should be the most valid genetic association results with very low false-positivity rates. Potential false positivity due to the stringency of statistical significance threshold may be an issue, but later meta-analyses may address this. Five GWAS yielded a number of results with relatively strong effect sizes (ORs around 3.0). The disappointing aspect of GWAS in anti-TNF response assessment is that there is not a single common association among the five completed studies, all among patients of European ancestry (Table 4). It is also noteworthy that no other race/ethnicity has been examined in GWAS for response to anti-TNF treatment by GWAS. Even the most recent study not yet listed in GWAS catalog [217] does not report any association that matches the previous GWAS results. Still more disappointing is the finding that none of the previous GWAS results reexamined in this largest study to date were conformed. It is, therefore, clear that GWAS have not been able to consistently identify a marker to be used to predict response to anti-TNF treatment.

Other biologics such as rituximab (a monoclonal antibody directed at the CD20 antigen on B-lymphocytes) or abatacept (an inhibitor of T-cell activation by selective binding to the CD80 and CD86 receptor) are considered in patients failing anti-TNF therapy. A number of studies also examined the potential predictors of response to these biologics. Generally small studies have generated some associations, but their full assessment is pending.

Besides genetic variants, peripheral blood [218–220] and synovium [221] gene expression profiles for prediction of response to anti-TNF treatment have also been examined. Although several different gene expression signatures have been observed, the results in these relatively small pilot studies lacked consistency, and no overwhelmingly significant result has been reported. In a study that has reexamined five previously reported gene expression signatures in 42 cases (18 good responders and 24 nonresponders) from the Netherlands [222], the sensitivity of previously identified signatures in this independent replication study ranged between 67 and 92 %, but with much lower specificity values (17–61 %).

These values are much lower than required from a good biomarker. The best result was that yielded by the 20 genes transcript set previously reported [218], which was able to classify the cases as anti-TNF responders and nonresponders with a sensitivity of 71 % and a specificity of 61 %. This replication study also included a transcriptomic assay and identified 113 genes that showed significantly different expression levels in responders and nonresponders to TNF blockers at baseline [222].

One of the promising markers for prediction of good response to anti-TNF treatment reported to date is a 24-marker set [223]. This profile utilizes a proteomics assay, arthritis antigen arrays, a multiplex cytokine assay, and a conventional ELISA. The multiparameter protein biomarker enabled the prediction of a good clinical response to etanercept in three different cohorts from the USA, Sweden, and Japan with positive predictive values 58–72 % and negative predictive values 63–78 %. No follow-up is available for the further development of this multimarker set into a biomarker. Even more promising results have been reported from a urine metabolomic study [224]. Although based only 16 cases, this study was able to define a set of metabolites detectable in the urine that will classify cases as good responders with a sensitivity of 89 % and a specificity of 86 %. These results are by far the most promising and if replicated in a larger study, should certainly be followed up in analytical and clinical validity studies to be assessed for clinical utility as a biomarker eventually.

Conclusions

There are a disproportionate number of associations with different aspects of RA compared with the number of biomarkers in use or in the pipeline. An association study reports a marker that reflects some correlation at the population level, but the value of the associated marker at the individual level for clinical prediction is almost always remains unexplored. Studies following up promising association results should make sure that the marker can act as a biomarker, that is, it can reclassify an individual's future risk better than existing conventional markers. For a biomarker to be clinically useful, it has to go through regulatory approvals (FDA in the USA), and it has to be documented that the availability of biomarkers leads to better clinical decision making and better patient outcomes especially compared to what is currently in use in clinical care – physician and patient-reported outcomes; to date this has not been shown with any candidate biomarkers. The common custom of calling any marker showing an association a biomarker is misleading. The development of a biomarker requires much more than the initial demonstration of an association, and the process is not too dissimilar from drug development. The multistep process of successful biomarker development requires a multidisciplinary team with extensive collaborative links. It is possible that in the near future, validated biomarkers will be available for use in clinical decision making thanks to the latest advancements in omics.

Electronic Resources

DRAP (Database of RA-associated Polymorphisms) by Group of Statistical Genetics, College of Bioinformatics Science and Technology, Harbin Medical University, China: http://210.46.85.180/DRAP/index.php/Metaanalysis

NIH NHGRI GWAS Catalog: http://www.genome.gov/gwastudies

GWAS Central: http://www.gwascentral.org

References

1. Katsavos S, Anagnostouli M. Biomarkers in multiple sclerosis: an up-to-date overview. Mult Scler Int. 2013;2013:340508.
2. Leidinger P, Backes C, Deutscher S, Schmitt K, Mueller SC, Frese K, Haas J, Ruprecht K, Paul F, Stahler C, et al. A blood based 12-miRNA signature of Alzheimer disease patients. Genome Biol. 2013;14:R78.
3. Sharma S, Moon CS, Khogali A, Haidous A, Chabenne A, Ojo C, Jelebinkov M, Kurdi Y, Ebadi M. Biomarkers in Parkinson's disease (recent update). Neurochem Int. 2013;63: 201–29.
4. Kelloff GJ, Sigman CC. Cancer biomarkers: selecting the right drug for the right patient. Nat Rev Drug Discov. 2012;11:201–14.
5. Lindstrom TM, Robinson WH. Biomarkers for rheumatoid arthritis: making it personal. Scand J Clin Lab Invest Suppl. 2010;242:79–84.
6. Isaacs JD, Ferraccioli G. The need for personalised medicine for rheumatoid arthritis. Ann Rheum Dis. 2011;70:4–7.
7. Kim SS, Paget SA. Biomarkers in RA: diagnostic, prognostic, and quantitative proteomic profiling of disease activity. Rheumatol Pract News. 2011:21–6.
8. Wilke W. Measures of disease activity in rheumatoid arthritis. Rheumatol Pract News. 2012;2012:18–22.
9. Miossec P, Verweij CL, Klareskog L, Pitzalis C, Barton A, Lekkerkerker F, Reiter S, Laslop A, Breedveld F, Abadie E, et al. Biomarkers and personalised medicine in rheumatoid arthritis: a proposal for interactions between academia, industry and regulatory bodies. Ann Rheum Dis. 2011;70:1713–8.
10. Willemze A, Toes RE, Huizinga TW, Trouw LA. New biomarkers in rheumatoid arthritis. Neth J Med. 2012;70:392–9.
11. Gallo V, Egger M, McCormack V, Farmer PB, Ioannidis JP, Kirsch-Volders M, Matullo G, Phillips DH, Schoket B, Stromberg U, et al. STrengthening the Reporting of OBservational studies in Epidemiology – Molecular Epidemiology (STROBE-ME): an extension of the STROBE Statement. PLoS Med. 2011;8:e1001117.
12. Robinson WH, Lindstrom TM, Cheung RK, Sokolove J. Mechanistic biomarkers for clinical decision making in rheumatic diseases. Nat Rev Rheumatol. 2013;9:267–76.
13. Glas AM, Floore A, Delahaye LJ, Witteveen AT, Pover RC, Bakx N, Lahti-Domenici JS, Bruinsma TJ, Warmoes MO, Bernards R, et al. Converting a breast cancer microarray signature into a high-throughput diagnostic test. BMC Genomics. 2006;7:278.
14. Marchionni L, Afsari B, Geman D, Leek JT. A simple and reproducible breast cancer prognostic test. BMC Genomics. 2013;14:336.
15. Ware JH. The limitations of risk factors as prognostic tools. N Engl J Med. 2006;355:2615–7.
16. Jakobsdottir J, Gorin MB, Conley YP, Ferrell RE, Weeks DE. Interpretation of genetic association studies: markers with replicated highly significant odds ratios may be poor classifiers. PLoS Genet. 2009;5:e1000337.

17. Trouw LA, Mahler M. Closing the serological gap: promising novel biomarkers for the early diagnosis of rheumatoid arthritis. Autoimmun Rev. 2012;12:318–22.
18. Eastman PS, Manning WC, Qureshi F, Haney D, Cavet G, Alexander C, Hesterberg LK. Characterization of a multiplex, 12-biomarker test for rheumatoid arthritis. J Pharm Biomed Anal. 2012;70:415–24.
19. MacGregor AJ, Snieder H, Rigby AS, Koskenvuo M, Kaprio J, Aho K, Silman AJ. Characterizing the quantitative genetic contribution to rheumatoid arthritis using data from twins. Arthritis Rheum. 2000;43:30–7.
20. van der Woude D, Houwing-Duistermaat JJ, Toes RE, Huizinga TW, Thomson W, Worthington J, van der Helm-van Mil AH, de Vries RR. Quantitative heritability of anti-citrullinated protein antibody-positive and anti-citrullinated protein antibody-negative rheumatoid arthritis. Arthritis Rheum. 2009;60:916–23.
21. Killock D. Genetic associations with RA expanded and strengthened. Nat Rev Rheumatol. 2013;9:4.
22. Frisell T, Holmqvist M, Kallberg H, Klareskog L, Alfredsson L, Askling J. Familial risks and heritability of rheumatoid arthritis: role of rheumatoid factor/anti-citrullinated protein antibody status, number and type of affected relatives, sex, and age. Arthritis Rheum. 2013;65:2773–82.
23. Klein K, Ospelt C, Gay S. Epigenetic contributions in the development of rheumatoid arthritis. Arthritis Res Ther. 2012;14:227.
24. Viatte S, Plant D, Raychaudhuri S. Genetics and epigenetics of rheumatoid arthritis. Nat Rev Rheumatol. 2013;9:141–53.
25. Grabiec AM, Reedquist KA. The ascent of acetylation in the epigenetics of rheumatoid arthritis. Nat Rev Rheumatol. 2013;9:311–8.
26. Wald NJ, Hackshaw AK, Frost CD. When can a risk factor be used as a worthwhile screening test? BMJ. 1999;319:1562–5.
27. Ioannidis JP. Is molecular profiling ready for use in clinical decision making? Oncologist. 2007;12:301–11.
28. Bueno-de-Mesquita JM, Linn SC, Keijzer R, Wesseling J, Nuyten DS, van Krimpen C, Meijers C, de Graaf PW, Bos MM, Hart AA, et al. Validation of 70-gene prognosis signature in node-negative breast cancer. Breast Cancer Res Treat. 2009;117:483–95.
29. Taylor JM, Ankerst DP, Andridge RR. Validation of biomarker-based risk prediction models. Clin Cancer Res. 2008;14:5977–83.
30. McShane LM. Statistical challenges in the development and evaluation of marker-based clinical tests. BMC Med. 2012;10:52.
31. Dancey JE, Dobbin KK, Groshen S, Jessup JM, Hruszkewycz AH, Koehler M, Parchment R, Ratain MJ, Shankar LK, Stadler WM, et al. Guidelines for the development and incorporation of biomarker studies in early clinical trials of novel agents. Clin Cancer Res. 2010;16: 1745–55.
32. Altman DG, McShane LM, Sauerbrei W, Taube SE. Reporting recommendations for tumor marker prognostic studies (REMARK): explanation and elaboration. PLoS Med. 2012;9: e1001216.
33. Teutsch SM, Bradley LA, Palomaki GE, Haddow JE, Piper M, Calonge N, Dotson WD, Douglas MP, Berg AO. The evaluation of genomic applications in practice and prevention (EGAPP) initiative: methods of the EGAPP Working Group. Genet Med. 2009;11:3–14.
34. Janssens AC, Ioannidis JP, van Duijn CM, Little J, Khoury MJ. Strengthening the reporting of genetic rIsk prediction studies: the GRIPS statement. PLoS Med. 2011;8:e1000420.
35. Moore HM, Kelly AB, Jewell SD, McShane LM, Clark DP, Greenspan R, Hayes DF, Hainaut P, Kim P, Mansfield EA, et al. Biospecimen reporting for improved study quality (BRISQ). Cancer Cytopathol. 2011;119:92–101.
36. Maksymowych WP, Landewe R, Boers M, Garnero P, Geusens P, El-Gabalawy H, Heinegard D, Kraus VB, Lohmander S, Matyas J, et al. Development of draft validation criteria for a soluble biomarker to be regarded as a valid biomarker reflecting structural damage endpoints in rheumatoid arthritis and spondyloarthritis clinical trials. J Rheumatol. 2007;34:634–40.

37. Pepe MS, Feng Z, Janes H, Bossuyt PM, Potter JD. Pivotal evaluation of the accuracy of a biomarker used for classification or prediction: standards for study design. J Natl Cancer Inst. 2008;100:1432–8.
38. Ransohoff DF. How to improve reliability and efficiency of research about molecular markers: roles of phases, guidelines, and study design. J Clin Epidemiol. 2007;60:1205–19.
39. Castaldi PJ, Dahabreh IJ, Ioannidis JP. An empirical assessment of validation practices for molecular classifiers. Brief Bioinform. 2011;12:189–202.
40. Tektonidou MG, Ward MM. Validity of clinical associations of biomarkers in translational research studies: the case of systemic autoimmune diseases. Arthritis Res Ther. 2010;12:R179.
41. Pepe MS, Janes H, Longton G, Leisenring W, Newcomb P. Limitations of the odds ratio in gauging the performance of a diagnostic, prognostic, or screening marker. Am J Epidemiol. 2004;159:882–90.
42. Janssens AC, Moonesinghe R, Yang Q, Steyerberg EW, van Duijn CM, Khoury MJ. The impact of genotype frequencies on the clinical validity of genomic profiling for predicting common chronic diseases. Genet Med. 2007;9:528–35.
43. Holmberg L, Vickers A. Evaluation of prediction models for decision-making: beyond calibration and discrimination. PLoS Med. 2013;10:e1001491.
44. Cook NR. Use and misuse of the receiver operating characteristic curve in risk prediction. Circulation. 2007;115:928–35.
45. Pencina MJ, D'Agostino Sr RB, D'Agostino Jr RB, Vasan RS. Evaluating the added predictive ability of a new marker: from area under the ROC curve to reclassification and beyond. Stat Med. 2008;27:157–72; discussion 207–12.
46. Pickering JW, Endre ZH. New metrics for assessing diagnostic potential of candidate biomarkers. Clin J Am Soc Nephrol. 2012;7:1355–64.
47. Steyerberg EW, Vickers AJ, Cook NR, Gerds T, Gonen M, Obuchowski N, Pencina MJ, Kattan MW. Assessing the performance of prediction models: a framework for traditional and novel measures. Epidemiology. 2010;21:128–38.
48. Wray NR, Yang J, Goddard ME, Visscher PM. The genetic interpretation of area under the ROC curve in genomic profiling. PLoS Genet. 2010;6:e1000864.
49. Mihaescu R, van Zitteren M, van Hoek M, Sijbrands EJ, Uitterlinden AG, Witteman JC, Hofman A, Hunink MG, van Duijn CM, Janssens AC. Improvement of risk prediction by genomic profiling: reclassification measures versus the area under the receiver operating characteristic curve. Am J Epidemiol. 2010;172:353–61.
50. Tzoulaki I, Liberopoulos G, Ioannidis JP. Use of reclassification for assessment of improved prediction: an empirical evaluation. Int J Epidemiol. 2011;40:1094–105.
51. Ioannidis JP. Biomarker failures. Clin Chem. 2013;59:202–4.
52. Thompson IM. PSA: a biomarker for disease. A biomarker for clinical trials. How useful is it? J Nutr. 2006;136:2704S.
53. Prensner JR, Rubin MA, Wei JT, Chinnaiyan AM. Beyond PSA: the next generation of prostate cancer biomarkers. Sci Transl Med. 2012;4:127rv3.
54. Keeling SO, Landewe R, van der Heijde D, Bathon J, Boers M, Garnero P, Geusens P, El-Gabalawy H, Inman RD, Kraus VB, et al. Testing of the preliminary OMERACT validation criteria for a biomarker to be regarded as reflecting structural damage endpoints in rheumatoid arthritis clinical trials: the example of C-reactive protein. J Rheumatol. 2007;34: 623–33.
55. Syversen SW, Landewe R, van der Heijde D, Bathon JM, Boers M, Bykerk VP, Fitzgerald O, Gladman DD, Garnero P, Geusens P, et al. Testing of the OMERACT 8 draft validation criteria for a soluble biomarker reflecting structural damage in rheumatoid arthritis: a systematic literature search on 5 candidate biomarkers. J Rheumatol. 2009;36:1769–84.
56. Maksymowych WP, Landewe R, Tak PP, Ritchlin CJ, Ostergaard M, Mease PJ, El-Gabalawy H, Garnero P, Gladman DD, Fitzgerald O, et al. Reappraisal of OMERACT 8 draft validation criteria for a soluble biomarker reflecting structural damage endpoints in rheumatoid arthritis, psoriatic arthritis, and spondyloarthritis: the OMERACT 9 v2 criteria. J Rheumatol. 2009;36: 1785–91.

57. Maksymowych WP, Fitzgerald O, Wells GA, Gladman DD, Landewe R, Ostergaard M, Taylor WJ, Christensen R, Tak PP, Boers M, et al. Proposal for levels of evidence schema for validation of a soluble biomarker reflecting damage endpoints in rheumatoid arthritis, psoriatic arthritis, and ankylosing spondylitis, and recommendations for study design. J Rheumatol. 2009;36:1792–9.
58. Taylor P, Gartemann J, Hsieh J, Creeden J. A systematic review of serum biomarkers anti-cyclic citrullinated Peptide and rheumatoid factor as tests for rheumatoid arthritis. Autoimmune Dis. 2011;2011:815038.
59. Trouw LA, Huizinga TW, Toes RE. Autoimmunity in rheumatoid arthritis: different antigens – common principles. Ann Rheum Dis. 2013;72 Suppl 2:ii132–6.
60. Shi J, Knevel R, Suwannalai P, van der Linden MP, Janssen GM, van Veelen PA, Levarht NE, van der Helm-van Mil AH, Cerami A, Huizinga TW, et al. Autoantibodies recognizing carbamylated proteins are present in sera of patients with rheumatoid arthritis and predict joint damage. Proc Natl Acad Sci U S A. 2011;108:17372–7.
61. Shi J, van de Stadt LA, Levarht EW, Huizinga TW, Toes RE, Trouw LA, van Schaardenburg D. Anti-carbamylated protein antibodies are present in arthralgia patients and predict the development of rheumatoid arthritis. Arthritis Rheum. 2013;65:911–5.
62. Stastny P. Association of the B-cell alloantigen DRw4 with rheumatoid arthritis. N Engl J Med. 1978;298:869–71.
63. Consortium WTCC. Genome-wide association study of CNVs in 16,000 cases of eight common diseases and 3,000 shared controls. Nature. 2010;464:713–20.
64. Bax M, van Heemst J, Huizinga TW, Toes RE. Genetics of rheumatoid arthritis: what have we learned? Immunogenetics. 2011;63:459–66.
65. Myouzen K, Kochi Y, Okada Y, Terao C, Suzuki A, Ikari K, Tsunoda T, Takahashi A, Kubo M, Taniguchi A, et al. Functional variants in NFKBIE and RTKN2 involved in activation of the NF-kappaB pathway are associated with rheumatoid arthritis in Japanese. PLoS Genet. 2012;8:e1002949.
66. Okada Y, Terao C, Ikari K, Kochi Y, Ohmura K, Suzuki A, Kawaguchi T, Stahl EA, Kurreeman FA, Nishida N, et al. Meta-analysis identifies nine new loci associated with rheumatoid arthritis in the Japanese population. Nat Genet. 2012;44:511–6.
67. Hu HJ, Jin EH, Yim SH, Yang SY, Jung SH, Shin SH, Kim WU, Shim SC, Kim TG, Chung YJ. Common variants at the promoter region of the APOM confer a risk of rheumatoid arthritis. Exp Mol Med. 2011;43:613–21.
68. Eleftherohorinou H, Hoggart CJ, Wright VJ, Levin M, Coin LJ. Pathway-driven gene stability selection of two rheumatoid arthritis GWAS identifies and validates new susceptibility genes in receptor mediated signalling pathways. Hum Mol Genet. 2011;20:3494–506.
69. Terao C, Yamada R, Ohmura K, Takahashi M, Kawaguchi T, Kochi Y, Okada Y, Nakamura Y, Yamamoto K, Melchers I, et al. The human AIRE gene at chromosome 21q22 is a genetic determinant for the predisposition to rheumatoid arthritis in Japanese population. Hum Mol Genet. 2011;20:2680–5.
70. Freudenberg J, Lee HS, Han BG, Shin HD, Kang YM, Sung YK, Shim SC, Choi CB, Lee AT, Gregersen PK, et al. Genome-wide association study of rheumatoid arthritis in Koreans: population-specific loci as well as overlap with European susceptibility loci. Arthritis Rheum. 2011;63:884–93.
71. Kochi Y, Okada Y, Suzuki A, Ikari K, Terao C, Takahashi A, Yamazaki K, Hosono N, Myouzen K, Tsunoda T, et al. A regulatory variant in CCR6 is associated with rheumatoid arthritis susceptibility. Nat Genet. 2010;42:515–9.
72. Stahl EA, Raychaudhuri S, Remmers EF, Xie G, Eyre S, Thomson BP, Li Y, Kurreeman FA, Zhernakova A, Hinks A, et al. Genome-wide association study meta-analysis identifies seven new rheumatoid arthritis risk loci. Nat Genet. 2010;42:508–14.
73. Gregersen PK, Amos CI, Lee AT, Lu Y, Remmers EF, Kastner DL, Seldin MF, Criswell LA, Plenge RM, Holers VM, et al. REL, encoding a member of the NF-kappaB family of transcription factors, is a newly defined risk locus for rheumatoid arthritis. Nat Genet. 2009;41: 820–3.

74. Raychaudhuri S, Remmers EF, Lee AT, Hackett R, Guiducci C, Burtt NP, Gianniny L, Korman BD, Padyukov L, Kurreeman FA, et al. Common variants at CD40 and other loci confer risk of rheumatoid arthritis. Nat Genet. 2008;40:1216–23.
75. Julia A, Ballina J, Canete JD, Balsa A, Tornero-Molina J, Naranjo A, Alperi-Lopez M, Erra A, Pascual-Salcedo D, Barcelo P, et al. Genome-wide association study of rheumatoid arthritis in the Spanish population: KLF12 as a risk locus for rheumatoid arthritis susceptibility. Arthritis Rheum. 2008;58:2275–86.
76. Plenge RM, Cotsapas C, Davies L, Price AL, de Bakker PI, Maller J, Pe'er I, Burtt NP, Blumenstiel B, DeFelice M, et al. Two independent alleles at 6q23 associated with risk of rheumatoid arthritis. Nat Genet. 2007;39:1477–82.
77. Plenge RM, Seielstad M, Padyukov L, Lee AT, Remmers EF, Ding B, Liew A, Khalili H, Chandrasekaran A, Davies LR, et al. TRAF1–C5 as a risk locus for rheumatoid arthritis–a genomewide study. N Engl J Med. 2007;357:1199–209.
78. Consortium TWTCC. Genome-wide association study of 14,000 cases of seven common diseases and 3,000 shared controls. Nature. 2007;447:661–78.
79. Knevel R, Grondal G, Huizinga TW, Visser AW, Jonsson H, Vikingsson A, Geirsson AJ, Steinsson K, van der Helm-van Mil AH. Genetic predisposition of the severity of joint destruction in rheumatoid arthritis: a population-based study. Ann Rheum Dis. 2012;71: 707–9.
80. Silman AJ, Newman J, MacGregor AJ. Cigarette smoking increases the risk of rheumatoid arthritis. Results from a nationwide study of disease-discordant twins. Arthritis Rheum. 1996;39:732–5.
81. Maxwell JR, Gowers IR, Moore DJ, Wilson AG. Alcohol consumption is inversely associated with risk and severity of rheumatoid arthritis. Rheumatology (Oxford). 2010;49: 2140–6.
82. Viatte S, Plant D, Bowes J, Lunt M, Eyre S, Barton A, Worthington J. Genetic markers of rheumatoid arthritis susceptibility in anti-citrullinated peptide antibody negative patients. Ann Rheum Dis. 2012;71:1984–90.
83. Jiang Y, Zhang R, Zheng J, Liu P, Tang G, Lv H, Zhang L, Shang Z, Zhan Y, Lv W, et al. Meta-analysis of 125 rheumatoid arthritis-related single nucleotide polymorphisms studied in the past two decades. PLoS One. 2012;7:e51571.
84. Song GG, Bae SC, Lee YH. Pathway analysis of genome-wide association studies on rheumatoid arthritis. Clin Exp Rheumatol. 2013;31:566–74.
85. Eyre S, Bowes J, Diogo D, Lee A, Barton A, Martin P, Zhernakova A, Stahl E, Viatte S, McAllister K, et al. High-density genetic mapping identifies new susceptibility loci for rheumatoid arthritis. Nat Genet. 2012;44:1336–40.
86. Cui J, Taylor KE, Destefano AL, Criswell LA, Izmailova ES, Parker A, Roubenoff R, Plenge RM, Weinblatt ME, Shadick NA, et al. Genome-wide association study of determinants of anti-cyclic citrullinated peptide antibody titer in adults with rheumatoid arthritis. Mol Med. 2009;15:136–43.
87. Gregersen PK, Silver J, Winchester RJ. The shared epitope hypothesis. An approach to understanding the molecular genetics of susceptibility to rheumatoid arthritis. Arthritis Rheum. 1987;30:1205–13.
88. du Montcel ST, Michou L, Petit-Teixeira E, Osorio J, Lemaire I, Lasbleiz S, Pierlot C, Quillet P, Bardin T, Prum B, et al. New classification of HLA-DRB1 alleles supports the shared epitope hypothesis of rheumatoid arthritis susceptibility. Arthritis Rheum. 2005;52:1063–8.
89. van der Helm-van Mil AH, Verpoort KN, Breedveld FC, Huizinga TW, Toes RE, de Vries RR. The HLA-DRB1 shared epitope alleles are primarily a risk factor for anti-cyclic citrullinated peptide antibodies and are not an independent risk factor for development of rheumatoid arthritis. Arthritis Rheum. 2006;54:1117–21.
90. Linn-Rasker SP, van der Helm-van Mil AH, van Gaalen FA, Kloppenburg M, de Vries RR, le Cessie S, Breedveld FC, Toes RE, Huizinga TW. Smoking is a risk factor for anti-CCP antibodies only in rheumatoid arthritis patients who carry HLA-DRB1 shared epitope alleles. Ann Rheum Dis. 2006;65:366–71.

91. Verpoort KN, van Gaalen FA, van der Helm-van Mil AH, Schreuder GM, Breedveld FC, Huizinga TW, de Vries RR, Toes RE. Association of HLA-DR3 with anti-cyclic citrullinated peptide antibody-negative rheumatoid arthritis. Arthritis Rheum. 2005;52:3058–62.
92. van der Woude D, Lie BA, Lundstrom E, Balsa A, Feitsma AL, Houwing-Duistermaat JJ, Verduijn W, Nordang GB, Alfredsson L, Klareskog L, et al. Protection against anti-citrullinated protein antibody-positive rheumatoid arthritis is predominantly associated with HLA-DRB1*1301: a meta-analysis of HLA-DRB1 associations with anti-citrullinated protein antibody-positive and anti-citrullinated protein antibody-negative rheumatoid arthritis in four European populations. Arthritis Rheum. 2010;62:1236–45.
93. Raychaudhuri S, Sandor C, Stahl EA, Freudenberg J, Lee HS, Jia X, Alfredsson L, Padyukov L, Klareskog L, Worthington J, et al. Five amino acids in three HLA proteins explain most of the association between MHC and seropositive rheumatoid arthritis. Nat Genet. 2012;44:291–6.
94. de Almeida DE, Ling S, Holoshitz J. New insights into the functional role of the rheumatoid arthritis shared epitope. FEBS Lett. 2011;585:3619–26.
95. Weyand CM, Hicok KC, Conn DL, Goronzy JJ. The influence of HLA-DRB1 genes on disease severity in rheumatoid arthritis. Ann Intern Med. 1992;117:801–6.
96. Weyand CM, Xie C, Goronzy JJ. Homozygosity for the HLA-DRB1 allele selects for extraarticular manifestations in rheumatoid arthritis. J Clin Invest. 1992;89:2033–9.
97. Mewar D, Marinou I, Coote AL, Moore DJ, Akil M, Smillie D, Dickson MC, Binks MH, Montgomery DS, Wilson AG. Association between radiographic severity of rheumatoid arthritis and shared epitope alleles: differing mechanisms of susceptibility and protection. Ann Rheum Dis. 2008;67:980–3.
98. Kunz M, Ibrahim SM. Non-major histocompatibility complex rheumatoid arthritis susceptibility genes. Crit Rev Immunol. 2011;31:99–114.
99. Criswell LA. Gene discovery in rheumatoid arthritis highlights the CD40/NF-kappaB signaling pathway in disease pathogenesis. Immunol Rev. 2010;233:55–61.
100. Takata Y, Inoue H, Sato A, Tsugawa K, Miyatake K, Hamada D, Shinomiya F, Nakano S, Yasui N, Tanahashi T, et al. Replication of reported genetic associations of PADI4, FCRL3, SLC22A4 and RUNX1 genes with rheumatoid arthritis: results of an independent Japanese population and evidence from meta-analysis of East Asian studies. J Hum Genet. 2008;53: 163–73.
101. Sigurdsson S, Padyukov L, Kurreeman FA, Liljedahl U, Wiman AC, Alfredsson L, Toes R, Ronnelid J, Klareskog L, Huizinga TW, et al. Association of a haplotype in the promoter region of the interferon regulatory factor 5 gene with rheumatoid arthritis. Arthritis Rheum. 2007;56:2202–10.
102. Padyukov L, Seielstad M, Ong RT, Ding B, Ronnelid J, Seddighzadeh M, Alfredsson L, Klareskog L. A genome-wide association study suggests contrasting associations in ACPA-positive versus ACPA-negative rheumatoid arthritis. Ann Rheum Dis. 2011;70:259–65.
103. Chakravarti A, Clark AG, Mootha VK. Distilling pathophysiology from complex disease genetics. Cell. 2013;155:21–6.
104. Bakir-Gungor B, Sezerman OU. A new methodology to associate SNPs with human diseases according to their pathway related context. PLoS One. 2011;6:e26277.
105. Nakano K, Whitaker JW, Boyle DL, Wang W, Firestein GS. DNA methylome signature in rheumatoid arthritis. Ann Rheum Dis. 2013;72:110–7.
106. Hindorff LA, Sethupathy P, Junkins HA, Ramos EM, Mehta JP, Collins FS, Manolio TA. Potential etiologic and functional implications of genome-wide association loci for human diseases and traits. Proc Natl Acad Sci U S A. 2009;106:9362–7.
107. So HC, Gui AH, Cherny SS, Sham PC. Evaluating the heritability explained by known susceptibility variants: a survey of ten complex diseases. Genet Epidemiol. 2011;35:310–7.
108. Slatkin M. Epigenetic inheritance and the missing heritability problem. Genetics. 2009;182: 845–50.
109. Flintoft L. Complex disease: adding epigenetics to the mix. Nat Rev Genet. 2010;11:94–5.
110. Visscher PM, Hill WG, Wray NR. Heritability in the genomics era – concepts and misconceptions. Nat Rev Genet. 2008;9:255–66.

111. Furrow RE, Christiansen FB, Feldman MW. Environment-sensitive epigenetics and the heritability of complex diseases. Genetics. 2011;189:1377–87.
112. Fraga MF, Ballestar E, Paz MF, Ropero S, Setien F, Ballestar ML, Heine-Suner D, Cigudosa JC, Urioste M, Benitez J, et al. Epigenetic differences arise during the lifetime of monozygotic twins. Proc Natl Acad Sci U S A. 2005;102:10604–9.
113. Javierre BM, Fernandez AF, Richter J, Al-Shahrour F, Martin-Subero JI, Rodriguez-Ubreva J, Berdasco M, Fraga MF, O'Hanlon TP, Rider LG, et al. Changes in the pattern of DNA methylation associate with twin discordance in systemic lupus erythematosus. Genome Res. 2010;20:170–9.
114. Baranzini SE, Mudge J, van Velkinburgh JC, Khankhanian P, Khrebtukova I, Miller NA, Zhang L, Farmer AD, Bell CJ, Kim RW, et al. Genome, epigenome and RNA sequences of monozygotic twins discordant for multiple sclerosis. Nature. 2010;464:1351–6.
115. Whitaker JW, Shoemaker R, Boyle DL, Hillman J, Anderson D, Wang W, Firestein GS. An imprinted rheumatoid arthritis methylome signature reflects pathogenic phenotype. Genome Med. 2013;5:40.
116. Miao CG, Yang YY, He X, Li J. New advances of DNA methylation and histone modifications in rheumatoid arthritis, with special emphasis on MeCP2. Cell Signal. 2013;25:875–82.
117. Maciejewska-Rodrigues H, Karouzakis E, Strietholt S, Hemmatazad H, Neidhart M, Ospelt C, Gay RE, Michel BA, Pap T, Gay S, et al. Epigenetics and rheumatoid arthritis: the role of SENP1 in the regulation of MMP-1 expression. J Autoimmun. 2010;35:15–22.
118. Ospelt C, Reedquist KA, Gay S, Tak PP. Inflammatory memories: is epigenetics the missing link to persistent stromal cell activation in rheumatoid arthritis? Autoimmun Rev. 2011;10: 519–24.
119. Arend WP, Firestein GS. Pre-rheumatoid arthritis: predisposition and transition to clinical synovitis. Nat Rev Rheumatol. 2012;8:573–86.
120. Lu Q. The critical importance of epigenetics in autoimmunity. J Autoimmun. 2013;41:1–5.
121. Oppermann U. Why is epigenetics important in understanding the pathogenesis of inflammatory musculoskeletal diseases? Arthritis Res Ther. 2013;15:209.
122. Bottini N, Firestein GS. Epigenetics in rheumatoid arthritis: a primer for rheumatologists. Curr Rheumatol Rep. 2013;15:372.
123. Brait M, Ford JG, Papaiahgari S, Garza MA, Lee JI, Loyo M, Maldonado L, Begum S, McCaffrey L, Howerton M, et al. Association between lifestyle factors and CpG island methylation in a cancer-free population. Cancer Epidemiol Biomarkers Prev. 2009;18:2984–91.
124. Terry MB, Ferris JS, Pilsner R, Flom JD, Tehranifar P, Santella RM, Gamble MV, Susser E. Genomic DNA methylation among women in a multiethnic New York City birth cohort. Cancer Epidemiol Biomarkers Prev. 2008;17:2306–10.
125. Christensen BC, Marsit CJ. Epigenomics in environmental health. Front Genet. 2011;2:84.
126. Wan ES, Qiu W, Baccarelli A, Carey VJ, Bacherman H, Rennard SI, Agusti A, Anderson W, Lomas DA, Demeo DL. Cigarette smoking behaviors and time since quitting are associated with differential DNA methylation across the human genome. Hum Mol Genet. 2012;21: 3073–82.
127. Sun YV, Smith AK, Conneely KN, Chang Q, Li W, Lazarus A, Smith JA, Almli LM, Binder EB, Klengel T, et al. Epigenomic association analysis identifies smoking-related DNA methylation sites in African Americans. Hum Genet. 2013;132:1027–37.
128. Lee KW, Pausova Z. Cigarette smoking and DNA methylation. Front Genet. 2013;4:132.
129. Shenker NS, Polidoro S, van Veldhoven K, Sacerdote C, Ricceri F, Birrell MA, Belvisi MG, Brown R, Vineis P, Flanagan JM. Epigenome-wide association study in the European Prospective Investigation into Cancer and Nutrition (EPIC-Turin) identifies novel genetic loci associated with smoking. Hum Mol Genet. 2013;22:843–51.
130. Zeilinger S, Kuhnel B, Klopp N, Baurecht H, Kleinschmidt A, Gieger C, Weidinger S, Lattka E, Adamski J, Peters A, et al. Tobacco smoking leads to extensive genome-wide changes in DNA methylation. PLoS One. 2013;8:e63812.
131. Sun YV, Lazarus A, Smith JA, Chuang YH, Zhao W, Turner ST, Kardia SL. Gene-specific DNA methylation association with serum levels of C-reactive protein in African Americans. PLoS One. 2013;8:e73480.

132. Richardson B, Scheinbart L, Strahler J, Gross L, Hanash S, Johnson M. Evidence for impaired T cell DNA methylation in systemic lupus erythematosus and rheumatoid arthritis. Arthritis Rheum. 1990;33:1665–73.
133. Liao J, Liang G, Xie S, Zhao H, Zuo X, Li F, Chen J, Zhao M, Chan TM, Lu Q. CD40L demethylation in CD4(+) T cells from women with rheumatoid arthritis. Clin Immunol. 2012;145:13–8.
134. Nile CJ, Read RC, Akil M, Duff GW, Wilson AG. Methylation status of a single CpG site in the IL6 promoter is related to IL6 messenger RNA levels and rheumatoid arthritis. Arthritis Rheum. 2008;58:2686–93.
135. Liu CC, Fang TJ, Ou TT, Wu CC, Li RN, Lin YC, Lin CH, Tsai WC, Liu HW, Yen JH. Global DNA methylation, DNMT1, and MBD2 in patients with rheumatoid arthritis. Immunol Lett. 2011;135:96–9.
136. Neidhart M, Rethage J, Kuchen S, Kunzler P, Crowl RM, Billingham ME, Gay RE, Gay S. Retrotransposable L1 elements expressed in rheumatoid arthritis synovial tissue: association with genomic DNA hypomethylation and influence on gene expression. Arthritis Rheum. 2000;43:2634–47.
137. Takami N, Osawa K, Miura Y, Komai K, Taniguchi M, Shiraishi M, Sato K, Iguchi T, Shiozawa K, Hashiramoto A, et al. Hypermethylated promoter region of DR3, the death receptor 3 gene, in rheumatoid arthritis synovial cells. Arthritis Rheum. 2006;54:779–87.
138. Karouzakis E, Gay RE, Michel BA, Gay S, Neidhart M. DNA hypomethylation in rheumatoid arthritis synovial fibroblasts. Arthritis Rheum. 2009;60:3613–22.
139. Karouzakis E, Rengel Y, Jungel A, Kolling C, Gay RE, Michel BA, Tak PP, Gay S, Neidhart M, Ospelt C. DNA methylation regulates the expression of CXCL12 in rheumatoid arthritis synovial fibroblasts. Genes Immun. 2011;12:643–52.
140. Nakano K, Boyle DL, Firestein GS. Regulation of DNA methylation in rheumatoid arthritis synoviocytes. J Immunol. 2013;190:1297–303.
141. Karouzakis E, Gay RE, Gay S, Neidhart M. Increased recycling of polyamines is associated with global DNA hypomethylation in rheumatoid arthritis synovial fibroblasts. Arthritis Rheum. 2012;64:1809–17.
142. de la Rica L, Urquiza JM, Gomez-Cabrero D, Islam AB, Lopez-Bigas N, Tegner J, Toes RE, Ballestar E. Identification of novel markers in rheumatoid arthritis through integrated analysis of DNA methylation and microRNA expression. J Autoimmun. 2013;41:6–16.
143. Liu Y, Aryee MJ, Padyukov L, Fallin MD, Hesselberg E, Runarsson A, Reinius L, Acevedo N, Taub M, Ronninger M, et al. Epigenome-wide association data implicate DNA methylation as an intermediary of genetic risk in rheumatoid arthritis. Nat Biotechnol. 2013;31: 142–7.
144. Joosten LA, Leoni F, Meghji S, Mascagni P. Inhibition of HDAC activity by ITF2357 ameliorates joint inflammation and prevents cartilage and bone destruction in experimental arthritis. Mol Med. 2011;17:391–6.
145. Miao CG, Yang YY, He X, Xu T, Huang C, Huang Y, Zhang L, Lv XW, Jin Y, Li J. New advances of microRNAs in the pathogenesis of rheumatoid arthritis, with a focus on the crosstalk between DNA methylation and the microRNA machinery. Cell Signal. 2013;25: 1118–25.
146. Chan EK, Ceribelli A, Satoh M. MicroRNA-146a in autoimmunity and innate immune responses. Ann Rheum Dis. 2013;72 Suppl 2:ii90–5.
147. Nell VP, Machold KP, Eberl G, Stamm TA, Uffmann M, Smolen JS. Benefit of very early referral and very early therapy with disease-modifying anti-rheumatic drugs in patients with early rheumatoid arthritis. Rheumatology (Oxford). 2004;43:906–14.
148. Korpela M, Laasonen L, Hannonen P, Kautiainen H, Leirisalo-Repo M, Hakala M, Paimela L, Blafield H, Puolakka K, Mottonen T. Retardation of joint damage in patients with early rheumatoid arthritis by initial aggressive treatment with disease-modifying antirheumatic drugs: five-year experience from the FIN-RACo study. Arthritis Rheum. 2004;50:2072–81.
149. de Rooy DP, van der Linden MP, Knevel R, Huizinga TW, van der Helm-van Mil AH. Predicting arthritis outcomes–what can be learned from the Leiden Early Arthritis Clinic? Rheumatology (Oxford). 2011;50:93–100.

150. Kuriya B, Cheng CK, Chen HM, Bykerk VP. Validation of a prediction rule for development of rheumatoid arthritis in patients with early undifferentiated arthritis. Ann Rheum Dis. 2009;68:1482–5.
151. Rantapaa-Dahlqvist S. What happens before the onset of rheumatoid arthritis? Curr Opin Rheumatol. 2009;21:272–8.
152. Tamai M, Kawakami A, Uetani M, Takao S, Arima K, Iwamoto N, Fujikawa K, Aramaki T, Kawashiri SY, Ichinose K, et al. A prediction rule for disease outcome in patients with undifferentiated arthritis using magnetic resonance imaging of the wrists and finger joints and serologic autoantibodies. Arthritis Rheum. 2009;61:772–8.
153. Willemze A, Trouw LA, Toes RE, Huizinga TW. The influence of ACPA status and characteristics on the course of RA. Nat Rev Rheumatol. 2012;8:144–52.
154. Rantapaa-Dahlqvist S, de Jong BA, Berglin E, Hallmans G, Wadell G, Stenlund H, Sundin U, van Venrooij WJ. Antibodies against cyclic citrullinated peptide and IgA rheumatoid factor predict the development of rheumatoid arthritis. Arthritis Rheum. 2003;48:2741–9.
155. Kokkonen H, Mullazehi M, Berglin E, Hallmans G, Wadell G, Ronnelid J, Rantapaa-Dahlqvist S. Antibodies of IgG, IgA and IgM isotypes against cyclic citrullinated peptide precede the development of rheumatoid arthritis. Arthritis Res Ther. 2011;13:R13.
156. Sokolove J, Bromberg R, Deane KD, Lahey LJ, Derber LA, Chandra PE, Edison JD, Gilliland WR, Tibshirani RJ, Norris JM, et al. Autoantibody epitope spreading in the pre-clinical phase predicts progression to rheumatoid arthritis. PLoS One. 2012;7:e35296.
157. Karlson EW, Chibnik LB, Tworoger SS, Lee IM, Buring JE, Shadick NA, Manson JE, Costenbader KH. Biomarkers of inflammation and development of rheumatoid arthritis in women from two prospective cohort studies. Arthritis Rheum. 2009;60:641–52.
158. Niu Q, Huang Z, Shi Y, Wang L, Pan X, Hu C. Specific serum protein biomarkers of rheumatoid arthritis detected by MALDI-TOF-MS combined with magnetic beads. Int Immunol. 2010;22:611–8.
159. van der Pouw Kraan TC, van Gaalen FA, Huizinga TW, Pieterman E, Breedveld FC, Verweij CL. Discovery of distinctive gene expression profiles in rheumatoid synovium using cDNA microarray technology: evidence for the existence of multiple pathways of tissue destruction and repair. Genes Immun. 2003;4:187–96.
160. Sokka T, Willoughby J, Yazici Y, Pincus T. Databases of patients with early rheumatoid arthritis in the USA. Clin Exp Rheumatol. 2003;21:S146–53.
161. Scott DL, Wolfe F, Huizinga TW. Rheumatoid arthritis. Lancet. 2010;376:1094–108.
162. Plant MJ, Williams AL, O'Sullivan MM, Lewis PA, Coles EC, Jessop JD. Relationship between time-integrated C-reactive protein levels and radiologic progression in patients with rheumatoid arthritis. Arthritis Rheum. 2000;43:1473–7.
163. Combe B, Dougados M, Goupille P, Cantagrel A, Eliaou JF, Sibilia J, Meyer O, Sany J, Daures JP, Dubois A. Prognostic factors for radiographic damage in early rheumatoid arthritis: a multiparameter prospective study. Arthritis Rheum. 2001;44:1736–43.
164. van der Helm-van Mil AH, Verpoort KN, Breedveld FC, Toes RE, Huizinga TW. Antibodies to citrullinated proteins and differences in clinical progression of rheumatoid arthritis. Arthritis Res Ther. 2005;7:R949–58.
165. van der Helm-van Mil AH, van der Kooij SM, Allaart CF, Toes RE, Huizinga TW. A high body mass index has a protective effect on the amount of joint destruction in small joints in early rheumatoid arthritis. Ann Rheum Dis. 2008;67:769–74.
166. Marinou I, Maxwell JR, Wilson AG. Genetic influences modulating the radiological severity of rheumatoid arthritis. Ann Rheum Dis. 2010;69:476–82.
167. Teare MD, Knevel R, Morgan MD, Kleszcz A, Emery P, Moore DJ, Conaghan P, Huizinga TW, Morgan AW, van der Helm-van Mil AH, et al. Allele-dose association of the C5orf30 rs26232 variant with joint damage in rheumatoid arthritis. Arthritis Rheum. 2013;65: 2555–61.
168. van der Linden MP, Feitsma AL, le Cessie S, Kern M, Olsson LM, Raychaudhuri S, Begovich AB, Chang M, Catanese JJ, Kurreeman FA, et al. Association of a single-nucleotide polymorphism in CD40 with the rate of joint destruction in rheumatoid arthritis. Arthritis Rheum. 2009;60:2242–7.

169. Maehlen MT, Nordang GB, Syversen SW, van der Heijde DM, Kvien TK, Uhlig T, Lie BA. FCRL3–169C/C genotype is associated with anti-citrullinated protein antibody-positive rheumatoid arthritis and with radiographic progression. J Rheumatol. 2011;38:2329–35.
170. Knevel R, de Rooy DP, Zhernakova A, Grondal G, Krabben A, Steinsson K, Wijmenga C, Cavet G, Toes RE, Huizinga TW, et al. Association of variants in IL2RA with progression of joint destruction in rheumatoid arthritis. Arthritis Rheum. 2013;65:1684–93.
171. Balsa A, Del Amo J, Blanco F, Caliz R, Silva L, Sanmarti R, Martinez FG, Tejedor D, Artieda M, Pascual-Salcedo D, et al. Prediction of functional impairment and remission in rheumatoid arthritis patients by biochemical variables and genetic polymorphisms. Rheumatology (Oxford). 2010;49:458–66.
172. Krabben A, Wilson AG, de Rooy DP, Zhernakova A, Brouwer E, Lindqvist E, Saxne T, Stoeken G, van Nies JA, Knevel R, et al. Genetic variants in the IL-4 and IL-4 receptor genes in association with the severity of joint damage in rheumatoid arthritis: a study in seven cohorts. Arthritis Rheum. 2013;65(12):3051–7.
173. Knevel R, Krabben A, Brouwer E, Posthumus MD, Wilson AG, Lindqvist E, Saxne T, de Rooy D, Daha N, van der Linden MP, et al. Genetic variants in IL15 associate with progression of joint destruction in rheumatoid arthritis: a multicohort study. Ann Rheum Dis. 2012;71:1651–7.
174. Ceccarelli F, Perricone C, Fabris M, Alessandri C, Iagnocco A, Fabro C, Pontarini E, De Vita S, Valesini G. Transforming growth factor beta 869C/T and interleukin 6–174G/C polymorphisms relate to the severity and progression of bone-erosive damage detected by ultrasound in rheumatoid arthritis. Arthritis Res Ther. 2011;13:R111.
175. de Rooy DP, Yeremenko NG, Wilson AG, Knevel R, Lindqvist E, Saxne T, Krabben A, Leijsma MK, Daha NA, Tsonaka S, et al. Genetic studies on components of the Wnt signalling pathway and the severity of joint destruction in rheumatoid arthritis. Ann Rheum Dis. 2013;72:769–75.
176. Knevel R, Krabben A, Wilson AG, Brouwer E, Leijsma MK, Lindqvist E, de Rooy DP, Daha NA, van der Linden MP, Tsonaka S, et al. A genetic variant in granzyme B is associated with progression of joint destruction in rheumatoid arthritis. Arthritis Rheum. 2013;65:582–9.
177. de Rooy DP, Zhernakova A, Tsonaka R, Willemze A, Kurreeman BA, Trynka G, van Toorn L, Toes RE, Huizinga TW, Houwing-Duistermaat JJ, et al. A genetic variant in the region of MMP-9 is associated with serum levels and progression of joint damage in rheumatoid arthritis. Ann Rheum Dis. 2014;73(6):1163–9.
178. Knevel R, Klein K, Somers K, Ospelt C, Houwing-Duistermaat JJ, van Nies JA, de Rooy DP, de Bock L, Kurreeman FA, Schonkeren J, et al. Identification of a genetic variant for joint damage progression in autoantibody-positive rheumatoid arthritis. Ann Rheum Dis. PMID: 23956247.
179. van Nies JA, Knevel R, Daha N, van der Linden MP, Gregersen PK, Kern M, le Cessie S, Houwing-Duistermaat JJ, Huizinga TW, Toes RE, et al. The PTPN22 susceptibility risk variant is not associated with the rate of joint destruction in anti-citrullinated protein antibody-positive rheumatoid arthritis. Ann Rheum Dis. 2010;69:1730–1.
180. Liu Z, Sokka T, Maas K, Olsen NJ, Aune TM. Prediction of disease severity in patients with early rheumatoid arthritis by gene expression profiling. Hum Genomics Proteomics. 2009; pii: 484351.
181. Zhu P, Lu N, Shi ZG, Zhou J, Wu ZB, Yang Y, Ding J, Chen ZN. CD147 overexpression on synoviocytes in rheumatoid arthritis enhances matrix metalloproteinase production and invasiveness of synoviocytes. Arthritis Res Ther. 2006;8:R44.
182. Andersson ML, Svensson B, Petersson IF, Hafstrom I, Albertsson K, Forslind K, Heinegard D, Saxne T. Early increase in serum-COMP is associated with joint damage progression over the first five years in patients with rheumatoid arthritis. BMC Musculoskelet Disord. 2013;14:229.
183. Syversen SW, Goll GL, van der Heijde D, Landewe R, Gaarder PI, Odegard S, Haavardsholm EA, Kvien TK. Cartilage and bone biomarkers in rheumatoid arthritis: prediction of 10-year radiographic progression. J Rheumatol. 2009;36:266–72.

184. Catrina AI, Lampa J, Ernestam S, af Klint E, Bratt J, Klareskog L, Ulfgren AK. Anti-tumour necrosis factor (TNF)-alpha therapy (etanercept) down-regulates serum matrix metalloproteinase (MMP)-3 and MMP-1 in rheumatoid arthritis. Rheumatology (Oxford). 2002;41: 484–9.
185. Houseman M, Potter C, Marshall N, Lakey R, Cawston T, Griffiths I, Young-Min S, Isaacs JD. Baseline serum MMP-3 levels in patients with rheumatoid arthritis are still independently predictive of radiographic progression in a longitudinal observational cohort at 8 years follow up. Arthritis Res Ther. 2012;14:R30.
186. Klimiuk PA, Sierakowski S, Latosiewicz R, Cylwik JP, Cylwik B, Skowronski J, Chwiecko J. Soluble adhesion molecules (ICAM-1, VCAM-1, and E-selectin) and vascular endothelial growth factor (VEGF) in patients with distinct variants of rheumatoid synovitis. Ann Rheum Dis. 2002;61:804–9.
187. Rioja I, Hughes FJ, Sharp CH, Warnock LC, Montgomery DS, Akil M, Wilson AG, Binks MH, Dickson MC. Potential novel biomarkers of disease activity in rheumatoid arthritis patients: CXCL13, CCL23, transforming growth factor alpha, tumor necrosis factor receptor superfamily member 9, and macrophage colony-stimulating factor. Arthritis Rheum. 2008;58: 2257–67.
188. Yamane S, Ishida S, Hanamoto Y, Kumagai K, Masuda R, Tanaka K, Shiobara N, Yamane N, Mori T, Juji T, et al. Proinflammatory role of amphiregulin, an epidermal growth factor family member whose expression is augmented in rheumatoid arthritis patients. J Inflamm (Lond). 2008;5:5.
189. Swanson CD, Akama-Garren EH, Stein EA, Petralia JD, Ruiz PJ, Edalati A, Lindstrom TM, Robinson WH. Inhibition of epidermal growth factor receptor tyrosine kinase ameliorates collagen-induced arthritis. J Immunol. 2012;188:3513–21.
190. Chambers RE, MacFarlane DG, Whicher JT, Dieppe PA. Serum amyloid-A protein concentration in rheumatoid arthritis and its role in monitoring disease activity. Ann Rheum Dis. 1983;42:665–7.
191. Johansen JS, Kirwan JR, Price PA, Sharif M. Serum YKL-40 concentrations in patients with early rheumatoid arthritis: relation to joint destruction. Scand J Rheumatol. 2001;30: 297–304.
192. Knudsen LS, Klarlund M, Skjodt H, Jensen T, Ostergaard M, Jensen KE, Hansen MS, Hetland ML, Nielsen HJ, Johansen JS. Biomarkers of inflammation in patients with unclassified polyarthritis and early rheumatoid arthritis. Relationship to disease activity and radiographic outcome. J Rheumatol. 2008;35:1277–87.
193. Dayer JM, Choy E. Therapeutic targets in rheumatoid arthritis: the interleukin-6 receptor. Rheumatology (Oxford). 2010;49:15–24.
194. Gonzalez-Alvaro I, Ortiz AM, Alvaro-Gracia JM, Castaneda S, Diaz-Sanchez B, Carvajal I, Garcia-Vadillo JA, Humbria A, Lopez-Bote JP, Patino E, et al. Interleukin 15 levels in serum may predict a severe disease course in patients with early arthritis. PLoS One. 2011;6:e29492.
195. Barrera P, Boerbooms AM, Janssen EM, Sauerwein RW, Gallati H, Mulder J, de Boo T, Demacker PN, van de Putte LB, van der Meer JW. Circulating soluble tumor necrosis factor receptors, interleukin-2 receptors, tumor necrosis factor alpha, and interleukin-6 levels in rheumatoid arthritis. Longitudinal evaluation during methotrexate and azathioprine therapy. Arthritis Rheum. 1993;36:1070–9.
196. Klein-Wieringa IR, van der Linden MP, Knevel R, Kwekkeboom JC, van Beelen E, Huizinga TW, van der Helm-van MA, Kloppenburg M, Toes RE, Ioan-Facsinay A. Baseline serum adipokine levels predict radiographic progression in early rheumatoid arthritis. Arthritis Rheum. 2011;63:2567–74.
197. Rho YH, Solus J, Sokka T, Oeser A, Chung CP, Gebretsadik T, Shintani A, Pincus T, Stein CM. Adipocytokines are associated with radiographic joint damage in rheumatoid arthritis. Arthritis Rheum. 2009;60:1906–14.
198. Lee SW, Park MC, Park YB, Lee SK. Measurement of the serum leptin level could assist disease activity monitoring in rheumatoid arthritis. Rheumatol Int. 2007;27:537–40.

199. Migita K, Maeda Y, Miyashita T, Kimura H, Nakamura M, Ishibashi H, Eguchi K. The serum levels of resistin in rheumatoid arthritis patients. Clin Exp Rheumatol. 2006;24:698–701.
200. Centola M, Cavet G, Shen Y, Ramanujan S, Knowlton N, Swan KA, Turner M, Sutton C, Smith DR, Haney DJ, et al. Development of a multi-biomarker disease activity test for rheumatoid arthritis. PLoS One. 2013;8:e60635.
201. Curtis JR, van der Helm-van Mil AH, Knevel R, Huizinga TW, Haney DJ, Shen Y, Ramanujan S, Cavet G, Centola M, Hesterberg LK, et al. Validation of a novel multibiomarker test to assess rheumatoid arthritis disease activity. Arthritis Care Res (Hoboken). 2012;64: 1794–803.
202. Bakker MF, Cavet G, Jacobs JW, Bijlsma JW, Haney DJ, Shen Y, Hesterberg LK, Smith DR, Centola M, van Roon JA, et al. Performance of a multi-biomarker score measuring rheumatoid arthritis disease activity in the CAMERA tight control study. Ann Rheum Dis. 2012;71:1692–7.
203. Hirata S, Dirven L, Shen Y, Centola M, Cavet G, Lems WF, Tanaka Y, Huizinga TW, Allaart CF. A multi-biomarker score measures rheumatoid arthritis disease activity in the BeSt study. Rheumatology (Oxford). 2013;52:1202–7.
204. Plenge RM, Greenberg JD, Mangravite LM, Derry JM, Stahl EA, Coenen MJ, Barton A, Padyukov L, Klareskog L, Gregersen PK, et al. Crowdsourcing genetic prediction of clinical utility in the Rheumatoid Arthritis Responder Challenge. Nat Genet. 2013;45:468–9.
205. Crews KR, Hicks JK, Pui CH, Relling MV, Evans WE. Pharmacogenomics and individualized medicine: translating science into practice. Clin Pharmacol Ther. 2012;92:467–75.
206. Giacomini KM, Yee SW, Ratain MJ, Weinshilboum RM, Kamatani N, Nakamura Y. Pharmacogenomics and patient care: one size does not fit all. Sci Transl Med. 2012;4: 153ps18.
207. Burgos PI, Danila MI, Kelley JM, Hughes LB, Bridges Jr SL. Understanding personalized medicine in rheumatoid arthritis: a clinician's guide to the future. Ther Adv Musculoskelet Dis. 2009;1:97–105.
208. van den Broek M, Visser K, Allaart CF, Huizinga TW. Personalized medicine: predicting responses to therapy in patients with RA. Curr Opin Pharmacol. 2013;13:463–9.
209. Romao VC, Canhao H, Fonseca JE. Old drugs, old problems: where do we stand in prediction of rheumatoid arthritis responsiveness to methotrexate and other synthetic DMARDs? BMC Med. 2013;11:17.
210. O'Rielly DD, Rahman P. Pharmacogenetics of rheumatoid arthritis: Potential targets from susceptibility genes and present therapies. Pharmgenomics Pers Med. 2010;3:15–31.
211. Fisher MC, Cronstein BN. Meta-analysis of methylenetetrahydrofolate reductase (MTHFR) polymorphisms affecting methotrexate toxicity. J Rheumatol. 2009;36:539–45.
212. Bohanec Grabar P, Rozman B, Tomsic M, Suput D, Logar D, Dolzan V. Genetic polymorphism of CYP1A2 and the toxicity of leflunomide treatment in rheumatoid arthritis patients. Eur J Clin Pharmacol. 2008;64:871–6.
213. Taniguchi A, Urano W, Tanaka E, Furihata S, Kamitsuji S, Inoue E, Yamanaka M, Yamanaka H, Kamatani N. Validation of the associations between single nucleotide polymorphisms or haplotypes and responses to disease-modifying antirheumatic drugs in patients with rheumatoid arthritis: a proposal for prospective pharmacogenomic study in clinical practice. Pharmacogenet Genomics. 2007;17:383–90.
214. Cui J, Saevarsdottir S, Thomson B, Padyukov L, van der Helm-van Mil AH, Nititham J, Hughes LB, de Vries N, Raychaudhuri S, Alfredsson L, et al. Rheumatoid arthritis risk allele PTPRC is also associated with response to anti-tumor necrosis factor alpha therapy. Arthritis Rheum. 2010;62:1849–61.
215. Plant D, Prajapati R, Hyrich KL, Morgan AW, Wilson AG, Isaacs JD, Barton A. Replication of association of the PTPRC gene with response to anti-tumor necrosis factor therapy in a large UK cohort. Arthritis Rheum. 2012;64:665–70.
216. O'Rielly DD, Roslin NM, Beyene J, Pope A, Rahman P. TNF-alpha-308 G/A polymorphism and responsiveness to TNF-alpha blockade therapy in moderate to severe rheumatoid arthritis: a systematic review and meta-analysis. Pharmacogenomics J. 2009;9:161–7.

217. Umicevic Mirkov M, Cui J, Vermeulen SH, Stahl EA, Toonen EJ, Makkinje RR, Lee AT, Huizinga TW, Allaart R, Barton A, et al. Genome-wide association analysis of anti-TNF drug response in patients with rheumatoid arthritis. Ann Rheum Dis. 2013;72:1375–81.
218. Lequerre T, Gauthier-Jauneau AC, Bansard C, Derambure C, Hiron M, Vittecoq O, Daveau M, Mejjad O, Daragon A, Tron F, et al. Gene profiling in white blood cells predicts infliximab responsiveness in rheumatoid arthritis. Arthritis Res Ther. 2006;8:R105.
219. Julia A, Erra A, Palacio C, Tomas C, Sans X, Barcelo P, Marsal S. An eight-gene blood expression profile predicts the response to infliximab in rheumatoid arthritis. PLoS One. 2009;4:e7556.
220. Meugnier E, Coury F, Tebib J, Ferraro-Peyret C, Rome S, Bienvenu J, Vidal H, Sibilia J, Fabien N. Gene expression profiling in peripheral blood cells of patients with rheumatoid arthritis in response to anti-TNF-alpha treatments. Physiol Genomics. 2011;43:365–71.
221. Lindberg J, Wijbrandts CA, van Baarsen LG, Nader G, Klareskog L, Catrina A, Thurlings R, Vervoordeldonk M, Lundeberg J, Tak PP. The gene expression profile in the synovium as a predictor of the clinical response to infliximab treatment in rheumatoid arthritis. PLoS One. 2010;5:e11310.
222. Toonen EJ, Gilissen C, Franke B, Kievit W, Eijsbouts AM, den Broeder AA, van Reijmersdal SV, Veltman JA, Scheffer H, Radstake TR, et al. Validation study of existing gene expression signatures for anti-TNF treatment in patients with rheumatoid arthritis. PLoS One. 2012; 7:e33199.
223. Hueber W, Tomooka BH, Batliwalla F, Li W, Monach PA, Tibshirani RJ, Van Vollenhoven RF, Lampa J, Saito K, Tanaka Y, et al. Blood autoantibody and cytokine profiles predict response to anti-tumor necrosis factor therapy in rheumatoid arthritis. Arthritis Res Ther. 2009;11:R76.
224. Kapoor SR, Filer A, Fitzpatrick MA, Fisher BA, Taylor PC, Buckley CD, McInnes IB, Raza K, Young SP. Metabolic profiling predicts response to anti-tumor necrosis factor alpha therapy in patients with rheumatoid arthritis. Arthritis Rheum. 2013;65:1448–56.

Outcome Measures in Rheumatoid Arthritis

Yusuf Yazici and Hilal Maradit Kremers

Outcome Measures in Rheumatoid Arthritis

Many quantitative measures such as joint examination, laboratory tests, radiographic imaging, and patient questionnaires have been used in the management of RA patients, either as single measures or as part of composite indices. The main reason for this is that no single "gold standard" measure has been identified for RA and, hence, can be applied to diagnosis, monitoring, prognosis, and assessment of outcomes in individual patients. Finally, it is particularly important to note that laboratory tests (i.e., RF, ACPA, erythrocyte sedimentation rate [ESR], and C-reactive protein [CRP]), while abnormal in the majority of patients with RA, are normal in at least 30–40 % of patients [1].

Up until the 1990s, there was no standardization of outcome measures in clinical trials and in everyday clinical care of RA patients, making it very difficult to determine how patients were fairing. The OMERACT network played and continues to play a significant role in standardization of outcome measures in rheumatology (http://www.omeract.org). The first OMERACT conference was in 1992 and focused exclusively on RA, with the term OMERACT meaning "Outcome Measures in Rheumatoid Arthritis Clinical Trials.". Since then, the OMERACT initiative has

Y. Yazici, MD (✉)
Division of Rheumatology, Department of Medicine, Seligman Center for Advanced Therapeutics and Behcet's Syndrome Center, NYU Hospital for Joint Diseases, New York University School of Medicine, New York University, 333 East 38th Street, New York, NY 10016, USA
e-mail: yusuf.yazici@nyumc.org

H.M. Kremers, MD
Departments of Health Sciences Research and Orthopedic Surgery, Mayo Clinic, 200 First St SW, Rochester, MN 55902, USA
e-mail: maradit@mayo.edu

H. Yazici et al. (eds.), *Understanding Evidence-Based Rheumatology*,
DOI 10.1007/978-3-319-08374-2_5

expanded into an international informal network with working groups on a number of outcome measurement issues in rheumatology. The first OMERACT conference and a series of subsequent meetings of the American and European rheumatology organizations resulted in consensus on the Core Data Set [2] that provides a standard set of measures to monitor disease status in RA patients. The Core Data Set includes 7 measures: 3 from patient history (physical function, pain, patient global estimate of status), 3 from physical examination (swollen joint count, tender joint count, physician/assessor patient global estimate of status), and one laboratory test (ESR or CRP). A radiograph is also used as the eighth measure in studies lasting longer than 1 year. Since then, the Core Data Set has become the de facto basis for the composite indices developed for monitoring RA.

Another significant development in management of RA is the concept of "treating to target." Over the last 15 years, the concept of "treating to target" has been accepted by the rheumatology community after a number of studies [3–5] showing that patients treated with a target value in mind (for low disease activity or remission) did better than those treated without a target value. The targets most widely used are composite indices, developed mainly from three to four items of the Core Data Set measures. Several of disease measures are currently recommended for monitoring RA activity. In sections below, we will focus on these, namely, the disease activity score (DAS28), clinical disease activity index (CDAI), simplified disease activity index (SDAI), and routine assessment of patient index data (RAPID3).

Finally, the issue of radiographic damage has also been studied in randomized controlled trials (RCTs) and routine clinical care, mostly with traditional radiographs of the hands and the feet. The newer tools such as ultrasonography and magnetic resonance imaging (MRI) have not been studied as extensively as radiographs, but data are accumulating that may better define their roles in RA patient management.

Core Data Set Measures and the ACR 20, 50 and 70 Responses

Up until the early 1990s, RA clinical trials and other research studies used several different outcome measures. Most of these measures were redundant, not comprehensive, insensitive to change, and rarely included patient-reported outcomes. Furthermore, the choice of outcome measures differed in the United States and Europe, making it impossible to compare results across studies. In early 1990s, the rheumatology community recognized the need for a standard core data set of measures for use in clinical trials and possibly in standard clinical care. Such well-defined measures would make it easier to compare different studies and treatment modalities [6]. A group of clinicians, rheumatologists, methodologists, and epidemiologists working together with rheumatology societies established a Core Data Set of measures for RA clinical trials [2]. Initially, candidate measures were identified and included the tender joint count, ESR, swollen joint count, physician global assessment, platelet count, grip strength, patient global assessment, pain, morning stiffness, hemoglobin, functional class, PIP circumference, walking time, quality of well-being, and digital joint size. These were further reviewed and the final set of 7 measures, 3 by an assessor (swollen joint count, tender joint count, and physician assessment of global status), 3 by patient self-report (physical function, pain, and global status on patient questionnaire), and one acute phase reactant – ESR or C-reactive protein CRP – were agreed upon as the Core Data Set. These measures were then utilized to develop the American College of Rheumatology (ACR) response thresholds [7] where improvement in at least 20 % in both the tender and swollen joint counts, as well as 3 of the 5 additional measures, came to be known as the "ACR 20."

While higher thresholds for improvement such as "ACR 50" and "ACR 70" were also described, the ACR 20 response was found to distinguish between active treatment with disease modifying antirheumatic drugs (DMARDs) versus placebo treatment more effectively than the ACR 50 and ACR 70 responses. These measures are currently reported in all contemporary clinical trials, enabling both the rheumatologists and regulatory agencies to interpret and compare treatment results across studies.

Although the ACR 20, 50, and 70 scores have been very useful for clinical trials where a change from baseline is needed to demonstrate efficacy, they are not necessarily useful in routine clinical care. Depending on where a patient has started, similar changes in the ACR scores can correspond to very different levels of disease activity. For example, a patient with 20 swollen joints before treatment would have an ACR50 response if the swollen joint count is 10 after treatment. Another patient who went from 6 swollen joints down to 3 after treatment would also have an ACR50 response. Despite having the same response as defined by ACR50, these are two very different patients and would likely require different next steps in disease management. Therefore, the ACR 20, 50, and 70 responses are not very helpful in routine clinical care. Instead, disease activity scores (which are discussed below) are used to capture such differences between patients. Another additional challenge is the classification of patients who are at the borders of categories, such as patients with responses of ACR 19, 21, 49, 51, 69, and 71. There would be very little clinical difference between an RA patient with an ACR49 and 51 response but they would be classified in different response categories (ACR20 vs. ACR50, respectively) and may be exposed to different treatment options. There has been some effort to address this issue but with little success so far. In response to the need to address the limitations of ACR response, a number of composite disease activity indices were developed. These indices provide a single number reflecting the current disease activity of the patient and are more comparable across different disease populations. Many such indices exist but four measures are the more commonly recommended and are part of the latest ACR recommendations on measures to use in clinical care [8].

Disease Activity Score (DAS)

Disease Activity Score (DAS) was developed in 1990 to combine single measures into an overall continuous measure of disease activity in RA [9]. It was originally developed to enable evaluation of patients with early-onset RA. It also showed a high predictive ability in discriminating "active RA" from "partial or complete remission" and between active drug and placebo-treated patients in clinical studies [10, 11].

DAS consists of the number of painful joints calculated by the Ritchie Articular Index (RAI), a 44 swollen joint count (44SJC), erythrocyte sedimentation rate (ESR), and a patient global assessment of disease activity (PtGA), or general health (GH) on a visual analog scale (VAS). CRP levels may also be used instead of ESR in later versions of the DAS.

Of the components of DAS, the RAI ranges from 0 to 78, 44SJC ranges from 0 to 44, ESR may range from 0 to 150, and GH can range from 0 to 100. These are put into a programmed calculator or computer, which can be accessed free of charge online at http://www.das-score.nl. The range for DAS is 0–10. The level of RA activity is classified as remission (DAS <1.6), low activity (1.6≤ DAS <2.4), moderate activity (2.4≤ DAS ≤3.7), and high disease activity (DAS >3.7) [12]. The European League Against Rheumatism (EULAR) classifies patients as good, moderate, or nonresponders based on changes in DAS scores.

The DAS is an extensively validated composite index. It can be calculated with three or four variables from the core set, and adding more variables in the DAS does not increase its validity [13]. DAS is also well correlated with the Health Assessment Questionnaire (HAQ). Various other versions of DAS have been developed. The most commonly used one is the DAS 28 joint count version (DAS28).

DAS28

DAS28 is a shorter version of DAS and is more practical for regular clinical use. It is also currently the most widely used disease activity index in clinical trials [14]. DAS28 was developed and validated to evaluate disease activity status in groups of patients with RA participating in clinical trials [15].

The DAS28 is calculated using four components of the Core Data Set: 28 tender joint count (28TJC), 28 swollen joint count (28SJC) both of which are performed by a physician, visual analogue scale (VAS) score of the patient's global health, and the laboratory parameter ESR. The level of disease activity is interpreted as remission (DAS28 <2.6), low (2.6≤ DAS28 <3.2), moderate (3.2≤ DAS28 ≤5.1), or high (DAS28>5.1) [12]. EULAR response states are classified as follows: good responders are patients with an improvement of 1.2 and a present score of 3.2; moderate responders are patients with an improvement of 0.6–1.2 and a present score of 5.1, or an improvement of 1.2 and a present score of 3.2; and nonresponders are any patients with an improvement of less than 0.6, or patients with an improvement of 0.6–1.2 and a DAS28 score of 5.1 or higher. DAS28-defined remission is classified as a score of 2.6 or less [16].

There is a strong linear relationship between DAS28-ESR and DAS28-CRP (correlation coefficient 0.946), suggesting that the DAS28-CRP can be used as an alternative to the DAS28-ESR and would be useful in situations in which only CRP values are available [17]. However, disease activity levels and their cutoff scores are not the same for DAS28 ESR and DAS28 CRP. This leads to confusion in some clinical trials where patients are classified as being in remission using the DAS28 CRP and a cutoff score of 2.6, but in fact, 2.6 is the remission cut off with the DAS28 ESR and not the DAS28 CRP.

Simple Disease Activity Index (SDAI)

SDAI was first published in 2003 to provide a simpler tool than DAS and DAS28 [14]. SDAI consists of a simple numerical addition of individual measures on their original scales. This overcomes the problems of transformations and weighting that are used in DAS and its derivatives with the consequent need for a calculator [18]. SDAI is endorsed by both the ACR and EULAR for RA disease activity measurement in clinical trials and for patient monitoring [12]. SDAI consists of a tender joint count (TJC), swollen joint count (SJC) based on 28 joint assessments, patient global assessment of disease activity (PtGA), and physician global assessment of disease activity (PhGA) both based on a VAS ranging from 0 to 10 cm and CRP [19]. 28SJC and 28TJC can range from 0 to 28, PtGA and PhGA range from 0 to 10, and CRP values can vary by laboratory where the test is done. The lower range of SDAI is 0 with the upper end resting on the upper limit of CRP level, often defined as 10 mg/dl, leading to a total upper limit of 86. CRP levels are included in SDAI instead of ESR levels because CRP is believed to be the most reliable measure of the acute phase response and is responsive to changes in tissue damage [18]. Time to complete the SDAI is about 10 s for patients and about 2 min for physicians but waiting time for CRP results can vary in individual institutions. Disease activity level is interpreted as remission (SDAI ≤3.3), low (3.3< SDAI ≤11), moderate (11< SDAI ≤26), or high (SDAI>26). The SDAI has good correlation with DAS28; the correlation of SDAI with functional impairment as evaluated by the Health Assessment Questionnaire (HAQ) or with radiographic progression is very similar to that of DAS28 [18].

Clinical Disease Activity Index (CDAI)

CDAI was developed in 2005 to be analogous to the Simplified Disease Activity Index (SDAI), but it does not include CRP. CDAI was developed as a simple calculation of disease activity for use in the clinic at the point of care. It does not include any lab measurements; therefore, all variables are easily available at the time of the patient visit. CDAI takes about 10 s for a patient to complete and less than 2 min for the physician [18].

CDAI consists of 28 swollen joint count (28SJC), 28 tender joint count (28TJC), PtGA on a scale of 10-cm visual analog scale (VAS), and PhGA on a 10-cm VAS. 28SJC and 28TJC can range from 0 to 28, and PtGA and PhGA range from 0 to 10. CDAI total can range from 0 to 76. High disease activity is defined at CDAI greater than 22, moderate activity is CDAI greater than 10 and less or equal to 22, low activity is less or equal to 10 and greater than 2.8, and remission is less or equal to 2.8 [12, 14].

The CDAI cutoff points reasonably reflect the absence of CRP in the score, which is also shown by the close correlation of CDAI scores with SDAI. DAS28 consists of three identical measures to CDAI and their correlation has been evaluated in five studies. Two of these studies found that 74 % of patients are classified in the same groups according to EULAR response [14, 20]. CDAI also shows a linear relationship with the HAQ and demonstrates the ability to discriminate degrees of ACR response.

Routine Assessment of Patient Index Data (RAPID3)

RAPID3 (Routine Assessment of Patient Index Data 3) is a pooled index of the three patient-reported Core Data Set measures – function, pain, and patient global estimate of disease activity. Each of the three individual measures is scored 0–10, for a total of 30. RAPID3 scores are correlated with DAS28 and CDAI in clinical trials and clinical care and are comparable to indices that distinguish active from control treatments in clinical trials. RAPID3 on a multidimensional health assessment questionnaire (MDHAQ) is scored in 5 s on a 0–30 scale, versus 90–94 s for a formal 28 joint count, 108 s for a CDAI, and 114 s for a DAS28 [21]. An MDHAQ can be completed by each patient at each visit in the waiting room, as a component of the infrastructure of routine care, to provide RAPID3 scores as well as additional valuable data with minimal effort of the rheumatologist and staff. RAPID3 can be included in the infrastructure of care of patients with RA and all rheumatic diseases to provide a baseline assessment and to monitor and document improvement or worsening over time, for all patients seen by a rheumatologist [22]. The capacity of RAPID3 to distinguish active from control treatments has been documented to be similar to that of DAS28 and CDAI in clinical trials of methotrexate, leflunomide, adalimumab, and abatacept [23]. Comparison of RAPID3 with DAS28 and CDAI indicated Spearman rank order correlation coefficients for DAS28 with RAPID3 of 0.66 and for CDAI with RAPID3 of 0.74, all highly significant ($p<0.001$) [24]. RAPID3 shares only 1 of the 4 measures with DAS28 and CDAI (patient global estimate of disease activity).

RAPID3 categories are established for high, moderate, and low disease activity and remission. Analysis of the 285 patients with RA seen in usual care on a 0–30 scale (differing from initial reports, as noted above) indicated classification criteria of high severity >12, moderate 6.1–12, low 3.1–6, and near-remission ≤3 [20].

Most patients who meet criteria for each of the four RAPID3 disease severity categories are found to meet similar activity categories of DAS28 scores, i.e., high >5.1, moderate 3.21–5.1, low 2.61–3.2, and remission ≤2.6, as well as four CDAI categories, >22, 10.1–22, 2.9–10, and ≤2.8, respectively. Overall, 81–84 % of patients who met DAS28 or CDAI moderate/high activity criteria met similar RAPID3 severity criteria and 68–70 % who met DAS28 or CDAI low activity/remission criteria met similar RAPID3 criteria. Again, RAPID3 was as informative as indices that included a physician/assessor joint count or physician/assessor global estimate [25].

ACR/EULAR Remission Criteria

Lastly, ACR/EULAR have recently proposed a new remission criteria [26]. One of the reasons behind the new remission criteria was the fact that it is possible to have a score less than 2.6 (i.e., cutoff value for remission in DAS28) but still have several swollen/tender joints, which is mostly an artifact of the algorithm used to calculate DAS28 scores. To rectify this problem, a more stringent definition of remission was deemed necessary. Working together, the ACR and EULAR developed a new Boolean definition for remission. The new definition states that swollen, tender joint counts, CRP, and patient global assessment of disease activity added together needs to be 1 or less. The authors state that "any definition of remission at a minimum has to include … tender, swollen joint counts and levels of an acute phase reactant." There are a number of concerns with the development methodology of the new remission criteria. First, very few options were considered for remission definition, such as swollen joint, patient, and physician global assessments, or an only patient-reported outcome derived index. Second, 3 of the 4 measures were predetermined. Third, an exercise of trying to determine the last measure to include was done by investigating the prediction of a good outcome in radiographic damage and function, by adding patient and physician global assessment, patient pain, and combinations of these to the 3 predetermined measures, as decided by the committee. Historically, physician-derived measures were regarded as the more "objective" measures compared to patient-reported measures. There are however data to suggest that patient-reported outcome measures may actually be more "objective" than physician-derived measures, in that patients are better at differentiating treatment from placebo and have better test-retest characteristics, making them more reliable and reproducible. Strand et al. examined the placebo responses in leflunomide trials for each of the individual disease activity scores and found the largest placebo response in swollen and tender joint counts, whereas laboratory tests and most of patient-derived measures had significantly less placebo response [27]. In a trial of tocilizumab, we had shown that at 1 week after the first infusion, patient measures were significantly better among those that received tocilizumab compared to placebo, whereas physician measures were not able to differentiate those who received the active drug versus placebo [28]. In another study looking at test-retest characteristics of individual measures and composite indices, authors found the highest correlations among patient measures rather than physician-derived measures [29].

A number of studies suggest that patient-reported measures are as good, if not better, than physician-derived measures in telling how patients are doing in clinical trials or the real world setting. Therefore, the commonly held belief among rheumatologists is that it is time to be more "evidence based" rather than "habit based" when making treatment decisions [30] and that it is hard to justify physician-based measures as the gold standard in any composite index. Second, a practical consideration is real world use. Even the best measure is of no value if it is unlikely to be adopted in routine clinical care. The measure has to have acceptance by both the physicians and patients. Most rheumatologists in the United States do not perform and/or record official joint counts. Hence, any measure that uses tender and swollen joint counts would be additional work for the already busy clinician and will likely not be done. However, a patient-reported disease activity index, such as the RAPID3, makes innate sense, as it is the patient who is experiencing the effects of the disease, would be a very good way of documenting response and a decision tool that can be used along with the physicians own assessment.

Heath Assessment Questionnaire (HAQ)

The Stanford Health Assessment Questionnaire (HAQ) is used in most clinical trials and outcome studies. HAQ has become the most common tool for measuring functional status in rheumatology and is the best predictor of mortality, work disability, joint replacement, and medical costs [31]. The HAQ was developed in 1980 by James Fries and his colleagues at Stanford University. The creation of the HAQ was based on studies of patient-centered health values on five generic outcome dimensions. Patients reported they wanted (1) to avoid disability, (2) to be free of pain and discomfort, (3) to avoid adverse effects of treatment, (4) to keep medical costs low, and (5) to postpone death. HAQ is one of the most cited and employed patient-reported outcome instrument [32, 33].

The HAQ is a measure of functional limitations where patients rate, on a scale of zero to three, zero meaning the person can normally complete the task with no difficulty, one meaning adequate completion of the task with some difficulty, two meaning limited completion, having much difficulty, and three meaning the person is unable to do the task. Patients rate the degree of difficulty they have experienced during the last week with 20 tasks grouped into the eight areas of dressing, rising, hygiene, reach, walking, eating, grip, and activities. Additional questions are asked relating to the use of companion aids and devices [34, 35]. The scores are then converted into an overall mean score ranging from 0 to 3, zero indicating no functional impairment and three indicating complete impairment. The HAQ is formatted into two sides of one page and consists of a complex scoring system [36]. After this initial work, other simpler versions of HAQ have been developed, to make the tool easier to use, and they have all been successful in clinical care. Modified HAQ (mHAQ) takes a question out of each of the eight categories of HAQ and creates a shorter index for function. MDHAQ (multidimensional HAQ) adds two more questions to the mHAQ to better differentiate those who are truly close to fully functional, as to address the floor effect seen with mHAQ. HAQ2 is yet another shorter version of HAQ.

Biomarkers

There is increasing interest in using biomarkers as outcome measures in RA. Biomarkers have the potential to provide objective measurement of the disease processes underlying RA, rather than external signs and symptoms. A promising biomarker is the multi-biomarker disease activity (MBDA) test. MBDA test is based on serum levels of 12 proteins associated with RA disease activity and combines them into a score between 1 and 100 [37].

Studies indicate that physicians have four main reasons for ordering the MBDA test: (1) facilitate a discussion with the patient regarding their treatment plan, (2) routine monitoring of disease activity, (3) assess disease activity in patients with comorbidity, and (4) confirm low disease activity. MBDA score can track response to treatment with biological and nonbiological DMARDs and is also a good indicator of risk for progressive joint damage in patients with RA [38].

A disease algorithm using the 12 serum protein biomarkers is applied to calculate the MBDA scores. This algorithm uses serum biomarkers concentrations to separately estimate 28 tender joint count (TJC28), 28 swollen joint count (SJC28), and a visual analog scale measuring general health (VAS-GH). The estimates for TJC28, SJC28 a VAS-GH are combined with a CRP result to calculate an overall MBDA score. The results are scaled and rounded to be integers on a scale of 1–100 such that an MBDA score of 1 is equivalent to a value of 0 on a DAS28-CRP scale and a score of 100 is equivalent to a value of 9.4 [37, 39]. RA remission is defined as MBDA score of ≤25, whereas scores of 26–29 indicate low, 30–44 indicate moderate, and >44 indicate high disease activity. MDBA scores have a significant correlation with DAS28-CRP. Since the MBDA score is calculated using a formula similar to DAS28-CRP, multiplying the DAS28-CRP value by 10.53 and adding 1 can calculate a MBDA score equivalent to DAS28-CRP value [40]. When CRP is removed from the panel, MBDA continues to correlate well with overall DAS28-CRP values and also with SDAI, CDAI, and RAPID3 [41]. The potential of MBDA in disease activity monitoring remains to be seen in the future. Although it performs very similar to available composite disease activity indices, it is expensive and the results are not available at the time of the office visit, when most treatment decisions are made.

Radiographs

Joint damage is one of the most important and impactful outcome of uncontrolled and untreated RA. Over the last 15 years, the advent of early and aggressive treatment and early use of methotrexate and combinations with biologic agents have led to a decrease in joint damage, as evidenced, for example, by the lower number of total joint replacements for RA [42]. Clinical trials have traditionally included radiographic joint damage as one of the RA efficacy outcomes and the Food and

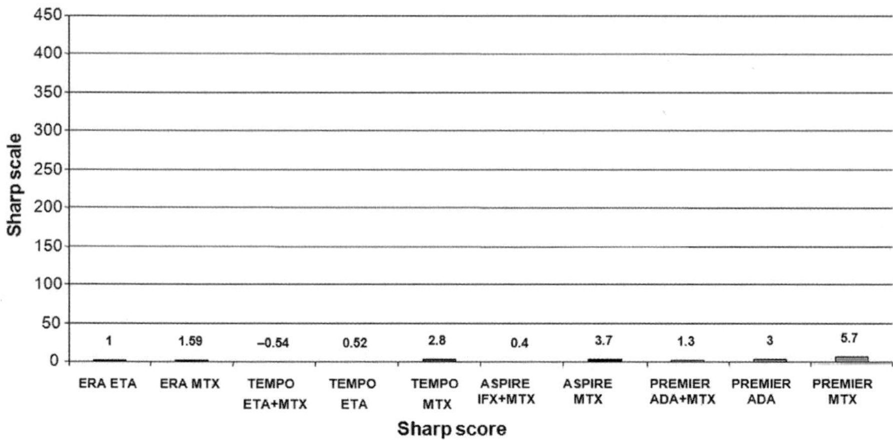

Fig. 1 Radiographic outcomes in randomized controlled trials with methotrexate-naïve patients. *TNF* tumor necrosis factor inhibitor, *MTX* methotrexate, *ETA* etanercept, *IFX* infliximab, *ADA* adalimumab, *ERA* early rheumatoid arthritis (From Yazici and Yazici [44])

Drug Administration seeks data on joint damage for approval of an agent as efficacious in stopping or slowing down radiographic progression. Initially the Larsen score and later the Sharp score and its modified versions, such as the van der Heijde and Genant, have been used [43]. The scale used for these measures ranges from 0–448 (van der Heijde) to 0–290 (Genant). However, the actual changes in scores in the RCTs are typically less than 20 units. These differences between treatment arms and placebo or control arms are usually statistically significant but not clinically relevant as less than 5 units is below the minimal detectable difference for these measures and clinically significant functional decrease happens at around 15–20 units, which is rarely if ever seen in RCTs [44] (Fig. 1). One of the reasons for this discrepancy of statistically significant but clinically irrelevant results is that fact that a very small minority of patients show progression and account for the difference. Over 80 % of the patients, regardless of which arm of the trial they are in, show no progression. As we have no current way of determining who the small minority who show progression will be, radiographic progression data does not help the clinician in everyday care of RA patients, and even if it did, the actual progression is very small for majority of patients. Hence, most rheumatologists don't advocate using radiographs for treatment decisions in clinical trials or routine care. There is potentially more promise with ultrasound and MRI measures and it is possible that these modalities may replace radiographs in the near future.

Conclusions

Use of standardized outcome measures in rheumatology increased significantly over the last decade and led to improvements in comparability of clinical studies across different settings and patient care. RA is the condition that drove the development of standardized outcome measures in rheumatology followed by other rheumatologic conditions. Many of the currently used standardized outcome measures in RA (i.e., DAS28, CDAI, SDAI, RAPID3, HAQ) are based on the Core Data Set that includes patient-reported (physical function, pain, patient global estimate of status), physical examination (swollen joint count, tender joint count, physician/assessor patient global estimate of status), and laboratory (ESR or CRP) measures. With increased understanding of the underlying disease processes in RA, there is growing interest in the development of imaging and biomarker-based measures that can be used in conjunction with patient-reported and physical examination measures to improve measurement of disease activity in RA.

References

1. Keenan RT, Swearingen CJ, Yazici Y. Erythrocyte sedimentation rate and C-reactive protein levels are poorly correlated with clinical measures of disease activity in rheumatoid arthritis, systemic lupus erythematosus and osteoarthritis patients. Clin Exp Rheumatol. 2008;26: 814–9.
2. Felson DT, Anderson JJ, Boers M, et al. The American College of Rheumatology preliminary core set of disease activity measures for rheumatoid arthritis clinical trials. Arthritis Rheum. 1993;36:729–40.
3. Grigor C, Capell H, Stirling A, et al. Effect of a treatment strategy of tight control for rheumatoid arthritis (the TICORA study): a single-blind randomised controlled trial. Lancet. 2004; 364:263–9.
4. Verstappen SM, et al. Intensive treatment with methotrexate in early rheumatoid arthritis: aiming for remission. Computer Assisted Management in Early Rheumatoid Arthritis (CAMERA, an open-label strategy trial). Ann Rheum Dis. 2007;66(11):1443–9.
5. Goekoop-Ruiterman YP, et al. Clinical and radiographic outcomes of four different treatment strategies in patients with early rheumatoid arthritis (the BeSt study): a randomized, controlled trial. Arthritis Rheum. 2005;52(11):3381–90.
6. Pincus T. The American College of Rheumatology (ACR) Core Data Set and derivative "patient only" indices to assess rheumatoid arthritis. Clin Exp Rheumatol. 2005;23 Suppl 39: S109–13.
7. Felson DT, Anderson JJ, Boers M, et al. American College of Rheumatology preliminary definition of improvement in rheumatoid arthritis. Arthritis Rheum. 1995;38:727–35.
8. Anderson J, Caplan L, Yazdany J, Robbins ML, Neogi T, Michaud K, Saag KG, O'Dell JR, Kazi S. Rheumatoid arthritis disease activity measures: American College of Rheumatology recommendations for use in clinical practice. Arthritis Care Res (Hoboken). 2012;64(5):640–7. doi:10.1002/acr.21649.
9. van der Heijde DMFM, van't Hof M, van Riel PLCM, van de Putte LBA. Development of a disease activity score based on judgment in clinical practice by rheumatologists. J Rheumatol. 1993;20:579–81.
10. Prevoo MLL, van't Hof MA, Kuper HH, van Leeuwen MA, van de Putte LB, van Riel PL. Modified disease activity scores that include twenty-eight-joint counts: development and validation in a prospective longitudinal study of patients with rheumatoid arthritis. Arthritis Rheum. 1995;38:44–8.
11. Fransen J, Stucki G, van Riel PL. Rheumatoid arthritis measures: Disease Activity Score (DAS), Disease Activity Score-28 (DAS28), Rapid Assessment of Disease Activity in Rheumatology (RADAR), and Rheumatoid Arthritis Disease Activity Index (RADAI). Arthritis Rheum. 2003;49 Suppl 9:S214–24.

12. Anderson JK, Zimmerman L, Caplan L, Michaud K. Measures of rheumatoid arthritis disease activity: patient (PtGA) and provider (PrGA) global assessment of disease activity, Disease Activity Score (DAS) and Disease Activity Score with 28-joint counts (DAS28), Simplified Disease Activity Index (SDAI), Clinical Disease Activity Index (CDAI), Patient Activity Score (PAS) and Patient Activity Score-II (PASII), Routine Assessment of Patient Index Data (RAPID), Rheumatoid Arthritis Disease Activity Index (RADAI) and Rheumatoid Arthritis Disease Activity Index-5 (RADAI-5), Chronic Arthritis Systemic Index (CASI), patient-based Disease Activity Score with ESR (PDAS1) and patient-based Disease Activity Score without ESR (PDAS2), and Mean Overall Index for Rheumatoid Arthritis (MOI-RA). Arthritis Care Res (Hoboken). 2011;63(Suppl):S14–36.
13. Prevoo ML, van Gestel AM, van't Hof MA, van Rijswijk MH, van de Putte LB, van Riel PL. Remission in a prospective study of patients with rheumatoid arthritis: American Rheumatism Association preliminary remission criteria in relation to the disease activity score. Br J Rheumatol. 1996;35:1101–5.
14. Gaujoux-Viala C, Mouterde G, Baillet A, Claudepierre P, Fautrel B, Le Loët X, et al. Evaluating disease activity in rheumatoid arthritis: Which composite index is best? A systematic literature analysis of studies comparing the psychometric properties of the DAS, DAS28, SDAI and CDAI. Joint Bone Spine. 2012;79(2):149–55.
15. Ton E, Bakker MF, Verstappen SM, et al. Look beyond the Disease Activity Score of 28 joints (DAS28): tender points influence the DAS28 in patients with rheumatoid arthritis. J Rheumatol. 2012;39:22–7.
16. Wells G, Becker JC, Teng J, Dougados M, Schiff M, Smolen J, et al. Validation of the 28-joint Disease Activity Score (DAS28) and European League Against Rheumatism response criteria based on C-reactive protein against disease progression in patients with rheumatoid arthritis, and comparison with the DAS28 based on erythrocyte sedimentation rate. Ann Rheum Dis. 2009;68:954–60.
17. Inoue E, Yamanaka H, Hara M, Tomatsu T, Kamatani N. Comparison of Disease Activity Score (DAS)28- erythrocyte sedimentation rate and DAS28- C-reactive protein threshold values. Ann Rheum Dis. 2007;66:407–9.
18. Aletaha D, Smolen J. The Simplified Disease Activity Index (SDAI) and the Clinical Disease Activity Index (CDAI): a review of their usefulness and validity in rheumatoid arthritis. Clin Exp Rheumatol. 2005;23(5 Suppl 39):S100–8.
19. Smolen JS, Breedveld FC, Schiff MH, Kalden JR, Emery P, Ederl G, et al. A simplified disease activity index for rheumatoid arthritis for use in clinical practice. Rheumatology. 2003;42: 244–57.
20. Pincus T, Swearingen CJ, Bergman M, Yazici Y. RAPID3 (Routine Assessment of Patient Index Data 3), a rheumatoid arthritis index without formal joint counts for routine care: proposed severity categories compared to disease activity score and clinical disease activity index categories. J Rheumatol. 2008;35(11):2136–47.
21. Yazici Y, Bergman M, Pincus T. Time to score quantitative rheumatoid arthritis measures: 28-Joint Count, Disease Activity Score, Health Assessment Questionnaire (HAQ), Multidimensional HAQ (MDHAQ), and Routine Assessment of Patient Index Data (RAPID) Scores. J Rheumatol. 2008;35(4):603–9.
22. Pincus T, Skummer PT, Grisanti MT, Castrejón I, Yazici Y. MDHAQ/RAPID3 can provide a roadmap or agenda for all rheumatology visits when the entire MDHAQ is completed at all patient visits and reviewed by the doctor before the encounter. Bull NYU Hosp Jt Dis. 2012;70(3):177–86.
23. Pincus T, Hines P, Bergman MJ, Yazici Y, Rosenblatt LC, Maclean R. Proposed severity and response criteria for Routine Assessment of Patient Index Data (RAPID3): results for categories of disease activity and response criteria in abatacept clinical trials. J Rheumatol. 2011;38(12): 2565–71.
24. Pincus T, Yazici Y, Bergman M, Swearingen C, Harrington T. A proposed approach to recognise "near-remission" quantitatively without formal joint counts or laboratory tests: a patient self-report questionnaire routine assessment of patient index data (RAPID) score as a guide to

a "continuous quality improvement" strategy. Clin Exp Rheumatol. 2006;24 Suppl 43: S60–73.
25. Pincus T, Bergman MJ, Maclean R, Yazici Y. Complex measures and indices for clinical research compared with simple patient questionnaires to assess function, pain, and global estimates as rheumatology "vital signs" for usual clinical care. Rheum Dis Clin North Am. 2009;35(4):779–86.
26. Felson DT, Smolen JS, Wells G, Zhang B, van Tuyl LH, Funovits J. American College of Rheumatology/European League Against Rheumatism provisional definition of remission in rheumatoid arthritis for clinical trials. Arthritis Rheum. 2011;63(3):573–86.
27. Strand V, Cohen S, Crawfrod B, et al. Patient-reported outcomes better discriminate active treatment from placebo in randomized controlled trails in rheumatoid arthritis. Rheumatology. 2004;43:640–7.
28. Yazici Y, Curtis JR, Ince A, Baraf HS, Lepley DM, Devenport JN, Kavanaugh A. Early effects of tocilizumab in the treatment of moderate to severe active rheumatoid arthritis: a 1- week sub-study of a randomised controlled trial (Rapid Onset and Systemic Efficacy [ROSE] Study). Clin Exp Rheumatol. 2013;31(3):358–64.
29. Uhlig T, Kvien TK, Pincus T. Test retest reliability of disease activity core set measures and indices in rheumatoid arthritis. Ann Rheum Dis. 2009;68:972–5.
30. Yazici Y. Rheumatoid arthritis: evidence-based rather than habit-based treatment options. Nat Rev Rheumatol. 2012;8(7):374–6. doi:10.1038/nrrheum.2012.79.
31. Anderson J, Sayles H, Curtis JR, Wolfe F, Michaud K. Converting modified health assessment questionnaire (HAQ), multidimensional HAQ, and HAQII scores into original HAQ scores using models developed with a large cohort of rheumatoid arthritis patients. Arthritis Care Res (Hoboken). 2010;62:1481–8.
32. Bruce B, Fries JF. The health assessment questionnaire (HAQ). Clin Exp Rheumatol. 2005;23(5 Suppl 39):S14–8.
33. Hawley DJ, Wolfe F. Sensitivity to change of the health assessment questionnaire (HAQ) and other clinical and. health status measures in rheumatoid arthritis: results of short term clinical trials and observational studies versus long term observational studies. Arthritis Care Res. 1992;5:130–6.
34. Ziebland S, Fitzpatrick R, Jenkinson C. Comparison of two approaches to measuring change in health status in rheumatoid arthritis: the health assessment questionnaire (HAQ) and modified HAQ. Ann Rheum Dis. 1992;51(350):1202–5.
35. Wolfe F, Michaud K, Pincus T. Development and validation of the health assessment questionnaire II: a revised version of the health assessment questionnaire. Arthritis Rheum. 2004;50: 3296–305.
36. Pincus T, Sokka T, Kautiainen H. Further development of a physical function scale on a multidimensional health assessment questionnaire for standard care of patients with rheumatic diseases. J Rheumatol. 2005;32:1432–9.
37. Bakkar MF, Cavet G, Bijlsma JW, Haney DJ, Shen Y, Hesterberg LL, Smith D, Centola M, Van Roon JAG, Lafeber FP, Welsing PM. Performance of a multi-biomarker score measuring rheumatoid arthritis disease activity in the CAMERA tight control study. Ann Rheum Dis. 2012;71:1692–7.
38. Li W, Sasso EH, Emerling D, Cavet G, Ford K. Impact of a multi-biomarker disease activity test on rheumatoid arthritis treatment decisions and therapy use. Curr Med Res Opin. 2013;29(1):85–92.
39. Hirata S, Dirven L, Shen Y, Centola M, Cavet G, Lems WF, Tanaka Y, Huizinga TWJ, Allaart CF. A multi-biomarker score measures rheumatoid arthritis disease activity in the BeSt study. Rheumatology (Oxford). 2013. doi:10.1093/rheumatology/kes362.
40. Curtis JR, van der Helm-van Mil AH, Knevel R, et al. Validation of a novel multi-biomarker test to assess rheumatoid arthritis disease activity. Arthritis Care Res. 2012;64(12):1794–803.
41. Wilke W. Measures of disease activity in rheumatoid arthritis. Rheumatol Pract News. 2012;2(1)18–22.
42. Khan NA, Sokka T. Declining needs for total joint replacements for rheumatoid arthritis. Arthritis Res Ther. 2011;13(5):130. doi:10.1186/ar3478.

43. Yazici Y, Sokka T, Pincus T. Radiographic measures to assess patients with rheumatoid arthritis: advantages and limitations. Rheum Dis Clin North Am. 2009;35(4):723–9.
44. Yazici Y, Yazici H. Tumor necrosis factor alpha inhibitors, methotrexate or both? An inquiry into the formal evidence for when they are to be used in rheumatoid arthritis. Clin Exp Rheumatol. 2008;26:449–52.

Issues in Setting Up a Study and Data Collection

Hilal Maradit Kremers and Banu Çakir

A successful start and the successful realization of any research activity depend upon the completion of certain rather well-defined chores before its embarkation. Several chapters in this book outline methodological principles that apply to different study designs. In this chapter, practical issues in setting up studies and data collection will be highlighted, with special emphasis to evidence-based rheumatology research.

Setting up a study involves tasks and activities that have to take place early in the development of a study, starting with protocol writing and funding application. These activities include literature searches, discussions of the research ideas with mentors and potential collaborators, preliminary feasibility assessment, identification of data resources, investigation of potential study designs, associated regulatory requirements, and, possibly, funding opportunities. Literature searches and discussions with coinvestigators and collaborators are particularly important in synthesizing the evidence and formulating the most relevant study questions. These discussions focus on previous efforts that address the same or related clinical questions, their strengths and weaknesses, and critical unknowns in the field.

H.M. Kremers, MD
Departments of Health Sciences Research and Orthopedic Surgery, Mayo Clinic,
200 First St SW, Rochester, MN 55902, USA
e-mail: maradit@mayo.edu

B. Çakir, MD, MPH, PhD (✉)
Department of Public Health, Hacettepe University Faculty of Medicine,
Bayindir Sokak Ismet Apt. 49/10 Kizilay, Ankara 06650, Turkey
e-mail: bcakir@hacettepe.edu.tr; banucakir4@gmail.com

H. Yazici et al. (eds.), *Understanding Evidence-Based Rheumatology*,
DOI 10.1007/978-3-319-08374-2_6

Setting up the study and data collection activities vary considerably depending on the study design (i.e., interventional or observational), the direction of data collection (prospective or retrospective), primary and secondary objectives, characteristics of the main exposure(s) and outcome(s) of interest, potential confounders and/or effect modifiers, and the study setting, whether it involves special data collection procedures, such as biospecimens or patient-reported outcomes, feasibility issues, and financial restrictions. Besides these, research in rheumatology is often prone to some unique challenges that tend to limit causal inference and, thus, shape design considerations. These unique challenges are (1) rare occurrence of many rheumatologic conditions, (2) long latency periods, (3) the need to apply classification criteria to define conditions, (4) genetic/hereditary effects, (5) comorbidities, (6) potential confounders, and (7) high likelihood of systematic errors in exposure and outcome measurement. All such issues need to be carefully evaluated in setting up the study and during data collection. They will also be further considered in statistical analyses and interpretation of the data. Thus, initial developmental stages in research activities is an iterative process and highly benefit from a multidisciplinary approach, involving epidemiologists and biostatisticians to provide input with respect to the technical feasibility of the conceptualized study design. Below, some practical issues are highlighted following an algorithm (Fig. 1), and with a special focus on study setup, protocol development, and data collection.

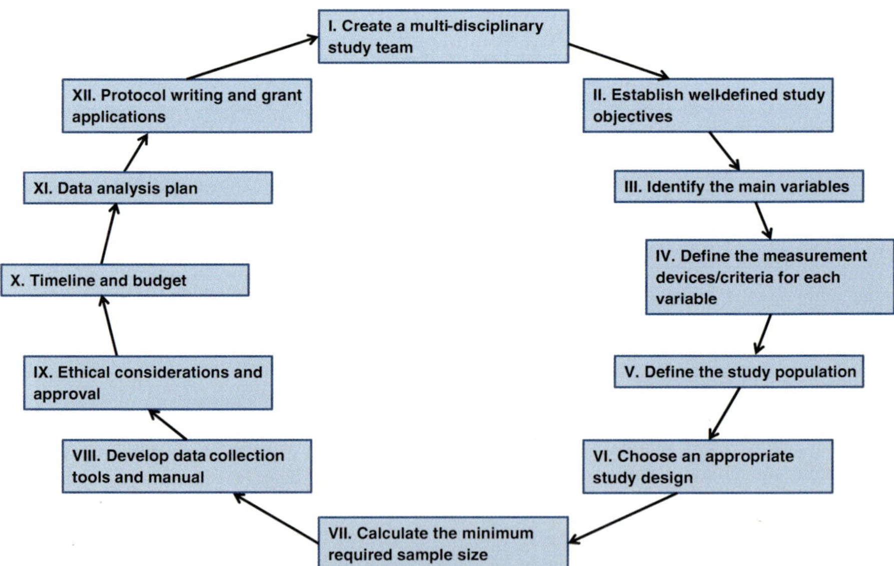

Fig. 1 Algorithm for setting up a rheumatology research project

Create a Multidisciplinary Study Team (i.e., Clinicians, Epidemiologists, Biostatisticians, Ethicists, Patient Representatives, and Others, as Needed)

Any rheumatology research is initiated by a problem in mind: this could be anything that the researcher seeks an answer for, a situation that s/he finds unsettled, with inconclusive evidence, or a condition/therapy/method that needs to be improved. Usually, research question is initially posed as a question, which serves as the focus of further investigation. Success in medical research is an end result of teamwork, with gathering of the research team early in the process. Any research project will significantly benefit from a well-balanced, multidisciplinary, complementary research team and avoid "reinventing the wheel."

Develop the Research Question

Research question is developed after a comprehensive review of the literature and careful feasibility evaluation. Literature review helps with shaping the study objectives and preventing unnecessary repetitions of work on already conclusive evidence. An effective literature review includes a review of all potential literature sources using targeted search terms, accessing and reviewing the articles and, if needed, accessing and reviewing the primary sources of referenced articles, and noting key points in these articles. Apart from Medline, OVID, and Embase databases, evidence-based research reviews can be identified through the Cochrane Collaboration topic reviews and Evidence-Based Medicine Reviews (EBMR). In reviewing the literature, it is important to consider the potential for publication bias: the published literature is typically limited to significant findings, and nonsignificant studies are not published. For example, Pocock et al. revealed that p values obtained from a systematic review of epidemiologic studies had a peak around p values greater than 0.01 and less than 0.05, rather than a normal distribution pattern, and concluded that statistically significant findings are more publishable [1]. Also, foreign language journals and publications can be difficult to access and review.

Once a study question is deemed worth pursing, then the next question is "feasibility" assessment in terms of study design, time frame, available resources (financial resources and manpower), and ethical implications. The types of study design typically fit under three headings (see Panel 1). Since each of these designs has different feasibility and resource implications, preliminary investigations are important. For example, for a clinical study, the preliminary counts of patients with the disease or surgical procedure of interest and the likelihood of participation (for prospective studies) will define the potential study population. Even for a registry or an existing database study, preliminary counts are informative in terms of the number of years to be included in the study. Since most rheumatologic conditions are rare, the minimum sample size requirements may necessitate multicenter studies. The study questions may also dictate whether population-based samples are needed (e.g., incidence, prevalence studies). Feasibility checks are repeated in other stages of study development.

Panel 1. Study Design

- Descriptive (incidence, prevalence studies)
- Hypothesis testing using an observational study design (e.g., case–control, cohort)
- Hypothesis testing using an interventional (experimental) study design, i.e., researcher decides who will get the "exposure" of interest

Identify the Main Exposure, Outcome, Potential Confounders, and Other Covariates

Detailed definition of the main exposure, outcome variables, potential confounders, and covariates determines what data need to be collected. Most studies attempt to estimate two types of parameters: the frequency of disease occurrence in a particular population and/or the effect size (if any) of a given exposure on disease occurrence. Some research questions do not focus on a relationship at all, and are simply descriptive, such as the prevalence of a particular rheumatologic condition in the population. In all situations, exposure and outcome definitions should be objective, standard, and comprehensive, including exclusion criteria (if any). For example, in a study examining the risk of rheumatoid arthritis associated with obesity, the main exposure variable is obesity and the outcome variable is rheumatoid arthritis. Yet, it is important to explain in detail what is meant by obesity, both in terms of body mass index cutoff values and exposure period in relation to the onset of rheumatoid arthritis (obesity during adolescence, during adulthood, past history of obesity, current obesity, etc.). The definition of rheumatoid arthritis is also specified as new onset, based on self-reported physician diagnosis or based on classification criteria.

In case of a hypothesis testing research design, all exposure and outcome variables are clearly defined, including whether they will be continuous measures or categorical measures and what to do in case of missing data. Some common mistakes are (a) improper grouping of quantitative exposure/outcome variables into several ordered groups, where the number of categories and justification of cut points are often unrealistic, such as, grouping age as below 15, 15–25, 25–35, 35, or above, where categories are overlapped and the group sizes are not similar or using a cut point of 130 mg/dl for identifying individuals with high fasting blood glucose, rather than using the widely accepted cut point of 126 mg/dl; (b) identification of confounders is often perceived as a task in statistical analysis stage and the requirements to be fulfilled for a variable to be a potential confounder is often ignored [2]. However, it is not possible to account for confounders in statistical analyses unless the relevant data are collected.

The selection of potential confounders is based on input from the clinicians and needs clarity, consistency, and explanation. At this stage, the investigator may also consider if there is any possibility for *effect modification*, i.e., effect of an exposure varies in subgroups of patients, such as men and women or young and old. If effect modification is likely, the subgroups of the effect modifier and the type of interaction (synergistic versus antagonistic, multiplicative versus additive) need to be defined, to the extent possible and power considerations, and sample size should be planned accordingly. As an example, Park et al. [3] found in their recent work that the risk of radiographic progression in rheumatoid arthritis was statistically significantly associated with LDL cholesterol and triglyceride levels (leading up to 5.6-fold risk in the third tertile of both groups). Moreover, LDL cholesterol synergistically increased the adjusted probability of radiographic progression in patients with high serum leptin levels but not in those without. In this situation, leptin is considered to modify the effect of LDL cholesterol on radiographic progression. The assessment of effect modification is important for properly specifying the predictors in statistical models, for making inferences about possible biological (causal) interactions between exposures (e.g., synergy), for generalizing the study findings to other populations, and also affect the minimum sample size requirement [4].

Define the Measurement Devices/Criteria to Be Used for Each Variable

All variables should be measurable, objective, and validated, as appropriate. All indices/questionnaires/inventories, etc., must (known to) be validated in the source population. Diagnostic/therapeutic/preventive thresholds, cutoff points, and "risk zones" should be comparable to those in the literature, unless needed/intended to be used otherwise. Issues related to data collection tools are further detailed below.

It is important to emphasize that the quality of data collection depends upon the measurement tools. Collection of diagnostic-classification criteria can be difficult, in particular, in chart review studies. In prospective studies involving multiple individuals, intra- and/or interobserver reliability can be significantly low, hampering the quality of data collection [5, 6]. Therefore, interobserver reliability studies are common in rheumatology, in particular, in studies involving imaging [7, 8].

Define the Study Population

Study population is typically a population-based sample (epidemiological studies), convenience sample (analytical studies), or volunteers (interventional studies, studies collecting biospecimens). If the goal is to estimate disease frequency in a particular population, such as the occurrence of new cases and/or deaths (incidence, mortality), or to study the presence of existing cases (prevalence), the base population of the study is the group of all individuals who, if they developed the disease, would become cases. In such situations, it is important that the study is conducted on an "adequate" size population, representatively chosen from the source population. Unfortunately, true population-based studies are feasible in only selected countries where routine healthcare data are available [9].

The investigator should attempt to clarify the rationale for selection of a particular population, the characteristics of the population, with emphasis on representativeness (if any), so that the generalizability (external validity) of the results could be estimated in advance. Representativeness depends upon the source of participants and the proportion participating, i.e., exclusions, refusals to participate, dropouts, or a discontinuity in preplanned follow-ups will hamper the generalizability of the final study findings. Due to some common sources of bias, representativeness is not always guaranteed. Studies in hospital settings may be prone to Berkson bias [10]. This type of selection bias arises in case–control studies in hospital settings. When both the exposure and disease/outcome under study increase the likelihood of admission to the hospital, then the exposure prevalence among hospital cases will be systematically higher than hospital controls and will in turn distort the odds ratio. Similarly, Neyman bias (synonyms: incidence–prevalence bias, selective survival bias) may distort the results of a rheumatologic study when a series of survivors is selected, if the exposure is related to prognostic factors or the exposure itself is a prognostic determinant, the sample of cases offers a distorted frequency of the exposure [11]. This bias can occur in both cross-sectional and case–control studies, if the risk factor influences mortality from the disease being studied. Detection bias may arise in cohort studies when exposed and unexposed individuals have different surveillance intensity to identify outcomes. For example, in a cohort study examining hypertension risk in rheumatic diseases, patients with rheumatic diseases may visit their doctor more frequently and may have a higher likelihood of hypertension being diagnosed than the comparison cohort of subjects without a rheumatic disease. Selection bias may distort findings also if study subjects or participants of a study are different than the pool of all potential diseased individuals. For example, volunteers who agree to participate in research studies are typically different than those who do not. Thus, it is important to carefully consider representativeness and appropriate procedures, where needed.

Choose an Appropriate Study Design

The study design is chosen based on the research questions. It can also be a combination of several designs:

In case–control studies, the focus is on selection of new onset cases and controls and matching, if needed. In cohort studies, the focus is defining exposure groups as accurately as possible, whereas in randomized interventional studies, the focus is on randomization methods and blinding. Irrespective of study design, selection bias can be a major threat to validity. The various study designs are outlined in other chapters, with emphasis on advantages and limitations of each. A few points are worth mentioning in this section. Randomized controlled trials (RCTs) provide the best scientific evidence but it is important to note that RCTs-based results are hampered in generalizability due to relatively small sample sizes and short follow-up periods of RCTs. Well-conducted observational studies can provide a wealth of epidemiologic information when randomized controlled trials are either not feasible or too expensive. Such observational studies are very useful in studying the real life effectiveness and/or safety of drugs. Post-marketing safety of many of the drugs commonly used in rheumatology is now being conducted using data from large administrative claims databases [12].

Calculation of the Minimum Required Sample Size

Sample size calculation should precede the study start. Sample size and power calculations are also required for grant applications to justify the proposed study size, unless a convenience sample is used, where the power of the study can be estimated backwards.

The minimum sample size will be the least number of individuals to be recruited for the study in order to reach robust estimates (prevalence, incidence, a particular effect size) for the population. Any sample size below the required minimum number will be prone to type II (beta) error, i.e., declaring a difference does not exist between the groups compared when in fact it does. Even in situations where an association is detected in a study with less than required number of study participants, its occurrence due to a type I error often cannot be ruled out. In other words, the authors may conclude by chance that a difference between the groups exist when in fact it does not.

A sample size calculation demands information on study design, the expected probability of the outcome in the source population, the minimum effect size in checking for an association, the desired precision in detecting an estimate, preset confidence interval/alpha error, the requested power (1-beta), ratio of controls to cases, number of hypotheses, and ad hoc analyses to be performed. There might still be other considerations. In calculation of sample sizes for rheumatologic studies, a common difficulty is the lack of knowledge of the standard deviation of the index variables. There are well-recognized tables established for calculating the sample size [13], yet the best approach will be a collaboration of a sampling expert and the clinician with a grasp of the related literature.

Sample size calculation is often conducted for the main hypothesis alone. Any *ad hoc* estimations (data dredging) or further control in multivariate analyses will lead to larger confidence intervals than initially aimed for, i.e., require adjustments in the minimum sample size. The minimum sample size calculated should also be inflated based on estimated completion rates (due to access problems, refusals), dropouts, etc.

Sample size calculation is a "must" to control for type I and type II errors. However, in rheumatologic studies, researchers should be aware of the clear distinction between the requirements for a "minimal sample size" and "representativeness" for a selected group of individuals (such as, cases/controls, cohort, the general population) for whom the study findings will be interpreted for. Studies conducted on sample sizes equal or above the required numbers do not always guarantee error-free estimations. Large simple trial designs, characterized by large sample sizes, are preferred study designs for drug safety research because it is considered as to control for biases inherent to observational research while still providing results that are generalizable to "real-world use" [14, 15]. Such studies often provide the investigator to control for many potential confounders that may be detected in a "large and heterogeneous" group of participants and maximize the benefit of using statistical models for robust estimations of adjusted risk estimates in studying potential associations. However, even in such situations, evaluations of the similarities between the study participants and all the eligible in the population will be needed to judge the representativeness of the study population. Thus, in gathering the "study population," the representativeness and sample size issues should be handled separately, but yet hand in hand. The expert support of the biostatistician is critical at this phase of study development.

A study is externally valid, or generalizable, if it can produce unbiased inferences regarding the target population (beyond the study participants). It is noteworthy that activities related to selection of study population (the sample) and completion of data collection from all selected cases are prone to a variety of biases that should be carefully evaluated and be controlled for, as much as possible [16–18]. These potential biases that hinder external validity of the study findings are listed in Table 1. These different forms of bias can create systematic errors that, even though the required sample size is achieved, results do not represent the general population because each eligible individual will not have a well-defined probability of selection chance to participate in a given study.

Table 1 Different types of selection bias

Referral bias	Common in case–control studies. Patient selection is influenced by exposure status. For example, patients taking NSAIDs and presenting with abdominal pain may be more likely to be suspected of having a gastric ulcer and referred for gastroscopy than those not taking NSAIDs. Therefore, a study using patients in the hospital may show a stronger and biased association between NSAIDs and mild non-bleeding GI ulcers
Self-referral/self-selection biases	Common in cohort studies. Subjects select themselves into a sample or a group or choose to visit hospital to seek care. Their exposure and disease characteristics may be different than those who did not
Nonrespondent bias	Common in surveys. The responses of subjects who participate in a survey are different than those who did not participate
Volunteer bias	In prospective studies (observational or interventional), subjects who volunteer to participate are different from the general population
Early/late comer bias	Similar to volunteer bias, subjects who participate early are different from nonparticipants or late participants
Loss to follow-up bias	Arises in cohort studies. Subjects lost from a cohort may have different health outcomes from subjects who remain under observation

(continued)

Table 1 (continued)

Withdrawal bias	Subjects who withdraw from a prospective follow-up study may have different outcomes than those who remain in the study
Berkson bias	Common in case–control studies in hospital settings. When both the exposure and disease outcome increase the likelihood of admission to the hospital, then the exposure prevalence among hospital cases is higher than in hospital controls
Neyman bias (prevalence–incidence bias)	Common in case–control studies and arises when prevalent cases are included, instead of incident (new onset) cases. Bias arises from selective survival among the prevalent cases (i.e., mild, clinically resolved, or fatal cases being excluded from the case group)
Centripetal bias	The hospital where the study is conducted attracts individuals with particular characteristics. Therefore, a study sample at that institution may not be representative of the population at large
Diagnostic access bias	Individuals with certain characteristics (such as healthcare professionals) may have greater access to healthcare and have a higher likelihood of certain diseases diagnosed
Ascertainment bias	A type of sampling bias where some subjects are more or less likely to be included than others, and therefore, the sample is not a random sample
Migratory bias	Bias arising from exclusion of subjects who have recently moved in or out of the study area

Develop Data Collection Tools and Data Collection Manual

Patient interviews, questionnaires, medical records, insurance records, physical examination and laboratory data, genetic analysis, quality of life indices, and other self-evaluation forms, etc., can be used in collecting individual data and/or could be merged/linked. In all such efforts, pretesting and pilot testing of both the data collection tool and data collecting personnel, reliability and validity evaluations are vital steps. Minimum number to be used in pilot testing can be determined by experts in epidemiology and biostatistics, but the rule of the thumb is "the number where no new information can be obtained upon repeated tests." A systematic difference between a true value and that actually observed (i.e., information bias) can appear in various stages of medical research, but the most common stage leading to information bias is during data collection.

Data collection method and instrument(s) can vary, yet all should be affordable, usable, acceptable (by the data collector and the study participants), objective, reliable, and valid. It is not often the case that all these requirements are fulfilled, yet the investigators should do their best to ensure these requirements as much as possible. Measurement scales to be used need to be clearly identified: this, in turn, will be important to be known for data analysis plans.

The data collection instrument must include comprehensive inquiries on personal information (re: both socio-demographic and health status) and potential confounders; time spans (of disease development, therapy course, remission periods, etc.) should be evaluated as much as possible, given the cumulative effects of risk factors and/or interactions over time.

There are two major data collection methods: (1) primary data collection with information obtained directly from the study participants; (2) secondary data collection based on existing data, such as those obtained from medical records, insurance records, and electronic patient files.

Questionnaires are standard forms used to collect medical history and exposure data from study subjects. Questionnaires are either self-administered or administered by an interviewer. Self-administered questionnaires are completed by the study subjects themselves, either at the clinic or mailed. This is typically a much cheaper option than interviewer-administered questionnaires and are often more effective in gathering personal and sensitive information. By contrast, face-to-face interviews are often valuable to minimize missing information due to illiteracy, physical problems, fatigue, and failure to follow skip patterns. Whatever the administration format, questionnaires need to be designed carefully and pretested before being administered to the study subjects. If standard and validated questionnaires were available, it would be best to use them instead of developing a new one. For example, there are several patient-reported outcome instruments in rheumatology to capture different dimensions of disease. Health Assessment Questionnaire (HAQ), modified HAQ, pain Visual Analog Scale (VAS), and patient global assessment by VAS are the most commonly used tools to assess function, pain, and global assessment of disease by the patient (see chapter "Outcome measures in rheumatoid arthritis").

The likelihood of response to questionnaires is higher if they are brief and each question is justified in terms of the objectives of the study. To the extent possible, open-ended questions (i.e., where subjects respond in their own words) should be reduced to a minimum to reduce response bias and ease data coding and processing. Also, wording should be simple and avoid direction of subjects to particular answers. Questions related to a particular topic can be grouped together branching of questions would avoid further responses to irrelevant questions, such as smoking details to be captured only for current or past smokers. When questions are presented with multiple choices, the researchers must further provide the options of "*I do not know*," "*I am not sure*," "*other* (*please specify*)," or "*not applicable*," as needed. In situations where more than one option could be appropriate, the participant should be informed that "more than one option can be marked." The ultimate goal is to gather the best evidence regarding the information requested in the simplest manner.

Questionnaire layout should be legible, pleasant, and with clear explanations, as needed. Once the first draft of a questionnaire is finalized, it should be tested and retested on a sample of potential study subjects to identify questions that are poorly understood. The final questionnaire will then need to be coded for future data entry and processing.

With increasing availability of electronic medical and other types of records, most studies these days rely on existing data sources to collect data. This type of data collection is typically cheaper, is faster and, depending on quality and level of details, may be more accurate. Yet, availability of data varies from one country or one hospital to another. For example, large population registries in Scandinavian countries offer unique research opportunities in terms of linkage of large numbers of subjects across registries.

Measurement, misclassification, and observational biases appear as common threats to data collection activities in rheumatologic studies. Questionnaire and interviewer biases are quite common systematic error that can be faced in rheumatologic research when self-reporting is an issue and several interviewers are needed to complete personal data. Standardization and pilot testing of the questionnaires is a standardized remedy for such situations, but even in such cases subject/observer, recall, faking good, faking bad, and/or obsequiousness biases could all limit the interviewer's ability to collect reliable and valid data. For example, even though SLE patients are generally consistent reporters of certain aspects of their histories, family history information provided is frequently not consistent with previous findings [19].

Similarly, measurement bias may arise if all measurement devices used are not comparable or not standardized initially and/or periodic calibration is not ensured. In situations where personal data need to be supported by other sources, medical data (such as hospital admission notes, discharge notes, family history) can also be retrieved as additional data. Comparability of study findings can be enhanced if established classification criteria/indices are used, such as the American College of Rheumatology/European Union League Against Rheumatism (ACR/EULAR) Rheumatoid Arthritis classification criteria in determining exposure and/or disease status of study participants.

In using secondary data, comprehensiveness and standardization of the data, coding errors, accessibility to health services, premature deaths, competing deaths, and spatial bias (in ecological studies) should all be evaluated as potential reasons for systematic errors. In current rheumatologic research activities, patient registries and administrative data bases are quite frequent resources for patient data. Observational and retrospective uses of such secondary data sources are highly prone to biases such as selection bias (in choosing controls),channeling bias, depletion of the susceptible bias, immortal time bias, mortality bias, and confounding by disease severity. It is important that the researcher(s) are aware of such bias potential in handling patient registry/administrative database data (see chapter "Limitations of traditional randomized controlled clinical trials in rheumatology").

In many rheumatology studies, participants are gathered from among those admitting to a hospital/clinic, which in turn makes data collected prone to a set of biases that arise when patients are either not representative of all eligible patients in the population or the disease status might have been diagnosed differently than all eligible patients due to reasons such as diagnostic suspicion and/or exposure suspicion.

Information bias may also appear due to inefficiencies and variations across use of data collection tool(s) by data collecting personnel. For example, the high interobserver variation in grading anteroposterior sacroiliac radiographs might be a cause of "sacroiliitis" reported in certain disease states [20]. Training of study personnel is perhaps the most important aspect of high-quality studies. Depending on the background of the study personnel, training involves both general training on ethics, GCP but also study-specific details. Regarding study-specific training, there may be a central training, with or without additional site training; the study manual should be thoroughly discussed and revised if needed; study personnel must be pilot tested (as needed) for data collection procedures; and initial training activities should be supported by regular monitoring and error checks as the study continues.

It is noteworthy that even when data tools and data collection activities are planned as standardized, individual involved in data gathering, data entry, data merging, and/or record linkage activities may lead to systematic errors. Study/field manuals are crucial in ensuring standardization in medical studies. Single-center studies are typically conducted based on the study protocol and a study manual, whereas large multicenter studies may require detailed standard operating procedures to be implemented at each of the participating sites. A study manual is needed even for the simplest studies. It documents the details of study-related procedures, including step-by-step instructions on how the questionnaires (if any) will be distributed, collected, and coded; definitions for variables; and collection and processing of biospecimens, etc. In order to maximize (inter- and intra-rate) reliability of data collection procedures, uses of such manuals are often of vital importance. These manuals help to minimize potential confusion on the content and context of the inquiries; they help to handle questions that may arise after the initial training of data collectors/sites and provide uniform explanations, such as for description of words used. These ultimately serve to minimize information bias. The manual should regularly be updated as well, based on needed changes while the study runs.

Almost all studies also have a (data) coding manual that outlines the conversion of data from questionnaires or data collection forms into a standardized format that is suitable for statistical analyses. For example, sex may be coded as 1 for females and 2 for males. Upfront definitions and a coding manual (precoding) can substantially reduce labor and increase efficiency during data editing, statistical analysis, and final interpretations.

Ethical Considerations and Approval

Irrespective of the study design, ethical issues are always a concern to the researcher. The basic question is: "will any physical, psychological or social harm come to anyone as a result of this particular study?" In general, ethical issues include protecting participants from harm, ensuring confidentiality of research data, informing participants of the objectives and content of the study, and getting informed consent from all participating parties. Where children are involved, further precautions are needed, such as parental consent and special counseling activities. Several national and international regulations define ethical considerations for the best interest of the patients/study participants. For prospective studies, informed consent, parental consent (if needed) is an integral and indispensable part of the study design. If a study involves direct patient contact or secondary use of patient data (physical, biological, genetic, etc.), the researcher probably will need to create an "*informed consent form*." The local ethics committee may provide consent forms from earlier studies and these may be used as templates. It is important to note that the consent form includes information about the investigators, study objectives in a plain language, expectations from participants, potential hazards (if any), potential benefits (if any), and related issues such as insurance, insurance/any other payments, means to protect confidentiality, and data security during and upon completion of the study. Ethical concerns also include whether the results will be shared with the participants and the preset rules on authorship rights in manuscript publications. Collection of biospecimens may require special procedures.

Timeline and Budget

Timeline and budget will vary, depending on the study design. Yet, it is important to plan a detailed and plausible study timeline and budget. Both the timeline and budget plan can be accompanied with milestones and deliverables. Budget plans typically include personnel costs (principal investigator and coinvestigators' salary and benefits), supplies, travel, data analysis costs, and renumeration of participants, if applicable.

Data Analysis Plan

Data analysis is often described broadly during study preparation. Yet, the type of variables to be studied, the type of analysis to be established (multivariate models, survival analysis, repeated measures, etc.), the number and type of control variables, the coding scheme to be used, and even the software to be used need to be well established prior to initiation of the study.

In studying the magnitude of a potential association between the exposure status and disease occurrence, the index and comparison groups are selected and compared in such a manner that the observed differences between them on the dependent (outcome) variables under study may, apart from sampling error, be attributed only to the hypothesized effect under investigation. This is called "internal validity." Internal validity of a study is a prerequisite and is more important than the external validity, as in the case of the important situation when we aim to get a valid estimate of the effect size (such as odds ratio or relative risk). In this case the generalizability of the results to the general population is a secondary aim. Even so, it is important also for internal validity to work on a heterogeneous population so that information can be obtained on potential confounders and other covariates of interest, which will directly affect the valid estimation of effect size in statistical modeling.

Certain measures of association, such as correlation coefficients and standardized regression coefficients, do not necessarily reflect "causal" relationships. Because the magnitude of these measures depends in part on the relative variance of the exposure and disease variable, which are influenced by the sampling strategy. Thus, the analyst must be aware of the details of the sampling technique and that information on potential confounders has been adequate for a meaningful analysis.

It is not rare that the epidemiologist/statistician is involved in the study team later in time to the sampling and data collection, is often not fully aware of the methodology used initially, and is unable to control for biases that may arise in data analysis stage. For example, it is often the case that matched case–control studies are analyzed using tests for unmatched situations, parametric and nonparametric tests are used interchangeably without attendance to the characteristics of the variables, multivariate models are frequently used without consideration of the default requirements, evaluation of effect modification and additive interactions are usually missing, use of unweighted estimates in situations where sampling is disproportionate to size, and/or complex samples are treated as simple random samples in statistical analysis. A quite common mistake is to provide prevalence estimates and/or effect size measures (odds ratio, relative risk, risk difference) without confidence intervals, which hinders usability of such information in comparisons across time or population settings.

It is noteworthy that several general problems in rheumatology research tend to limit validity of causal inferences and, thus, shape design decisions. Among these, long latency periods (i.e., time from onset of symptoms to diagnosis) could arise from nonspecificity of the symptoms, limitations of medical diagnostic technology, and limited access to experts, besides the prolonged induction period in which years are needed for a disease process to become manifest. Long latency periods constraint researchers' ability to estimate relative effects of exposures and comorbid situations. Retrospective evaluations are limited with availability of medical records, standardization of measurements, recall bias, and good biological indicators of exposure levels. Low prevalence of rheumatologic diseases/conditions, together with long latency periods, makes cohort studies difficult, thus compromises causal inferences seriously.

Protocol Writing and Grant Applications

A research proposal communicates the intentions of the researcher: conveys the purpose of the study and justification of the resources, together with a step-by-step plan for conducting the study. Study protocol should include a draft for report writing stage, including the plan to share activities across investigators, with a tentative timeline. In the report, problems are identified, questions or hypotheses are stated, variables are identified, and terms are defined. The subjects to be included in the sample, the sampling technique (if any), the instrument(s) and the measurement scales to be used, the study design, and the procedures to be followed will be detailed, including how the data will be analyzed. When possible, connections are needed to be established with previous related research. A written proposal will allow interested parties (including the funding agencies, if any) to evaluate the worth of the proposed study and to make suggestions for improvement. Also, this material will be used at the completion of the study to check whether all aimed objectives are fulfilled successfully.

Preparation of a study protocol is typically an iterative process that involves frequent discussions with collaborators, mentors, and statisticians. A frequently forgotten aspect of a successful protocol is that it should be as simple as is reasonably possible or as is needed. Careful protocol development and writing will minimize potential mistakes and necessary modifications. If the researcher(s) aims to apply for funding, it is advisable that the protocol should follow the format of the funding agency, as requirements may vary substantially. Nevertheless, some aspects of protocol writing are universal and are outlined in Panel 2.

Grant Application

If the proposed project is small, it can be conducted using local resources. Yet, most studies require external financial support. Obtaining funding can be a long and iterative process. Potential funding agencies vary depending on the disease area. Furthermore, funding agencies typically have different deadlines and grant application forms. It is advisable to review grant application deadlines carefully and contact the agencies to confirm whether proposed research would be of interest to the agency. Furthermore, before applying for funding, it is advisable to show the study protocol to experienced investigators (mentors, colleagues) and ask them for a critical review of your proposal, so that you can address potential problems before submission.

Panel 2. Protocol Components

Abstract or executive summary is meant to serve as a short and accurate description of the proposed study. The most important things to include are (a) what the issue/question is, (b) why the issue is important, (c) how the issue will be addressed, and (d) what the clinical relevance of the issue is. For all studies but in particular, for clinical trials, this section should clearly state the exposure(s), outcome(s), and hypotheses, if applicable.

Specific aims section describes what the study is intends to accomplish and how it will be achieved. Specific aims may range from one to many in number, but typically well thought-out research projects have no more than three or four specific aims and hypotheses, if applicable. Specific aims and hypotheses should be stated in clear, simple statements and should also include a concise description of the exposure(s) or intervention(s) to be studied and the outcome(s) of interest.

Background section is a critical summary of existing literature, highlighting the magnitude of the problem and the knowledge gaps that the project is intended to fill. It is important to keep this section focused to the literature that is relevant to the research and not a broad literature review of the disease area. This section should convey the significance and relevance of the research for the field.

Research design and methods is perhaps the most detailed and longest section of any protocol. Researcher must carefully plan his/her study methodology, with special emphasis on the study design, sample size calculation, the need for covariate data, random errors and systematic errors (bias), and potential means to control for bias and confounding. The quality of measurements must be secured and maximized by effective initial planning, standardization and calibration, and timely and on-site monitoring.

It is best to follow a standard format (e.g., funding agency guidelines, previous protocols) to include information on preliminary studies (any similar research that you have already done), inclusion/exclusion criteria, diagnostic methods, recruitment procedures and materials, diagnostic tests, data elements and definitions, statistical methods, and power. It is always a good idea to work with a statistician in development of the study methods and statistical analyses. Methods section should also include a realistic time frame and an explicit assessment of strengths, limitations, and potential problems of proposed research.

Human subjects section is mainly targeted for the ethics review committees and includes a detailed description of the proposed involvement of human subjects in the study, with details on their characteristics, anticipated number, age range, and health status. It is advisable to provide rationale for the involvement of special groups of subjects, e.g., pregnant women or children. This section should outline the sources of research materials (medical records, questionnaires, biospecimens), potential risks to subjects, and procedures for minimizing potential risks. If the study involves prospective recruitment, it is important to describe circumstances under which consent will be obtained, the nature of the information to be provided to prospective subjects and the method of documenting consent.

Budget is broadly divided into personnel costs (salaries), equipment and supplies, and, if applicable, travel and subcontracting costs. Depending on the duration of the study, it is advisable to take into account inflation. Some funding agencies do not cover overheads (e.g., telephone, mailing costs), whereas others will pay only up to a certain percent.

References

1. Pocock SJ, Collier TJ, Dandreo KJ, de Stavola BL, Goldman MB, Kalish LA, Kasten LE, McCormack VA. Issues in the reporting of epidemiological studies: a survey of recent practice. BMJ. 2004;329:883.
2. Cakir B. Do not get confused by the confounders: identification and control of confounders. Turk J Public Health. 2004;2:34–43.

3. Park YJ, Cho CS, Emery P, Kim WU. LDL cholesterolemia as a novel risk factor for radiographic progression of rheumatoid arthritis: a single-center prospective study. PLoS One. 2013;8:e68975.
4. Morgenstern H, Thomas D. Principles of study design in environmental epidemiology. Environ Health Perspect. 1993;101 Suppl 4:23–38.
5. Seror R, Bootsma H, Bowman SJ, Dorner T, Gottenberg JE, Mariette X, Ramos-Casals M, Ravaud P, Theander E, Tzioufas A, Vitali C. Outcome measures for primary Sjogren's syndrome. J Autoimmun. 2012;39:97–102.
6. Yazici H. A critical look at diagnostic criteria: time for a change? Bull NYU Hosp Jt Dis. 2011;69:101–3.
7. Micu MC, Serra S, Fodor D, Crespo M, Naredo E. Inter-observer reliability of ultrasound detection of tendon abnormalities at the wrist and ankle in patients with rheumatoid arthritis. Rheumatology. 2011;50:1120–4.
8. Taylor WJ, Porter GG, Helliwell PS. Operational definitions and observer reliability of the plain radiographic features of psoriatic arthritis. J Rheumatol. 2003;30:2645–58.
9. Kremers HM, Myasoedova E, Crowson CS, Savova G, Gabriel SE, Matteson EL. The Rochester Epidemiology Project: exploiting the capabilities for population-based research in rheumatic diseases. Rheumatology. 2011;50:6–15.
10. Westreich D. Berkson's bias, selection bias, and missing data. Epidemiology. 2012;23: 159–64.
11. Hill G, Connelly J, Hebert R, Lindsay J, Millar W. Neyman's bias re-visited. J Clin Epidemiol. 2003;56:293–6.
12. Winthrop KL, Chen L, Fraunfelder FW, Ku JH, Varley CD, Suhler E, Hills WL, Gattey D, Baddley JW, Liu L, Grijalva CG, Delzell E, Beukelman T, Patkar NM, Xie F, Herrinton LJ, Fraunfelder FT, Saag KG, Lewis JD, Solomon DH, Curtis JR. Initiation of anti-TNF therapy and the risk of optic neuritis: from the safety assessment of biologic ThERapy (SABER) Study. Am J Ophthalmol. 2013;155:183–9.e181.
13. Bellamy N, Carette S, Ford PM, Kean WF, le Riche NG, Lussier A, Wells GA, Campbell J. Osteoarthritis antirheumatic drug trials. II. Tables for calculating sample size for clinical trials. J Rheumatol. 1992;19:444–50.
14. Reynolds RF, Lem JA, Gatto NM, Eng SM. Is the large simple trial design used for comparative, post-approval safety research? A review of a clinical trials registry and the published literature. Drug Saf. 2011;34:799–820.
15. Wright NC, Warriner AH, Saag KG. Study design considerations for a large simple trial of bisphosphonates. Curr Opin Rheumatol. 2013;25:517–23.
16. Choi BC, Noseworthy AL. Classification, direction, and prevention of bias in epidemiologic research. J Occup Med. 1992;34:265–71.
17. Greenland S, Lash TL. Bias analysis. In: Rothman KJ, Greenland S, Lash TL, editors. Modern epidemiology. 3rd ed. Philadelphia: Lippincott Williams & Wilkins; 2008. p. 345–80.
18. Maclure M, Schneeweiss S. Causation of bias: the episcope. Epidemiology. 2001;12:114–22.
19. Yazici Y, Erkan D, Harrison MJ, Peterson MG, Yazici H. Reporting consistency in systemic lupus erythematosus patients: how reliable are patient histories? Lupus. 2002;11:46–8.
20. Yazici H, Turunc M, Ozdogan H, Yurdakul S, Akinci A, Barnes CG. Observer variation in grading sacroiliac radiographs might be a cause of sacroiliitis reported in certain disease states. Ann Rheum Dis. 1987;46:139–45.

The Randomized Controlled Trial: Methodological Perspectives

Emmanuel Lesaffre

Introduction

A *clinical trial* is any form of planned experiment in medicine, which involves patients and is designed to elucidate the most appropriate treatment for future patients with a given medical condition. In the *randomized clinical trial* (RCT), the subjects are randomly assigned to two or more healthcare interventions. The results from this limited sample of patients are exploited to get insight about what treatment should be given in the general population of patients. In the famous pyramid of evidence-based medicine (see, e.g., Chapter 2 of [1]), the RCT scores the second highest (immediately below meta-analyses of RCTs) with respect to the hard evidence it provides about the tested intervention. In fact, the RCT is the only single study design which allows the researcher to draw causal relationships between a risk factor (absence or presence of experimental treatment) and outcome (improvement of the patient's condition).

RCTs have been widely used in health care starting only in the second half of the twentieth century with the British Medical Research Council trial of streptomycin for treatment of tuberculosis as the landmark study [2]. However, despite the inherent strength of the RCT, its conclusions are only to be trusted when it is set up and conducted properly. In this chapter, we review the essential concepts, steps in setting up, conducting, analyzing, and reporting as related to the RCT.

E. Lesaffre, Dr. Sc. (✉)
Department of Biostatistics, Erasmus MC, Dr. Molewaterplein, 50-60, Rotterdam 3015 GE, The Netherlands

L-Biostat, KU Leuven, Leuven, Belgium
e-mail: e.lesaffre@erasmusmc.nl

H. Yazici et al. (eds.), *Understanding Evidence-Based Rheumatology*,
DOI 10.1007/978-3-319-08374-2_7

The National Institutes of Health (NIH) classifies the trials into six different types: (1) prevention trials, which aim to prevent people from disease via, e.g., lifestyle changes; (2) screening trials to detect, e.g., diseases; (3) diagnostic trials, which look for better diagnostic procedures; (4) treatment trials to test experimental treatments based on drugs, surgical techniques, etc.; (5) quality-of-life trials, which test new strategies to improve the quality of life of patients; and (6) compassionate use trials that offer experimental (but not yet approved) therapeutics to patients for whom there is no effective therapy and who have no other realistic options. In this chapter, we focus on drug treatment trials in rheumatology, but most of the topics discussed apply also to the other types of interventional studies. Furthermore, what we discuss is not limited to rheumatology.

Phases of Clinical Research

Drug research is typically classified into the following stages:

- *Preclinical phase*: These are studies on animals to provide Information about efficacy, toxicity, and pharmacokinetics.
- *Phase 0*: This is to find out whether the drug behaves as expected. Subtherapeutic doses are administered to a small number of people (10–20 subjects).
- *Phase I* (Is the drug safe?): These are dose-ranging studies to find the maximally tolerated dose on healthy volunteers or patients (between 20 and 100 subjects), often done in an adaptive manner. In addition, initial information on adverse events is collected, together with pharmacokinetics and pharmacodynamics parameters.
- *Phase II* (Does the drug work?): This is about testing the drug on about 100–300 patients to obtain a better idea of efficacy and safety. This phase determines whether one should move on to phase III studies and are referred to as "proof of concept" studies.
- *Phase III* (Is the drug better than what is on the market?): Here, the formal testing of the therapeutic dose of the drug on patients takes place, involving typically at least 500–1,000 patients. This phase is decisive for the registration of the drug by regulatory agencies like the U.S. Food and Drug Administration (FDA, http://www.fda.gov/) and European Medicines Agency (EMEA, http://www.emea.europa.eu/).
- *Phase IV* (Are there other uses of/problems with the drug?): These are postmarketing surveillance studies to determine infrequent adverse events.
- *Phase V*: This phase is about translational research and is done on already collected data.

Sometimes, a further subdivision into phases IIa, IIb, IIIa, IIIb, etc. is made [3]. In [4] phase 0 to phase II, trials are referred to as *learning* (or exploratory) phase trials, while phase III trials are called *confirmatory* (also pivotal). Nowadays, there is a trend to shorten the entire regulatory process of an experimental drug by combining, especially, phase II and phase III trials in the so-called adaptive designs [5]. From above, it is evident that the aims are different in the different phases of clinical research. The topics discussed in this chapter primarily concern phase II and III trials.

Asking the Appropriate Scientific Question

A well-formulated scientific question is an essential condition for a successful clinical trial. While it sounds almost as an obvious requirement, in practice, there is always the temptation to verify a great variety of (definitely interesting) clinical hypotheses in one RCT. There is now overwhelming evidence that the identification of an unambiguous *primary scientific question* has enormous benefits for all aspects of the trial. Less important research questions (but still within the scope of the trial) can then be classified as *secondary questions*. By focusing the design and implementation of the trial to address the needs of the primary question, one maximizes the chances of obtaining a definitive answer. Obviously, the nature of the primary and secondary questions depends on the phase of the trial.

The general principles of formulating scientific questions for RCTs of all phases are described below using the *PICO system* (http://www.usc.edu/hsc/ebnet/ebframe/PICO.htm), which specifies that a "well-built" question should identify: (1) the population, (2) the intervention and control treatment, and (3) the outcome.

The Population

A detailed description of the study *population* is a necessary part of the scientific question. The RCT population is defined by *inclusion* and *exclusion criteria*. The inclusion criteria specify what kind of patients one wishes to treat. For instance, the inclusion criteria for patients with systemic sclerosis treated with a disease-modifying intervention might be (1) older than 18 years of age, (2) clinically apparent involvement of the skin on the extremities proximal to the elbows or knees or on the trunk, and (3) disease duration <2 years from the first symptom; see [6]. On the other hand, exclusion criteria aim to reduce the heterogeneity of the population. For instance, an often used exclusion criterion is "drug or alcohol abuse," but also "pregnant women." In reference [6], the investigators excluded also patients with kidney malfunction. Exclusion criteria also address ethical considerations. For instance, by excluding pregnant women, embryos are not exposed to unknown risks. Another typical exclusion criterion is the administration of concomitant medication that might interfere with the trial treatments. This is to avoid adverse events originating from sources other than those from the trial treatment.

Strict eligibility criteria will make the RCT population more homogeneous, which in general will reduce the variability of the outcome measure and hence the necessary study size. The drawback of strict criteria is that they limit the extrapolation of the trial results to the general patient population and thus affect the *generalizability*, also called the *external validity*, of the trial. For instance, by excluding pregnant women from the trial, no claim can be made on the efficacy and safety of the experimental treatment on this subpopulation. Note also that strict eligibility criteria may harden patient recruitment. Therefore, establishing appropriate inclusion and exclusion criteria is often a difficult process balancing between homogeneity and external validity. See also the section on "RCTs versus observational studies" for a further discussion on external validity. Different eligibility criteria across studies with the same experimental treatment can throw light of the generalizability of the estimated efficacy and safety of the drug. However, when eligibility criteria vary wildly across RCTs with different experimental treatments, the comparability of the effects across the treatments will become difficult. In reference [6], a list of proposed guidelines for specifying eligibility criteria in systemic sclerosis is given.

Choice of Intervention and Control Treatment

The choice of the interventional treatment is often quite clear from the start of the RCT, except for some possibly important details. Indeed, the RCT is set up to evaluate the effect of that intervention. That does not, however, mean that it is a fait accompli. For instance, in drug trials, it may be clear what the experimental medication is, but it still needs to be decided what the mode of delivery (tablet, solution, intravenous, or subcutaneous injection), dose, frequency, and timing of administration of the intervention will be.

Placebo treatment is often the preferred control treatment by regulatory agencies, unless there is an established accepted active treatment for the disease in which case it is unethical to administer a placebo treatment. It goes without saying that placebo treatment does not imply absence of treatment but rather that the standard care has been provided to the patient. Since standard care improves over time, the need for a "placebo" also evolves with time. The choice of the control (active or placebo) arm may impact the type of significance test; see section "Superiority and non-inferiority tests."

More than one intervention or control treatment may be considered. For instance, in phase I *dose escalation studies*, patients are allocated to one of several different doses of a drug with the goal of identifying the dose with an optimal trade-off between a desired biological action and unwanted side effects. Multiple group designs may also arise when combinations of interventions are tested, which occurs in the *factorial design* (see section "Factorial Designs").

Superiority and Non-inferiority Tests

The classical statistical tests described in chapter "A review of statistical approaches for the analysis of data in rheumatology" aim to show that one treatment is superior to the other treatment, either a placebo or an active control. However, in many therapeutic areas, it becomes harder to improve upon current medication and one will be contented if the experimental drug has about the same efficacy as the control drug but shows better properties in other respects. This leads to non-inferiority tests explained below.

For a long time, clinical trials were only *superiority trials*; namely, they were set up to show that the experimental (E) treatment was superior to a control (C) treatment. The statistical tests used to analyze such trials are *superiority tests*. Recall that E is statistically significantly better than C at $\alpha = 0.05$ when $P < 0.05$, or equivalently that the 95 % confidence interval for the true difference (or ratio, odds ratio, etc.) does not include zero (or one in case of a relative measure).

It is, however, increasingly difficult to come up nowadays with new drugs that improve upon the existing ones in efficacy. For instance, thrombolytic agents have been developed over the last five decades to treat patients with an acute myocardial infarction. The initial 30-day mortality rates (percent of patients dying within 30 days after the onset of attack) were around 15 % but then dropped to about 6–7 % a decade later. It became clear that a further reduction in mortality rate may not be hoped for so that the focus turned into improving secondary objectives such as the mode of administration of the thrombolytic agent while preserving the achieved 30-day mortality rates. This requires other types of statistical tests, i.e., equivalence and non-inferiority tests, which will now be illustrated via fictive examples.

An example of a superiority trial in RA could be where one aims to show that $\Delta_S = 10$ % more patients who go into a remission after 6 months for the experimental treatment E compared to the placebo control. In another RCT, the aim might be to show that this experimental treatment has the same efficacy as a standard control treatment C. However, proving that E and C are equally effective is not possible in classical statistics, as we discussed in chapter "A review of statistical approaches for the analysis of data in rheumatology". In fact, we can only show that treatments are practically equivalent, say, that they differ in efficacy by at most, say, 2 %, in absolute value. Such a test is called an *equivalence test* and is used to show that generic drugs have similar properties as the original patented drugs. A one-sided version of such a test is a *non-inferiority test* and the associated trial a *non-inferiority trial*. Namely, a treatment E is called *non-inferior* to treatment C, when it is either better or not much worse than C where "not much worse" is defined by the *non-inferiority boundary* here denoted as Δ_{NI}. This value should be chosen small enough so that it does not create ethical difficulties. Let us assume that for the above RA trial, $\Delta_{NI} = 2$ % is a good choice. Then one way to prove non-inferiority is to show that the 95 % confidence interval does not include $\Delta_{NI} = 2$ %. Since Δ_{NI} should be considerably smaller than Δ_S, the required sample size with a non-inferiority study is often much larger than that of a superiority trial. The choice of the appropriate non-inferiority boundary is often subjective and requires a balanced choice between ethical, practical, statistical, and regulatory considerations. This may render the comparison of non-inferiority trials with different boundaries hard. Another flaw of the non-inferiority trial is that there is no standard analysis set, in contrast to a superiority trial where the intention-to-treat population is usually the default analysis set (as discussed below in the section on "Intention-to-treat versus per-protocol analysis"). An illustrative example of the difference between a superiority and non-inferiority trial can be found in [7]. Briefly, this study consists of two studies comparing etoricoxib 30 mg qd (ET) and celecoxib 200 mg qd (CE) to placebo (PL), which is the superiority part of the trial. In the second part of the trial, two studies were conducted to compare the relative performance of ET and CE with a non-inferiority design. The two randomized three-arm double-blinded clinical trials described in [7] each contains a non-inferiority assessment of ET versus CE for the treatment of osteoarthritis of the knee and hip using a time-weighted average (TWA) change from baseline over 12 weeks in (a) the WOMAC pain subscale (WOMACPA), (b) the WOMAC physical function subscale (WOMACPH), and (c) the patient global assessment of disease status (PGADS). All three scales are scored on a visual analogue scale. The experimental treatment CE was defined to be non-inferior to ET when the upper bound of the two-sided 95 % CIs for the difference between CE and ET was not more than 10 mm for the three primary endpoints WOMACPA, WOMACPH, and PGADS. Thus, in order that non-inferiority is shown, all three conditions had to be satisfied. In [7], it is shown that for the two studies, these conditions were satisfied (95 % CIs entirely below upper bound), and the authors' conclusion was therefore that "etoricoxib 30 mg is comparable to celecoxib 200 mg in osteoarthritis." At first glance, the authors used a tough criterion for "non-inferiority," only it is not clear how they chose $\Delta_{NI} = 10$ mm.

We refer to [8] for a more detailed nontechnical introduction to non-inferiority studies, while a more technical and a broader discussion of the subject can be found in [9].

Study Outcomes

The outcome, also called the *endpoint*, is the third component of the PICO system, and its characteristics determine many other aspects of the RCT. That is, the choice of the primary endpoint has a large impact on the size and the conduct of the study. *Hard endpoints*, such as mortality, leave no room for interpretation. However, when we choose for cardiac mortality, subjectivity creeps in since now the clinical judgement of the treating physician is required and this makes it a softer endpoint. *Soft endpoints* suffer from intra- and interobserver variability, and their use will therefore increase the necessary study size. Examples of (relatively) soft endpoints are, e.g., the EULAR response criteria (DAS and DAS28) and the ACR response criteria (ACR20, ACR50, ACR70); see also chapter "Outcome measures in rheumatoid arthritis." The use of many different criteria in European and US clinical trials to measure the rheumatic disease outcomes makes it difficult to compare and combine results in a meta-analysis (chapter "Systematic reviews and meta-analyses in rheumatology"). This was the trigger to establish the OMERACT network in 1992 [10]. Through regular meetings, the network aims to improve the outcome measures in rheumatology.

Clinical considerations may be in conflict with statistical requirements. For instance, it may be clinically more relevant to take the binary endpoint remission defined as DAS28 <2.6. However, from a statistical viewpoint, binarizing the endpoints implies a loss of information and hence a decrease in power. In addition, a statistical comparison between treatments based on DAS28 measurements only at the study end may suffer a lot from intersubject variability. This variability can be drastically reduced by taking the improvement from baseline as an endpoint instead, as in the ACR criteria.

Prior to the study, it may feel unconformable to bet on one endpoint, so there is often the temptation to select several endpoints and then to choose the one that demonstrates best the efficacy of the experimental treatment. However, this leads to an inflation of the Type I error rate as we discussed in chapter "A review of statistical approaches for the analysis of data in rheumatology". An alternative approach is to make use of a *composite endpoint*, which is a clinical combination of different endpoints. Many of the responses in rheumatology trials are composite. Composite endpoints are also popular when the primary endpoint of interest exhibits a too low frequency, thereby increasing the necessary study size. An example in cardiovascular research is the binary composite endpoint MACE (major adverse cardiac events), which can be 0 or 1. While there are several definitions of MACE, the common definition is an outcome of death, having a myocardial infarction or a stroke. However, interpretation difficulties will occur when, e.g., a better result for MACE is seen under treatment A, while under treatment B, mortality is lower. Finally, we note that multiple endpoints can also be combined in a statistical manner (subject to the same issues as the above clinical composite endpoints) using a factor analysis technique; see chapter "A review of statistical approaches for the analysis of data in rheumatology" and [11].

Patient-centered outcomes, i.e., outcomes that represent a tangible benefit or harm to the patient, are especially most relevant in phase III trials. But because it may take too long to record the patient-centered endpoint, it might be necessary to choose for a *surrogate* endpoint, also called *disease-centered outcomes*. Such an outcome represents a measure of the disease process that is believed/hoped to be strongly related to a tangible patient benefit or harm. However, often such a relation is believed to exist purely from lower level studies, e.g., from animal studies. For example, in oncology, progression-free survival (PFS), which is the time to progression of the tumor, is often used in clinical trials as a surrogate outcome for overall survival. While there is a growing use of PFS as a primary outcome, there is no clear evidence of such a strong relationship (see, e.g., [12]), which therefore puts serious doubts on the usefulness of this outcome. We conclude that there are no specific statistical issues involved with using a surrogate endpoint; rather, the problem lies in the clinical interpretation of the study results. See also [13] for considerations on patient- and disease-centered outcomes.

Finally, in some studies, it may be of interest to express the benefit of an experimental treatment by the whole longitudinal profile of the primary endpoint or a summary measure of the profile. For instance, one might be interested in the rate with which DAS28 decreases over time. In that case, the average profiles need to be compared between the treatment arms, or at least the averages of the summary measure. This requires the use of longitudinal models as we saw in chapter "A review of statistical approaches for the analysis of data in rheumatology". In other studies, one might be interested in the time to an event. For instance, one might be interested in the time to remission (DAS28 <2.6). In that case, survival analysis techniques are required; see again chapter "A review of statistical approaches for the analysis of data in rheumatology".

Randomization and Blinding

Random allocation of patients to treatments together with blinding enables one to draw a causal relationship between the administered treatment and the status of the patient at completion of the RCT. Randomization guarantees balance of the treatment arms with respect to the recorded covariates but also to all unmeasured covariates. Such a balance can never be achieved by any epidemiological study, irrespective of the analysis tricks used (e.g., with regression models).

Several randomization schemes are in use. The simplest randomization technique, e.g., by using a toss of a coin, is only practical for small study sizes, as in phase II studies, but even then, it is rarely used nowadays. Nowadays, the majority of phase III RCTs involve many centers often with a small number of patients from each center. In this case, simple randomization implies too much risk for imbalance in the treatment arms, and this could compromise the conclusions of the study. Therefore, a *blocked randomization* is often used in each center. Block randomization is not a pure stochastic allocation procedure anymore, but rather allocates patients to treatments such that balance is created within blocks of consecutive patients usually sized 6 to 10. To mask the block size (to avoid the investigator can predict the next treatment to administer), the block size is often taken random. Note that any randomization procedure that allocates patients within a center is called a *stratified randomization procedure* with center as stratum.

The with *adaptive randomization*, also discussed in the section on "Adaptive designs," the probability of allocation to one of the treatment arms may change over time. *Minimization* is an example of an adaptive allocation procedure that allocates subjects to treatments such that in a dynamic way, the imbalance of a set of a priori chosen covariates is minimized. For example, when the gender distribution is aimed to be balanced, the next male will be allocated to treatment B when the proportion of males is higher in the treatment arm A. The method is basically deterministic but can be given a stochastic flavor by adding a random component. Adaptive randomization can also be based on the response. In that case, more patients will be dynamically allocated to the winning treatment arm.

Note that randomization guarantees only that there is balance between the treatment groups for large samples. But, there is always the possibility of a random imbalance. Covariate adjustment, via using a regression model containing baseline covariates, can then, besides increasing the power, also remove the random imbalance and thereby improve the interpretability of the results.

Further, note that it does not make sense to statistically compare two randomized treatment groups at baseline with *P*-values since at baseline the patients are only different in the label they received from the trialist (A or B).

In practice, patients are allocated using any of the above procedures in combination with an automated (computerized) allocation system connected to either the Internet or a telephone. For example, the interactive voice response system (IVRS) is a multi-language automated telephone system that allocates patients to different treatments, which can accommodate stratified randomization.

While randomization ensures balanced treatment arms at the start, blinding the treatment allocation to all parties of the RCT will avoid bias due to knowledge of which treatment was delivered. The terms "single blind" and "double blind" are often used to indicate that only the patient (single blind) or both the patient and clinician (double blind) are masked, but double blinding often means that basically everyone involved in the study is blinded during the conduct of the study. While double-blinded studies are the gold standard procedure, for some interventions, any blinding may be hard to achieve. For example, suppose that two knee-replacement surgical techniques are compared in one RCT, then blinding the surgeons will be impossible. On the other hand, there is a way out by appointing an evaluator (different from the treating surgeons) who is blinded to the administered treatment.

Study Designs

In this section, various designs for RCTs are discussed. Focus will be on superiority trials, but what is discussed equally applies to non-inferiority trials.

Single-Center Versus Multicenter Studies

A multicenter trial is a clinical trial conducted at more than one medical center or clinic. Most large clinical trials, particularly phase III trials, are conducted in several clinical research centers. The organizational aspects with single-center studies are considerably simpler than with multicenter studies. A simple illustration of this is that stratified randomization is required for multicenter studies, while simple randomization may readily work for single-center studies. Multicenter studies are recommended whenever it takes too much time for a single center to recruit the necessary number of patients. Such studies may also considerably increase the external validity of the RCT. Statistical methods for multicenter studies are somewhat more involved. While they should incorporate the stratification factor center, in practice, it is often and wrongly ignored. With a small number of centers, a Mantel-Haenszel-type test (see chapter "Methodological issues relevant to observational studies, registries, and administrative health databases in rheumatology") could be used or a regression model with each center as binary covariate (called fixed effects model). With many centers, a mixed effects model may be used with center represented by a random intercept, but there is no consensus on which model is preferable [14].

Parallel-Group Versus Cross-Over Designs

Most popular is the *parallel-group design* whereby patients are randomly assigned to one of two (or more) treatment regimens and are followed up in time. It is a simple design, which is almost always possible to implement. The statistical analysis is often also straightforward involving only standard statistical tests such as the chi-square test for binary outcomes, the unpaired *t*-test for continuous outcomes, a *log-rank test* for survival outcomes, etc.; see chapter "A review of statistical approaches for the analysis of data in rheumatology".

On the other hand, in a *cross-over design* involving treatments A and B, each patient receives more than one treatment in a random order. Namely, one group of patients receives the treatment sequence A-B and the other group receives treatment sequence B-A. More complex allocations with more switches such as ABBA, BABA, etc. and more than two treatment arms are possible. This design has the advantage over the parallel group design in that within-patient treatment comparisons become possible by this method. This, in turn, removes a major portion of the intersubject variability and therefore commonly achieves a higher power than the parallel-arm design (with equal number of patients recruited). However, the cross-over design is only applicable in diseases where the patients return to their initial condition upon withdrawal of the study medication. This happens, for instance, when examining the effect of beta-blockers in treating hypertensive patients. An important issue with cross-over designs is that the effect of the first period treatment may leak into the second period and cause a *carry-over effect* (also called *cross-over effect*). In drug trials, this problem can be solved by inserting a *washout* period between the two treatment periods.

Cross-over designs are typically used in phase II trials, while parallel group designs are regularly applied in phase II and phase III studies. Both designs can be used in a single- and multicenter setting, but single-center cross-over studies are more frequent. Finally, we note that the statistical tests for the analysis of cross-over trials are extensions of the tests seen in chapter "A review of statistical approaches for the analysis of data in rheumatology" for paired data. A comprehensive treatment of cross-over designs can be found in [15].

Factorial Designs

Factorial designs aim to examine the effects of two interventions simultaneously. In [16], an RCT with a factorial design was set up to examine the effect of patient-administered assessment tools for pain and disability, on the one hand, and an unsupervised home-based exercise program alone, on the other hand, or their combination on the symptoms of osteoarthritis. In that trial, the rheumatologists were assigned to four groups according to the treatment given to the patient: (1) patient-administered assessment tools, (2) or more exercises, (3) both tools and exercises, or (4) usual care. The aim was to check whether exercises have an impact on the symptoms and also whether the assessment tools gave a better insight to the necessary treatment to also reduce symptoms. In addition, it was of interest to know whether the two or more interventions work synergistically when combined. Factorial designs are analyzed using 2-way ANOVA approaches when the response is continuous or with logistic regression models for binary or ordinal responses with interaction terms (see chapter "Evidence-based medicine in rheumatology: how does it differ from other diseases?").

The Cluster-Randomized Design

In the abovementioned study [16], the rheumatologists and not the patients were randomized to treatments. In the case of the *cluster-randomized design*, all patients in a center are randomly assigned to the same treatment with the expectation that in another center all patients will be randomized to the alternative medication by other doctors. This design may be needed when it is not practical or ethical to randomize patients within a center, which was the case in [16]. In that study, the cluster-randomized design was chosen because the investigators were convinced that one could not insist that one physician advises one patient to do physical exercises and not give the same advice to other patients. Therefore, each rheumatologist was to enroll four patients with osteoarthritis. Since the response of the four patients assigned to a rheumatologist is more alike than for the patients assigned to another rheumatologist, there is more clustering in the data as compared to what is seen in standard multicenter studies. This almost inevitable clustering must be taken into account at the design stage (increasing the sample size compared to a design without clustering) and at the analysis stage. Specialized statistical methodology has been developed for cluster-randomized designs [17, 18] to account for the correlation between outcomes within a cluster.

Group Sequential Designs

It may be of interest for ethical and/or commercial reasons to evaluate the results of an RCT at an interim time. However, such interim analyses cannot be done ad hoc; there are statistical issues with repeated testing (multiple testing), and it would be impractical not to know in advance when cleaned data ready for inspection should be available. Regulatory authorities require indeed a correction for multiple testing. However, not all interim analyses deserve a statistical penalty. There are three types of interim analyses: (1) administrative interim analyses, (2) interim analyses for safety, and (3) interim analyses for efficacy. Such analyses are typically evaluated by an external committee called the Data Monitoring Committee (DMC) (also called Data and Safety Monitoring Board (DSMB)) consisting of two to four clinicians and one independent statistician. The purpose of an *administrative interim analysis* is to evaluate whether the study, up to that time point, has been conducted according to the plan. If the number of patients enrolled has been too few, the DMC may suggest including more centers in the study or to relax the inclusion and exclusion criteria. With an administrative interim analysis, there is no statistical penalty.

Interim analyses for safety are necessary for RCTs where there is a risk for life-threatening adverse events. In such an interim analysis, the DMC reviews safety and other data (e.g., demographic data, data on past medication use, etc.) in a semi-blinded (only the labels A and B are given, not the actual treatments) or unblinded manner. Again, no correction for multiple testing is required, since the treatments are not compared for efficacy.

Interim analyses for efficacy involve repeated statistical comparisons between the administered treatments with the aim to see whether the study can be stopped early for efficacy. A correction for multiple testing is required to avoid producing spurious conclusions. Correction for multiple testing is done with dedicated procedures that devote at each interim analysis a part of the overall significance level α (often equal to 0.05) such that together they amount to α. The methods look similar to the Bonferroni correction, but here, they capitalize on the staggered data presented at the DMC meetings. They are therefore called *group sequential designs,* but in contrast to Bonferroni correction, their global significance level is exactly the a priori defined α. A group sequential design allows stopping the study when the results become convincing enough. In that case, the number of patients needed enroll will be less than originally planned. However, the originally planned (maximal) sample size will be larger with planned interim analyses because the correction for multiple testing inflates the sample size. Pocock's method [19] was one of the first group sequential designs. The procedure specifies an equal, more stringent, significance level at each interim analysis, e.g., for $\alpha = 0.05$ and 5 analyses (4 interim and one final analysis), the study can only be stopped when the *P*-value is smaller than 0.016. Nowadays, the O'Brien-Fleming [14] design is more popular. For this design, a very stringent significance level is used in the early part of the study making it hard to stop early, but is then relaxed towards the end of the study. The timing of the repeated analyses with group sequential designs can be *calendar-driven* or *event-driven*; they must however be specified at the start of the study. A more flexible design was proposed by Lan and DeMets [14], which allows flexible timing and number of analyses, called the *alpha spending approach*. This is now the most popular approach because of its flexibility and has been extended in various ways, e.g., to non-inferiority studies, to cluster-randomized designs, etc. Note that these designs can be also used to monitor safety.

The second type of interim analysis for efficacy checks whether there is a reasonable chance that the study will be positive at the end. Such an analysis, called *futility analysis*, aims to avoid wasting financial resources in a study that has little chance to show a beneficial effect of the experimental treatment. The need for correction for multiple testing is, in this instance, negligible, since now the trial cannot be stopped when at interim the experimental arm shows much better efficacy than the control arm.

Adaptive Designs

Adaptive designs are generalizations of the group sequential designs. Examples of adaptive designs are (1) determination of the maximum tolerated dose in a phase I oncology trial, (2) adaptive randomization, (3) sample size reestimation, and (4) adaptive seamless designs. Below, we briefly elaborate on some of these examples but refer to [5, 20] for more details and references. Adaptive designs are sometimes referred to as flexible designs, but the latter incorporate both planned and unplanned features, while the first must be described in detail at the start of the study and must ensure that the probability for a Type 1 error is addressed.

In phase I oncology trials, there is the *continual reassessment method* (CRM) [5, 28], which is a Bayesian approach to determine the maximum tolerated dose of the test drug. It involves assuming a model for the relationship between the dose and the probability of an unacceptable side effect. The maximal dose that a new patient can be administered is determined via the (Bayesian posterior) probability of causing an unacceptable adverse effect.

Adaptive randomization is an allocation rule whereby the allocation probabilities depend on covariate imbalance and/or response imbalance (see section "Randomization and blinding" for more details).

Establishing the sample size of a study is not an easy task, always prone to misjudgment. In section "Sample size calculations," we show how sample size estimation is done in practice and indicate possible difficulties in establishing a well-motivated choice. It seems reasonable to roughly guess the sample size of a pilot portion of the trial data and then reestimate the sample size for the whole trial based on this. This is done in a calibrated *internal pilot design*, which is a two-stage design with no interim testing for efficacy but only estimating the nuisance parameters (say common standard deviation for an unpaired *t*-test) from the first-stage data. This approach does not necessitate a correction in the projected Type I error rate.

Traditionally, phase II and phase III trials are set up in two distinct stages. Since this may delay regulatory approval, statisticians have looked for ways to speed up the approval of experimental treatments. One way is to rapidly move from phase II to phase III studies, in fact in a seamless manner. This is done in an *adaptive seamless design* that combines the data of the two stages for the final analysis. For example, one trial could consist in choosing between two doses of a drug in the first stage, while in the second stage, the chosen dose is compared to a control group.

Adaptive designs have recently gained a lot of popularity. However, they are considerably more complex not only from a statistical viewpoint but also from an organizational viewpoint, needing a much more sophisticated clinical trial infrastructure.

Sample Size Calculations

The sample size calculation is an essential part of any RCT. It attempts to minimize the risk of not detecting the aimed effect (if present) of the experimental treatment vis-à-vis the control treatment. Ultimately, a statistical test determines the necessary sample size and is a quite technical job that most often requires a computer program. The computation of the sample size for a classical (superiority) unpaired *t*-test goes as follows: (1) fix the overall significance (two-sided) level α (usually=0.05) and the power (at least 0.80); (2) choose the clinically relevant difference Δ_S (not the difference that we expect but the difference that we aim for); (3) make an educated guess about the common standard deviation σ; and (4) the sample size in each treatment arm is then the result of the equation $n=\left(t_{2n-2,a/2}+t_{2n-2,a/2}\right)^2/\Delta_S^2$, with $t_{2n-2,-/2}$ is the $\alpha/2$ quantile of a t-distribution with $2n-2$ degrees of freedom.

These steps illustrate a few important things for computing the sample size:

- Clinicians must have a good idea of the effect they aim to show, i.e., what value for Δ_S to choose, but they do not need to guess what the true effect might be.
- Extra information to perform the computations is usually required. Here, it is the common standard deviation. For the comparison of two proportions, it is the proportion of the control arm.
- The computation of the sample size is in general quite technical, varies from test to test, and usually requires a dedicated computer program.

Note that for a non-inferiority test, Δ_S needs to be replaced by Δ_{NI} and the statistical test needs to be adapted accordingly. For group sequential designs, dedicated programs have been written not only to compute the sample size but also to compute the intermediate significance levels. For more complicated statistical tests, such as for mixed models (see chapter "A review of statistical approaches for the analysis of data in rheumatology") and adaptive designs, often only a simulation computer program may throw light on the required study size. A comprehensive, but technical, reference for sample size calculation is given in [21].

Intention-to-Treat Versus Per-Protocol Analysis

The eligibility criteria specify which of the screened patients will be included in the statistical analysis. However, during the conduct of the study, a lot of deviations from the initial plan may take place. For instance, it may happen that due to an administrative error, a patient who should have been randomized to treatment A in fact received treatment B, or that a patient violates the protocol (takes forbidden concomitant medication), or even drops out from the study, etc. What to do with such patients? One approach is to take in the analysis only the "pure patient population," i.e., only patients who strictly adhere to the instructions. This set of patients is called the *per-protocol (PP) set* and is preferred by many clinicians because it is believed to express best what the effect of the treatment is on the patients. That is true for the patients still included at the end of the study, but not necessarily for all patients randomized. It is rather the *intention-to-treat (ITT) set* that is the standard in RCTs. The ITT principle states that all patients who have been randomized in the study should be included in the analysis according to the planned treatment irrespective of what happened during the conduct of the trial. This principle may appear logical at first but may have some unexpected implications. For instance, patients wrongly allocated to B will be analyzed as if they received treatment A; protocol violators are in the ITT analysis set, also patients dropping out the study will be part of the ITT population, etc. FDA and EMEA prefer the ITT analysis in a superiority trial, because it delivers a conservative result in case of the abovementioned problems during the conduct of the study. While the ITT principle is clear, in practice, it may not always be easy to implement and consequently several versions of an ITT analysis exist. For example, it is not immediately clear how to include patients in an ITT analysis with missing values on the primary endpoint. In that case, the ITT analysis cannot include all randomized subjects. But if some values of the primary response are available, then techniques for imputing missing values allow for including such dropouts. Statistical methods that can deal appropriately with missing data are quite important to guarantee the *internal validity* of the RCT, i.e., that the RCT estimates the true treatment effect in an unbiased manner. An imputation technique that was quite popular for many years but now recognized as problematic is *the last-observation-carried-forward (LOCF) approach*. This imputation technique imputes the last observed value for the missing primary outcome. For example, suppose the total treatment period is 2 years and every 6 months the primary outcome is measured. Then, when a patient drops out at year 1, the imputed value with the LOCF method for the primary outcome at years 1.5 and 2 is equal to the value observed at year 1. The problem with the LOCF approach is that it imputes an unrealistic value for the outcome (not taking into account the natural pattern of the disease and/or of the curing process) and it underestimates the natural variability of the outcome. In [22], more appropriate imputation techniques are discussed.

In an equivalence or non-inferiority study, the ITT analysis is not the primary analysis anymore since the ITT analysis will bias the results and the conclusions towards the desired hypothesis (equivalence or non-inferiority). Because also the PP analysis does not guarantee to provide an unbiased estimate, regulatory agencies require that an ITT and a PP analysis are performed in an equivalence/non-inferiority RCT and that they show consistent results.

RCT and Some Practical Aspects

The *protocol* is the reference manual for the RCT containing the background of the intervention, the reason and motivation for conducting the trial, a review of the phase I and phase II results, the justification of the sample size, the eligibility criteria, and the primary and secondary endpoints. In addition, it contains details of the randomization procedure, the informed consent document, the administration of the interventions, etc.

Furthermore, NIH developed a document, called the *Manual of Procedures* (MOP) (http://www.ninds.nih.gov/research/clinical_research/policies/mop.htm), that transforms a protocol into an operational research project that ensures compliance with federal law and regulations. The MOP typically describes in detail all key ingredients of the conduct of the study, for instance, how data capture will be done, how the patients will be followed up in order to maximize data collection, etc. For example, a list of all eligible patients is never available at the start of an RCT, so the process by which potential trial participants are identified needs to be explicitly stated at the start. In practical terms, this implies that it needs to be specified which countries and centers will be involved in the RCT and what characteristics the involved centers should have.

The protocol also specifies which statistical tests will be chosen for analysis. This can be tricky since many statistical tests depend on distributional assumptions. For instance, the unpaired *t*-test assumes that there is normality in each of the two treatment arms and that the variances are equal. But, one can only test these assumptions when the results roll in. This rigid requirement does not leave much room for creativity, but is needed to preserve the Type I error rate. As an example, suppose that the protocol dictates to choose the unpaired *t*-test but that this test does not yield a significantly better result for the experimental arm while a nonparametric Wilcoxon rank-sum test (see chapter "A review of statistical approaches for the analysis of data in rheumatology") does. Hand switching from one statistical test to another only on the basis of the obtained *P*-value is an example of a data dredging exercise, which is known to produce many spurious results. In a RCT, all statistical activities should be described in even more detail than discussed in *the statistical analysis plan* (SAP). The SAP is typically finalized prior to locking the database to avoid speculative choices of statistical procedures.

Trial participants must be fully aware of the risks and benefits of participation and therefore must fill in an *informed consent* form. This document is also part of the trial protocol.

Finally, each protocol of a RCT needs to be approved by the *Medical Ethical Committee* of the centers where the study is conducted; they are also called *Institutional Review Boards* in the United States. In addition, in order to avoid difficulties when applying for registration, protocols are nowadays often discussed with the regulatory bodies to obtain approval (not the drug!) prior to the start of the RCT.

Reporting the Results of a RCT

The statistical analysis plan specifies in detail which statistical tests need to be chosen. No doubt this is accordingly reported in the registration file for the experimental drug, but this is not necessarily the case for the scientific paper written after the study is finalized. Indeed, most referees of medical journals do not check the consistency of the technical report with the submitted paper. Hence, in principle, the reader cannot be sure that the analysis described in the scientific paper is an exact reflection of what has been specified in the protocol. For example, a recently published phase III trial compared pazopanib with sunitinib with respect to progression-free survival in renal-cell carcinoma patients [23]. In that paper, the authors state that "the results of the progression-free survival analysis in the per-protocol population were consistent with the results of the primary analysis" without providing further details. However, from the technical report, one can infer that the predefined margin of non-inferiority (<1.25) was only met for the ITT population and not for the PP population. This is in conflict with the requirement that in both analysis sets, non-inferiority must be claimed (see also [24]).

Subgroup analyses have been a topic of discussion already for many years. Next to the global analysis, clinicians wish to know which patients (if any) may benefit most from the experimental treatment (if any). Therefore, subsequent to a global primary analysis, often the treatments are compared in a variety of subgroups, e.g., within the group of patients (a) below 65 years of age, (b) above 65 years of age, (c) males, (d) females, etc. This is a typical example of data dredging, especially because there is often no strong clinical background why in a particular subgroup the experimental treatment should do much better. Subgroup analyses are sometimes prespecified in the protocol, but that does not alleviate the problem much. Subgroup analyses can be thought provoking, but should always be considered as exploratory analyses for which the conclusions need to be verified with a new study or in a meta-analysis.

RCTs Versus Observational Studies

In chapter "Methodological issues relevant to observational studies, registries, and administrative health databases in rheumatology" it is seen that the major difference of the observational study with the RCT is that in the observational study, the groups are self-selected. This causes the groups to be different at baseline. The problem is now that there is no way to guarantee that the difference in disease outcome may not be a result of an existing difference at the start of the study. Hence, it is said that an observational study has in general a relatively low internal validity. Regression methods (including the method of propensity scores, see chapter "Methodological issues relevant to observational studies, registries, and administrative health databases in rheumatology") may improve the internal validity by correcting for baseline imbalance, but one can never rule out a residual imbalance caused by unobserved characteristics of the patients. On the other hand, randomization and blinding alone do not guarantee that an RCT has a high internal validity. Indeed, the internal validity can be highly affected by missing values and dropouts. For example, if in one treatment group, patients drop out because of inefficacy of the treatment, while in the other treatment group patients drop out because of safety concerns, then the estimated treatment effect at the end of the RCT is likely not to be a good estimate of the true treatment effect based on all patients who should have been treated.

In an observational study, a heterogeneous group of subjects is included. This is in contrast to an RCT where a homogeneous group of patients is aimed at. This implies that an observational study has a higher external validity than a RCT.

In [25], the factors that cause the low external validity of the RCT are discussed; see also [26]. The author discusses the impact of the general settings of the trial (e.g., the country or countries in which the study is executed), the eligibility criteria of the patients, the difference between the trial protocol and routine practice, etc. Further, the author recommends a thorough consideration of factors which might interfere with the generalizability of the RCT findings to the clinical practice (see also chapter "Limitations of traditional randomized controlled clinical trials in rheumatology").

The Bayesian Approach to RCTs

In chapter "A review of statistical approaches for the analysis of data in rheumatology" the Bayesian approach to inference was introduced. The main difference with the classical (also called frequentist) approach is that the posterior distribution and its summary measures make up the inference, instead of the *P*-value. For instance, in the frequentist approach, the conservation of the overall Type I error is the motivation to develop the group sequential designs that allow for interim analyses in a calibrated manner. A Bayesian approach in this case consists in repeatedly evaluating the posterior probability that the experimental treatment is better than the control treatment and stops either when the planned number of patients was recruited or that posterior probability was, say, greater than 0.975. An alternative Bayesian approach is to let the stopping rule based on the posterior predictive probability, generate future samples (combined with the already sampled subjects), and determine the predictive probability of a significant result (with a classical test), as was done in [27]. Yet another example of a Bayesian approach is an interim analysis that exploits prior information on the drug (say from phase II and III studies) when monitoring the safety of the drug for a rare event in a phase III study.

The *Bayesian adaptive approach*, i.e., counterpart of the frequentist adaptive approach, is gaining much popularity. While the frequentist approach aims to maintain the overall Type I error rate, the Bayesian approach monitors the more intuitive posterior probabilities (which could be a few in a complex design). We refer to [28] for a recent but a technical review of this topic.

The Bayesian approach has been widely accepted in phase I studies, as mentioned above, and is becoming increasingly popular in phase II studies. Yet in a phase III study, this approach is more used for interim and auxiliary analyses, and there is great resistance against its use for the primary analysis. However, I predict that when combined with non-informative priors, the Bayesian approach will likely become one of the options for a phase III study if the investigator can show its good frequentist properties. Note that in medical device trials, it has now become one of the standard approaches. See the NIH website on guidelines for the use of Bayesian methods for medical devices:http://

www.fda.gov/medicaldevices/deviceregulationand guidance/guidancedocuments/ucm071072.htm

Conclusions

After its introduction in the 1940s, the RCT remains the only study type that allows for causal relationships between risk factors and disease outcome. However, that does not mean it is the only study type useful for this. The often limited external validity, and the difficulty to keep the internal validity high, requires considering alternative study types more explored in chapter "Methodological issues relevant to observational studies, registries, and administrative health databases in rheumatology" in the context of using registries and administrative data bases.

There are many excellent textbooks on RCTs. For an accessible introduction for clinicians, there is the standard book of Pocock [29] and the more recent book by Senn [30].

References

1. Lesaffre E, Feine J, Leroux B, Declerck D, editors. Statistical and methodological aspects of oral health research. New York: Wiley; 2009.
2. Medical Research Council. Streptomycin treatment of pulmonary tuberculosis. Br Med J. 1948;2:769–82.
3. Spilker BL. Guide to clinical studies and developing protocols. New York: Raven; 1984.
4. Pong A, Chow S-C, editors. Handbook of adaptive designs in pharmaceutical and clinical development. Boca Raton: CRC Press; 2011.
5. Chin R. Adaptive and flexible clinical trials. Boca Raton: CRC Press; 2012.
6. White B, Bauer EA, Goldsmith LA, et al. Guidelines for clinical trials in systemic sclerosis (sleroderma). Arthritis Rheum. 1995;38:351–60.
7. Bingham III CO, Sebba AI, Rubin BR, et al. Efficacy and safety of etoricoxib 30 mg and celecoxib 200 mg in the treatment of osteoarthritis in two identically designed, randomized, placebo-controlled, non-inferiority studies. Rheumatology. 2007;46:496–507.
8. Lesaffre E. Superiority, equivalence and non-inferiority trials. Bull NYU Hosp Jt Dis. 2008; 66(2):150–4.
9. Rothmann MD, Wiens BL, Chan ISF. Design and analysis of non-inferiority trials. Boca Raton: CRC Press; 2012.
10. Tugwell P, Boers M, Brooks P, Simon L, Strand V, Idzerda L. OMERACT: an international initiative to improve outcome measurement in rheumatology. Biomed Cent. 2007;8:38. 1–6.
11. Pillemer SR, Tilley B. Clinical trials, outcome measures, and response criteria. J Rheumatol. 2004;31:407–10.
12. Booth CM, Eisenhauer EA. Progression-free survival: meaningful or measurable. J Clin Oncol. 2012;30(10):1030–3.
13. Lassere MN, Johnson KR, Boers M, et al. Definitions and validation criteria for biomarkers and surrogate endpoints: developments and testing of a quantitative hierarchical levels of evidence schema. J Rheumatol. 2007;34:607–15.

14. Senn S. Some controversies in planning and analyzing multi-centre trials. Stat Med. 1998;17: 1753–65.
15. Byron J, Kenward MG. Design and analysis of cross-over trials. 2nd ed. Boca Raton: Chapman and Hall/CRC; 2003.
16. Ravaud P, Giraudeau B, Logaert I, et al. Management of osteoarthritis (OA) with an unsupervised home based exercise programme and/or patient administered assessment tools. A cluster randomized controlled trial with a 2×2 factorial design. Ann Rheumatol Dis. 2004;63:703–8.
17. Donner A, Klar N. Design and analysis of cluster randomization trials in health research. London: Arnold; 2000.
18. Murray DM. Design and analysis of group-randomized trials. New York: Oxford University Press; 1998.
19. Jennison C, Turnbull BW. Group sequential methods with applications to clinical trials. Boca Raton: CRC Press; 2000.
20. Kairalla JA, Coffey CS, Thomann MA, Muller KE. Adaptive trial designs: a review of barriers and opportunities, Biomed Cent. 2012;13:145. http://www.trialsjournal.com/content/13/1/145.
21. Julious SA. Sample sizes for clinical trials. Boca Raton: CRC Press; 2009.
22. Molenberghs G, Kenward MG. Missing data in clinical studies. Chichester: Wiley; 2007.
23. Motzer RJ, Hutson TE, Cella D, et al. Pazopanib versus sunitinib in metastatic renal-cell carcinoma. N Engl J Med. 2013;369:722–31.
24. Casper J, Schumann-Binarsch B, Köhne C-H: Letter to the Editor to Motzer RJ, Hutson TE, Cella D, et al. Pazopanib versus sunitinib in metastatic renal-cell carcinoma. N Engl J Med. 2013;369:1969.
25. Rothwell PM. External validity of randomized controlled trials: "to whom do the results of this trial apply?". Lancet. 2005;365:82–93.
26. Pincus T, Sokka T. Should contemporary rheumatoid arthritis clinical trials be more like standard patient care and vice versa. Ann Rheum Dis. 2004;63(Suppl II):ii32–9.
27. Buzdar AU, Ibrahim NK, Francis D, et al. Significantly higher pathologic complete remission rate after neoadjuvant therapy with trastuzumab, paclitaxel, and epirubicin chemotherapy: results of a randomized trial in human epidermal growth factor receptor 2–positive operable breast cancer. J Clin Oncol. 2005;23(16):3676–85.
28. Berry SM, Carlin BP, Lee JJ, Müller P. Bayesian adaptive methods for clinical trials. Boca Raton: CRC Press; 2011.
29. Pocock SJ. Clinical trials: a practical approach. Chichester: Wiley; 1987.
30. Senn S. Statistical issues in drug development. 2nd ed. New York: Wiley; 2008.

Limitations of Traditional Randomized Controlled Clinical Trials in Rheumatology

Theodore Pincus

Introduction

The randomized controlled clinical trial is appropriately regarded as the most rigorous method to document the efficacy of a therapy compared to another therapy or a placebo. A clinical trial allows isolation of a single variable, the test therapy, mimicking a laboratory "scientific experiment" [1]. This approach conforms to a "biomedical model" [2], the dominant paradigm of contemporary medicine. In recent years, the randomized controlled clinical trial often has been regarded in the medical literature as the *only* approach to assess the value of a new therapy according to "evidence-based medicine" [3]. However, randomized trials have many limitations, some of which are summarized in this chapter.

The earliest randomized controlled trials were conducted in the 1940s in infectious diseases such as tuberculosis [4, 5]. Clinical trials in infectious diseases have advantages over those in many other diseases, particularly chronic diseases, for several reasons. First, the target of the medication involves simple unicellular pathogens such as bacteria or fungi, rather than complex mammalian cells. Therefore, any efficacious antibiotic medication without an adverse effect is likely to benefit *all* individuals infected by the pathogen that is the target of the medication. By contrast, much greater variation is seen in responses of individuals to medications which affect mammalian cells, as seen in chronic rheumatic diseases. Second, results of a therapy in an infectious disease generally are apparent over days, weeks, or sometimes months, in contrast to years and even decades in chronic rheumatic diseases. For example, superior efficacy of penicillin versus placebo for a streptococcal sore throat can be documented definitively after 10–14 days of treatment in

T. Pincus, MD (✉)
Division of Rheumatology, Rush University Medical Center,
1611 West Harrison Street, Chicago, IL 60612, USA
e-mail: tedpincus@gmail.com

H. Yazici et al. (eds.), *Understanding Evidence-Based Rheumatology*,
DOI 10.1007/978-3-319-08374-2_8

all infected individuals, while treatment effects in a chronic rheumatic disease vary among individuals and even may indicate efficacy or no differences from placebo in groups after 6–24 months, but different outcomes after 5–10 years, as discussed in detail below.

Rheumatic diseases, as well as most noninfectious diseases, do not involve "foreign" cells as in infectious disease or chemicals that require eradication to restore homeostasis. Rheumatic diseases involve a dysregulation of normal cells and/or chemicals which may be over- or underproduced due to faulty internal signals. Similar pathogenetic mechanisms based on dysregulations are seen in many common chronic diseases such as hypertension, hyperlipidemia, or diabetes. The natural history of an untreated dysregulation is organ damage to blood vessels, kidneys or joints, or other organs.

Infectious diseases are "curable" through eradication of a foreign pathogen. By contrast, dysregulatory diseases are *incurable*, based on current knowledge. However, *control* of the dysregulation retards or prevents organ damage and indirectly prevents or reduces premature mortality associated with these diseases [6–12]. Nonetheless, long-term indefinite ongoing medication generally is required, since no therapy to eradicate the etiology of the dysregulation is available at this time.

While rheumatic diseases are similar to hypertension, hyperlipidemia, or diabetes in a pathogenesis involving dysregulation of normal components leading to organ damage [13], rheumatic diseases differ from the other diseases in several features. One important difference is that rheumatic diseases are not characterized by a single "gold standard" biomarker such as blood pressure, hemoglobin A1c, bone density, etc., that can be applied to diagnosis, assessment, prognosis, and monitoring of *all individual* patients [14]. Therefore, an index of multiple measures is needed to assess and estimate changes in the clinical status of patients with rheumatic diseases.

The discovery in the 1940s of rheumatoid factor [15, 16] in rheumatoid arthritis (RA), antinuclear antibodies (ANA) [17] in systemic lupus erythematosus (SLE), and other biomarkers led to hopes that laboratory tests could be used effectively for diagnosis and management of all individual patients with RA, SLE, and other rheumatic diseases, similar to other diseases in a traditional "biomedical model." However, more than one-third of patients with RA have a negative test for rheumatoid factor, or anti-cyclic citrullinated peptide (anti-CCP) antibodies (ACPA) [18–21], and more than 40 % have a normal erythrocyte sedimentation rate (ESR) or C-reactive protein (CRP) at presentation [21]. More than one-third of patients with SLE have no detectable anti-DNA antibodies, anti-Smith (anti-Sm), and anti-ribonucleoprotein (anti-RNP), while a positive ANA test is found in least 10 % of the normal population [22–24].

In the absence of a single gold standard measure, as noted, a pooled index [25] is applied to most rheumatic diseases. Formal indices have been developed for RA [26–31], SLE [32–39], vasculitis [40–45], psoriatic arthritis [46–48], ankylosing spondylitis [49–53], and other rheumatic diseases. These indices generally include three types of measures from patient self-report, physical examination, and laboratory tests; data may be included in some indices, particularly in longer studies. The formal indices are used in clinical trials and other clinical research, but not widely in routine clinical care [54, 55].

Inclusion of patient history information and specific physical examination findings, e.g., joint counts, reflects that a patient history and physical examination are more significant in clinical decisions in rheumatic diseases than in many other types of chronic diseases [56]. Information from a patient history may be captured as standardized, "scientific" quantitative data, according to validated self-report questionnaires [57]. Patient questionnaires may be used effectively to guide management, document change in status, assess outcomes, and improve the quality of care in rheumatic diseases, analogous to laboratory tests in other diseases [58]. Inclusion of a specific patient questionnaire at every visit of every patient ensures that some quantitative data are collected at each encounter with minimum effort on the part of the doctor and staff [59].

A contemporary view of "evidence-based medicine" recognizes limitations of clinical trials, as presented in the chapter "Evidence-based medicine in rheumatology: how does it differ from other diseases?" and described in a number of thoughtful reports by several observers [1, 3, 60–81], as well as in some of the author's own commentaries [82–88]. A recent report from the Oxford Centre for Evidence-Based Medicine [60] noted that "While they are simple and easy to use, early hierarchies that placed randomized trials categorically above observational studies were criticized [3] for being simplistic [61]. In some instances, observational studies give us the 'best' evidence [3]. For example, there is a growing recognition that observational studies – even case-series [62] *and anecdotes* [63] can sometimes provide definitive evidence."

Recognition of limitations of clinical trials in no way denies their value as the optimal method to distinguish short- and medium-term treatment effects of a medication from another medication or placebo. Indeed, it might be optimal if most patients with a chronic rheumatic disease would have an opportunity to participate in a randomized controlled clinical trial, because of the largely "experimental" nature of most available treatments. Since a "best" therapy for an individual patient usually is not identified, a health professional must "guess" at the best treatment for most patients. In this situation, the most ethical approach might appear to randomize the patient to one of several treatments, so the individual patient has a chance to experience the "best" treatment for herself/himself [89].

Therefore, it is recognized that the methodology of the randomized controlled clinical trial often provides a framework of an optimal method to evaluate the efficacy of a therapy. However, it also is important to recognize limitations of randomized controlled clinical trials, just as there are limitations to any method to acquire knowledge in medicine or any field. The author's recognition of limitations of clinical trials is based in large part on experience in conducting more than 35 randomized clinical trials.

Limitations of clinical trials are grouped into two categories. Those resulting from issues in practical implementation in modern clinical research are termed *pragmatic* limitations. Other limitations would exist even if all pragmatic limitations could be overcome, but are weaknesses of the methodology (as exist for any methodology, as noted, but often overlooked for clinical trials) and are termed *intrinsic* limitations (Table 1).

Table 1 Pragmatic and intrinsic limitations of clinical trials in chronic rheumatic diseases

Pragmatic limitations of clinical trials	
1	A relatively short time frame in chronic diseases – sometimes too short to identify important clinical benefits or to recognize loss of efficacy
2	Inclusion and exclusion criteria may restrict eligibility to fewer than 10 % of patients with a particular diagnosis who may be considered eligible for a clinical trial
3	Differences between a medication and a placebo are required to be statistically significant but not necessarily robust – statistical significance may indicate only marginal clinical benefit
4	Clinically important differences may not be statistically significant due to insufficient numbers of patients for statistical power
5	Important variables affecting outcomes other than whether a patient was randomized to a medication versus another medication or placebo may be seen – but generally ignored in clinical trial reports
6	Traditional clinical trials with parallel designs have inflexible dosage schedules and restrict concomitant medications, although a flexible dosage schedule toward a target with multiple medications may provide optimal results
7	Surrogate markers and indices used in clinical trials may be suboptimal measures to detect changes in clinical status or predict important clinical outcomes
8	Rare side effects cannot be identified in most trials
Intrinsic limitations of clinical trials	
1	The design can greatly influence results – availability of a control group does not eliminate bias
2	Data are reported in groups – ignore possible substantial variation in groups
3	No absolute criteria for the balance of risk and benefit for the therapy – different individuals may interpret very differently and all be "correct"
4	Loss of a placebo effect in a clinical trial (although gain of more extensive care which may offset and even surpass the usual "placebo effect")

Eight Pragmatic Limitations of Randomized Clinical Trials in Chronic Diseases

Eight types of pragmatic limitations in chronic diseases are summarized below:

1. *The relatively short time frame of clinical trials in chronic diseases.*
   A prominent limitation of clinical trials in chronic diseases involves too short a time frame of observation to recognize meaningful clinical trends that develop only over longer periods. For example, a randomized controlled clinical trial in RA was conducted over 48 weeks to compare results of 3 regimens – methotrexate monotherapy, auranofin (oral gold) monotherapy, and a combination of methotrexate and auranofin [90]. No significant differences were found between results with any of these three regimens (Fig. 1) [90].

   A similar conclusion was reported from a far more extensive meta-analysis of 66 clinical trials reported in 1990 concerning the efficacy of disease-modifying antirheumatic drugs (DMARDs) in the treatment of RA [91] (Fig. 2). This meta-analysis included 117 treatment groups: 11 for antimalarial drugs

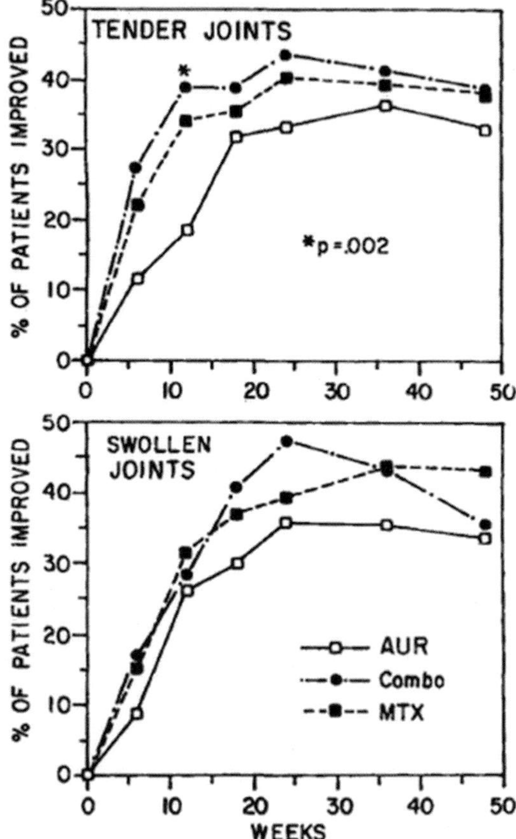

Fig. 1 Results of a randomized clinical trial in 297 patients with rheumatoid arthritis treated with auranofin (*AUR*), methotrexate (*MTX*), or auranofin plus methotrexate (*Combo*) [90]. The figure illustrates percentages of patients with ≥50 % meaningful improvement in tender or swollen joints. Final results showed no significant differences between the three groups over one year

(e.g., hydroxychloroquine), 23 for auranofin, 29 for in efficacy injectable gold, 7 for methotrexate, 19 for d-penicillamine, 6 for sulfasalazine, and 22 for placebo. The meta-analysis indicated no significant differences in efficacy between sulfasalazine, d-penicillamine, methotrexate, and injectable gold (Fig. 2) [91], i.e., that the efficacy of methotrexate for RA was equivalent to hydroxychloroquine, sulfasalazine, d-penicillamine, and injectable gold.

Results of the meta-analysis did not appear translated into actual clinical practice over 5 years in an observational study of duration of treatment courses of DMARDs in 7 rheumatology practices reported in 1992 [92] (Fig. 3, Panel a). Duration of treatment courses in an incurable chronic disease such as RA can serve as a composite measure of effectiveness and safety of a medication. A formal analysis of estimated duration of continuation of 1,083 courses of 6 DMARDs over 60 months in 477 patients with RA indicated that approximately 80 % of methotrexate courses were continued after 2 years, compared to 50 % of courses of hydroxychloroquine, penicillamine, parenteral gold, and azathioprine and only 20 % of courses of oral gold (Fig. 3, Panel a). After 5 years, approximately

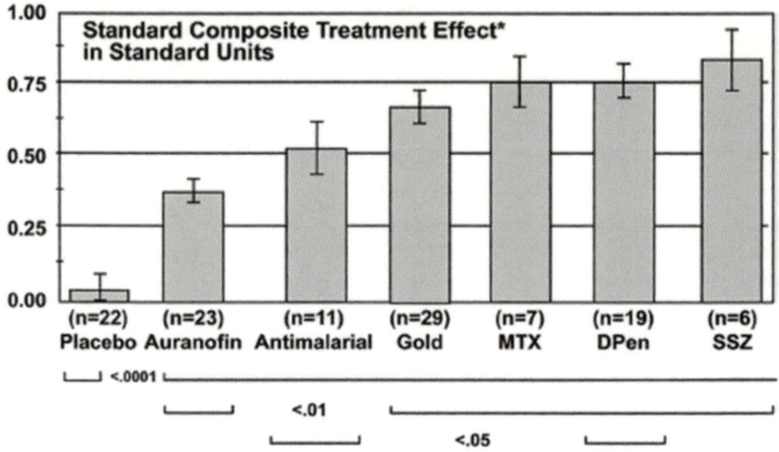

Fig. 2 Standard composite treatment effect (in standard units). Meta-analysis of 66 clinical trials reported in 1990 concerning the efficacy of DMARDs in the treatment of RA [91]. This meta-analysis included 117 treatment groups: 11 for antimalarial drugs (e.g., hydroxychloroquine), 23 for auranofin, 29 for injectable gold, 7 for methotrexate, 19 for d-penicillamine, 6 for sulfasalazine, and 22 for placebo. All drugs have greater efficacy than placebo in the management of RA, determined according to a composite of grip strength (a measure of effectiveness of grip), tender joint count, and erythrocyte sedimentation rate, adjusted for disease duration, trial length, initial tender joint count, and blinding. In these analyses, no significant differences were seen between sulfasalazine, d-penicillamine, methotrexate, and injectable gold (From Felson et al. [91] with permission)

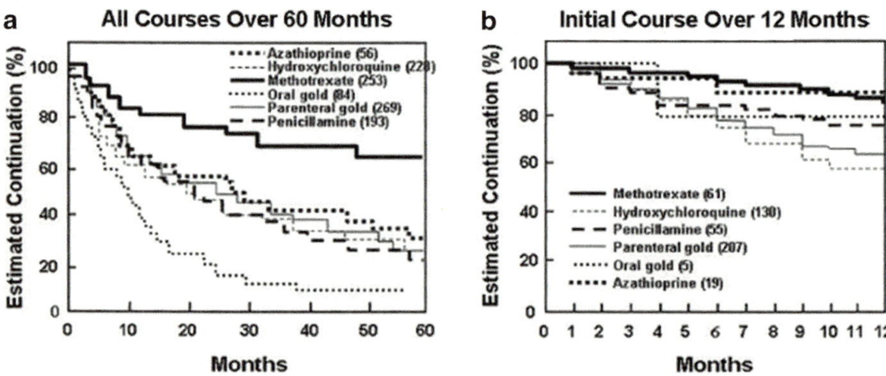

Fig. 3 (**a**) Estimated continuation of all 1,083 courses of DMARDs in 532 patients with rheumatoid arthritis over *60 months*. Differences between methotrexate and all other drugs, as well as between oral gold (auranofin) and all other drugs, are statistically significant ($P<0.001$), while differences among other drugs are not significant. (**b**) Estimated continuation of 477 courses of the *initial* DMARD used in the same 532 patients over *12 months*. Differences between methotrexate versus oral gold (auranofin) are not statistically significant and are considerably less apparent than in A, in which estimated continuation was studied for *all* courses over *60 months* [92]

60 % of the methotrexate courses were continued versus approximately 20 % of the hydroxychloroquine, penicillamine, parenteral gold, and azathioprine courses, and virtually no course of oral gold (Fig. 3, Panel a) [92].

The data from the observational study were analyzed over only *1 year* for the *initial* 447 DMARD courses, conditions that mimic clinical trials (Fig. 3, Panel b), in contrast to the above analyses of *all* DMARD courses over *5 years* (Fig. 3, Panel a) [92]. Continuation rates of courses of all 6 DMARDs were similar, including no difference between methotrexate versus parenteral versus oral gold (auranofin) (Fig. 3, Panel b), as seen in the clinical trial (Fig. 1).

The absence of statistically significant differences between DMARD courses over 1 year (seen in Fig. 3b) mimics results of clinical trials in Figs. 1 and 2 but differs considerably from the results seen in actual clinical care over 5 years (Fig. 3a). Therefore, results of both the clinical trials and observational study are accurate and "correct." However, the accurate data in the clinical trials and meta-analysis were not translated into long-term clinical care over 5 years, and the clinical trial results were *not* applicable to routine clinical care.

These observations suggest caution in interpretation of data from clinical trials to physicians for routine care. Nonetheless, in 2008 (16 years after publication of the report of differences between results of clinical trials and clinical care [90]), a "systematic review" of DMARDs in the principal journal for internists, *Annals of Internal Medicine*, concluded that there was "moderate evidence that sulfasalazine, leflunomide, and methotrexate were equivalent in efficacy, with no obvious major differences in adverse events and discontinuation rates among these three DMARDs" [93].

This conclusion differs from contemporaneous clinical care in the international QUEST-RA database of many countries (Table 2), in which methotrexate was taken by 83 % of patients, sulfasalazine by 43 %, leflunomide by 21 %, and biological agents by 23 % [94]. These patterns were seen in countries in which patients do not pay for medications [94], so they could be explained only in small part on the basis of costs. A strict methodologist may conclude that the clinicians were in error and not practicing "evidence-based medicine," since the systematic review concluded that the three agents were similar in efficacy and adverse events. However, if the conclusion of the systematic review were accurate, comparable usage of the 3 DMARDs might be expected in routine care, but that is not seen. These findings again indicate that data from short-term clinical trials may provide less accurate information about long-term results of therapies than long-term observational studies, as a result of limitations of the clinical trial methodology [87].

Limitations of a short time frame also are seen in a trial conducted in patients with polymyositis to compare therapeutic efficacy of a combination of prednisone plus azathioprine versus prednisone monotherapy (plus placebo) [95, 96]. The initial report concerning this clinical trial indicated no differences between the two groups after 3 months of treatment, according to three measures, i.e., days to normalize the creatinine phosphokinase (CPK) muscle enzyme, change in the muscle strength score, and reduction of inflammation on the muscle biopsy

Table 2 The use of disease-modifying antirheumatic drugs (DMARDs) in the QUEST-RA countries

Country	Delay to start DMARDS, months, median	DMARD exposure years, mean	Selected DMARDs ever taken; percentage of patients in the QUEST-RA study per country					
			Prednisone (%)	MTX (%)	HCQ (%)	SSZ (%)	LEF (%)	Any biological agent (%)
Argentina	13	3.7	83	68	49	***6***	16	3
Denmark	10	7.9	43	85	39	64	11	23
Finland	7	14.4	74	85	**74**	**84**	21	17
France	8	9.9	83	86	55	49	**42**	**53**
Germany	15	8.4	54	78	30	36	25	29
Ireland	11	6.3	71	**92**	***15***	33	24	41
Italy	9	7.1	69	79	42	14	31	26
The Netherlands	5	8.1	***26***	91	28	35	6	19
Poland	4	7.2	69	87	34	60	18	8
Serbia	11	6.6	**88**	69	55	17	7	***2***
Spain	14	7.3	67	82	43	29	34	27
Sweden	12	8.8	66	83	34	62	9	31
Turkey	12	8.9	69	88	27	61	22	7
UK	12	7.9	51	***67***	39	46	***4***	16
USA	9	7.9	77	85	49	12	19	33
Total	9	8.1	66	83	41	43	21	23

Adapted from Sokka et al. [94]
The highest percentage for each drug is indicated in bold and the lowest in bold italics
DMARD disease-modifying antirheumatic drug, *HCQ* hydroxychloroquine, *LEF* leflunomide, *MTX* methotrexate, *QUEST-RA* Quantitative Standard Monitoring of Patients with Rheumatoid Arthritis, *SSZ* sulfasalazine

Table 3 Comparison of results in treatment of polymyositis with prednisone + azathioprine versus prednisone + placebo over 3 years according to functional grade disability [96]

Treatment	Functional grade disability		
	Onset	1 Year*	3 Years*
Prednisone + azathioprine	4.5	3.0	2.1
Prednisone only	4.1	3.6	3.0

Adapted from: Bunch [96]
*$p < 0.01$

[95]. The authors concluded that "in a controlled, prospective, randomized, double-blind study…azathioprine does not afford any therapeutic advantage when used in addition to accepted prednisone dosages in the initial management of polymyositis" [95].

The randomized controlled trial was then continued further to 3 years. After 3 years (Table 3), improvement according to functional grade disability was significantly greater for patients treated with the combination of prednisone plus

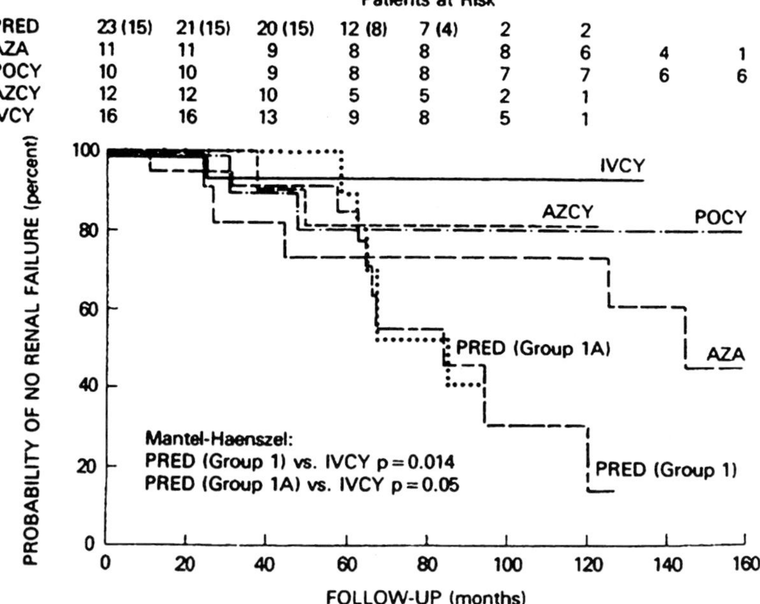

Fig. 4 Probability of maintaining life-supporting renal function in long-term randomized clinical trials of 72 high-risk patients with active SLE nephritis, according to treatment group: *PRED* prednisone, *AZA* azathioprine, *POCY* oral cyclophosphamide, *AZCY* combined oral azathioprine and cyclophosphamide, *IVCY* intravenous cyclophosphamide [97]

azathioprine versus those treated with prednisone monotherapy. In retrospect, differences were seen after 1 year according to functional status, but not according to CPK, muscle strength, or muscle biopsy. The authors concluded that "longer follow-up (3 years) has shown that the group given prednisone plus azathioprine has improved more with respect to functional disability; this group also requires less prednisone for disease control" [96].

These observations illustrate two important principles regarding analyses of treatments in a rheumatic disease: (*a*) Recognition of the possible advantages of combination second-line therapy may require periods of years, rather than months. (*b*) Differences in results of two treatments may be apparent according to measures of functional disability, rather than laboratory or biopsy data, as discussed below (see point 7 concerning surrogate markers). These principles may be relevant to studies of all rheumatic diseases.

A striking example of the importance of a long time frame in a clinical trial to assess treatment of a chronic disease is seen in a trial designed to prevent renal failure in patients with SLE nephritis using several treatment regimens, including prednisone monotherapy versus combinations of prednisone with azathioprine and/or cyclophosphamide (Fig. 4) [97]. Substantial advantages to cyclophosphamide plus prednisone were seen over 10 years, with preservation of renal function in about 90 % of patients versus only about 30 % of patients treated with prednisone monotherapy (Fig. 4). These results established cyclophosphamide as the standard of care for SLE nephritis for at least two decades in the 1980s and 1990s. It is not widely recognized, however, that even after 4 years, renal function was preserved in more than 90 % of patients in all groups, i.e., prednisone monotherapy appeared as effective as the combination with cyclophosphamide (Fig. 4).

As a result of this clinical trial, combination therapy with cyclophosphamide plus prednisone became the standard of cate for SLE nephritis over the next two decades. However, if this trial had been conducted over only a 3-year period or less, *as is the case in more than 98 % of randomized controlled trials in rheumatology*, it would have been concluded that no advantage is seen to the combination of prednisone plus cyclophosphamide over prednisone monotherapy! Only a clinical trial conducted in relatively asymptomatic individuals with support from the intramural program of the United States National Institutes of Health (NIH) allowed 10 years of observation, which would not be possible at most clinical settings to establish a new standard of care.

2. *Inclusion and exclusion criteria may restrict eligibility to fewer than 10 % of patients with a particular diagnosis who may be considered eligible for a clinical trial.*

   In theory, all individuals with a particular diagnosis should be eligible to participate in a clinical trial. This goal is more likely to be met in a short-term trial of an antibiotic to eradicate an infectious agent, rather than for a longer-term (but usually not long enough) trial of a medication that affects primarily mammalian cells. In practice, however, all clinical trials have inclusion and exclusion criteria, designed to ensure that a relatively homogeneous group of patients with sufficient disease activity and without severe confounding comorbidities are studied to document improvement.

   In many, if not most, instances, inclusion criteria are rather stringent, so that only a small fraction of patients are eligible for the trial. For example, inclusion criteria in the Anti-TNF therapy in RA with concomitant therapy (ATTRACT) trial of infliximab – the first trial reported of a biological agent in RA – were found to exclude 95 % of patients seen in 2000 in the author's clinical setting [98] (Fig. 5). The three inclusion criteria were six swollen and six tender joints, met by only about one-third of patients; morning stiffness of 45 min and elevated ESR or CRP (2 of 3), met by only half the patients who had six tender and swollen joints; and a methotrexate dose greater than 12.5 mg per week which was met by only one-third of these patients. Cumulatively, these three basic inclusion criteria allowed only 5 % of RA patients to be eligible for this trial [98] (Fig. 5). Similar data have been reported in other reports [99, 100].

   All clinical trials also list exclusion criteria, as many variables other than assignment to an intervention or a placebo may affect possible outcomes, such as high age, low education level, low or high disease severity, comorbidities, organ damage, fibromyalgia, previous and concomitant interventions, and many others. Exclusion criteria also restrict entry into the trial to certain possible subjects,

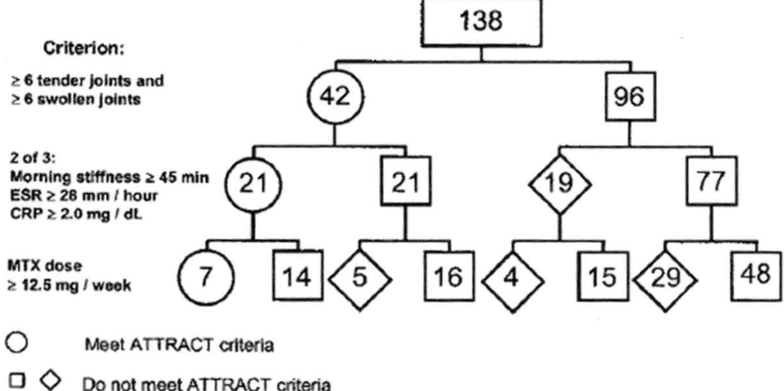

Fig. 5 Analysis of patients with rheumatoid arthritis (RA) who were potential participants in the ATTRACT (anti-tumor necrosis factor α trial in rheumatoid arthritis with concomitant therapy) trial of infliximab plus methotrexate versus methotrexate monotherapy. Of the 152 patients in this consecutive patient cohort, 12 did not have a joint count recorded and another 2 patients were taking etanercept or infliximab at the time of the first joint count and would therefore have been ineligible for the ATTRACT study. Thus, 138 patients were analyzed for meeting the inclusion criteria of the ATTRACT trial: ≥6 tender joints and ≥6 swollen joints; 2 of the following 3 – morning stiffness of ≥45 min, ESR of ≥28 mm/h, or CRP of ≥2 mg/dl; and methotrexate (MTX) dose of ≥12.5 mg/week [98] (From Sokka and Pincus [98] with permission)

in an effort to isolate observed differences to the treatment, and reduce effects of confounding variables.

In theory, the process of randomization should allow adjustment for other variables that might affect the results of a clinical trial. However, in practice, extensive exclusion criteria are common – and compromise the generalizability of results to all patients. For example, many clinicians would treat a patient with RA who is older than 80 years and has a history of breast cancer in remission for 20 years with a biological agent, the efficacy of which was documented in a clinical trial that excluded people who met both criteria for age and comorbidity.

3. *Differences between a medication and a placebo are required to be statistically significant but not necessarily robust – statistical significance may indicate only marginal clinical significance.*

A clinical trial that includes large numbers of patients may indicate that marginal clinical differences are statistically significant. For example, hundreds of clinical trials conducted during the 1970s and early 1980s indicated that various nonsteroidal anti-inflammatory drugs (NSAIDs), such as ibuprofen, naproxen, piroxicam, and diclofenac, led to improvement in RA patients in the number of tender or swollen joints.

The data were highly statistically significant in clinical trials which included relatively large numbers of patients. However, NSAIDs provided only marginal benefits to most patients [101], although a few individual patients experienced great benefit with each of the medications. NSAIDs often are not used at all, or only on an "as needed" basis in contemporary management of RA, although efficacy was documented in dozens of clinical trials.

4. *Clinically important differences may not be statistically significant due to insufficient numbers of patients for statistical power.*
Many important rheumatic conditions are seen in relatively small numbers by any individual health professional. Furthermore, enrollment in a clinical trial may be limited by inclusion and exclusion criteria. For example, during the early 1970s, four randomized controlled clinical trials were conducted in patients with SLE nephritis to compare mortality with combinations of prednisone plus azathioprine versus prednisone monotherapy (plus placebo). Two trials of Donadio et al. [102] and Hahn et al. [103] indicated no significant differences with combination versus prednisone monotherapy, while two others of Sztejnbok et al. [104] and Cade et al. [105] indicated lower mortality in patients treated with a combination of prednisone and azathioprine versus prednisone monotherapy (Table 4). Differences in results may be explained in part by differences in patients selected for the trials, as the two studies in which an advantage was seen to the combination included more patients with diffuse proliferative glomerulonephritis, the type of SLE nephritis with the poorest prognosis.
Many individual trials in rheumatic diseases do not have sufficient statistical power to provide statistically significant conclusions. Such limitations in individual clinical trials in SLE nephritis have been overcome in part by a pooled analysis performed by Felson et al. (Fig. 6) [106]. The pooled analysis of eight studies indicated clear statistically significant advantages to combinations of corticosteroids plus immunosuppressive therapy versus corticosteroids alone in treatment of SLE nephritis (Fig. 6). Enhanced statistical power provided by a pooled analysis may overcome in part limitations of small numbers in individual clinical trials.

Table 4 Analysis of mortality in four randomized controlled clinical trials in SLE nephritis in which treatment with prednisone + azathioprine was compared to prednisone only

	Randomized controlled trials			
Trial characteristics/results	Sztejnbok et al. (1971) [104]	Cade et al. (1973) [105]	Donadio et al. (1974) [102]	Hahn et al. (1975) [103]
Period of observation	3 years	4 years	3 years	2 years
Prednisone monotherapy: % 4-year mortality (in *N* patients)	32 % (19)	73 % (15)	0 % (9)	30 % (13)
Prednisone + azathioprine: % 4-year mortality (in *N* patients)	0 % (16)	46 % (13)	0 % (9)	18 % (11)
Difference statistically significant?	Yes	Yes	No	No
Number with diffuse proliferative glomerulonephritis/total number	24/35	28/28	7/16	14/24

Adapted from Sztejnbok et al. [104], Cade et al. [105], Donadio et al. [102], and Hahn et al. [103]

Fig. 6 Rate of renal deterioration in SLE nephritis patients treated with steroids alone and in those treated with a combination of immunosuppressive drugs and steroids. Each point represents 1 of 8 studies in a pooled analysis performed by Felson et al. [106]

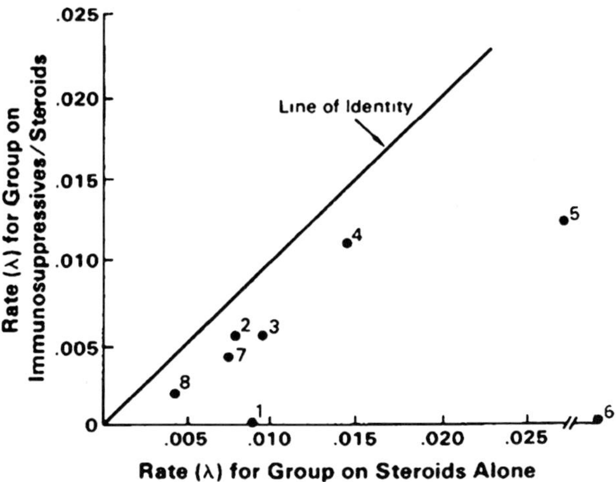

Although "power calculations" are based on sophisticated mathematical computations, implying substantial precision, in actual fact, they must be based on estimates, which may involve incorrect assumptions. Furthermore, many rheumatic diseases are quite unusual, and it may be difficult to identify a sufficient number of patients to participate in the study, even if power calculations are valid. Therefore, many clinical trials may not show an effect simply because there is insufficient statistical power. Enhanced statistical power may be provided by a meta-analysis of many clinical trials, which may overcome in part limitations of small numbers in individual clinical trials [91], but even meta-analysis cannot overcome a short time frame, exclusion criteria, etc., as noted above.

5. *Important variables affecting outcomes other than whether a patient was randomized to a medication versus another medication or placebo may be seen – but usually ignored in reporting of the clinical trial.*

   The basic design of the randomized controlled clinical trial is focused on identifying differences in results using one intervention versus another or a placebo, and reports of results naturally emphasize this comparison. However, in some trials, outcomes are affected more by variables other than whether a patient was randomized to a drug versus another medication or placebo.

   One example of this phenomenon is seen in the Beta-Blocker Heart Attack Trial (BHAT) study, designed to compare treatment with a beta-blocker medication, propranolol, versus placebo, to prevent death from a second heart attack in people who had suffered a recent heart attack [107]. The trial documented that propranolol was more effective than placebo (Fig. 7). However, the patients' level of formal education – a surrogate for self-management, life stress, and social support – was associated with greater differences than medication versus placebo (Fig. 7) [108]. Of note, recognition of differences according to educational level is not nearly as widely known as differences according to the medication versus placebo.

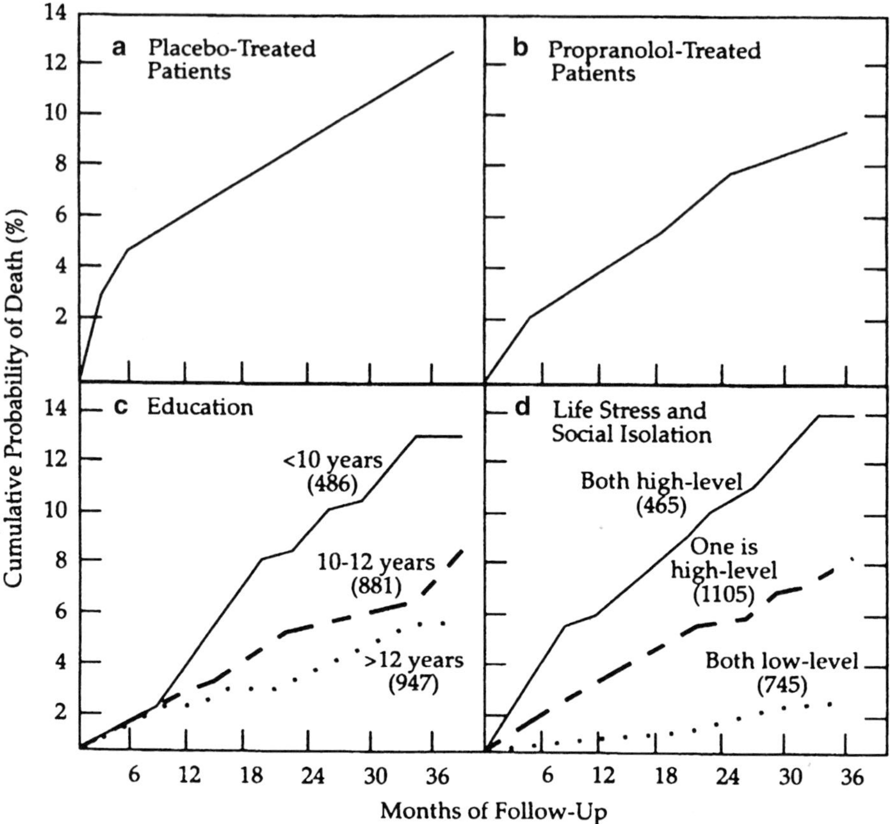

Fig. 7 Life-table cumulative mortality curves in the Beta-Blocker Heart Attack Trial (BHAT) according to (**a**) placebo treatment, (**b**) propranolol treatment, (**c**) education level, and (**d**) life stress and social isolation [108]

Another example of a clinical trial in which other variables were more significant than differences between the medication and placebo involved analysis of clofibrate versus placebo to reduce lipid levels in cardiovascular disease [109]. The 5-year mortality of patients treated with clofibrate was 20 % compared to 21 % in patients treated with placebo, a nonsignificant difference [109] (Table 5). However, 5-year mortality of patients randomized to clofibrate who adhered to their prescriptions was 15 % versus 24 % in nonadherents and virtually identical in patients randomized to placebo 15 % in adherents to placebo versus 28 % in nonadherents (P <0.0001 for adherent vs. nonadherent within each treatment arm) (Table 5). These data indicate that adherence to a treatment regimen was far more powerful to explain a reduction in mortality than whether or not patients were assigned to a lipid-lowering medication versus a placebo.

Table 5 Five-year mortality in patients given clofibrate or placebo, according to cumulative adherence to protocol prescription [109]

	Treatment group			
	Clofibrate		Placebo	
Adherence[a]	*N*	% mortality[b]	*N*	% mortality[b]
<80 %	357	24.6 ± 2.3 % (22.5 %)	882	28.2 ± 1.5 % (25.8 %)
≥80 %	708	15.0 ± 1.3 % (15.7 %)	1,813	15.1 ± 0.8 % (16.4 %)
Total study group	1,065	18.2 ± 1.2 % (18.0 %)	2,695	19.4 ± 0.8 % (19.5 %)

[a]A patient's cumulative adherence was computed as the estimated number of capsules actually taken as a percentage of the number that should have taken according to the protocol during the first 5 years of follow-up or until death (if death occurred during the first 5 years)
[b]The figures in parentheses are adjusted for 40 baseline characteristics. The figures given as percentages ±1 SE are unadjusted figures whose SEs are correcting to within 0.1 unit for the adjusted figures

6. *Traditional clinical trials with a parallel design have inflexible dosage schedules and restrict concomitant medications, although a flexible dosage schedule toward a target with multiple medications may provide optimal results.*
   Contemporary trials designed for registration of new therapies require that a new medication have statistically significantly greater efficacy than a placebo, with an acceptable profile for adverse events, in a parallel design [110]. This type of clinical trial may provide unequivocal documentation that a therapy under study is superior to placebo.

   However, this parallel design does not allow testing combinations of therapies, which are recognized increasingly as optimal for most patients with inflammatory rheumatic diseases [111]. One approach to overcome this limitation involves a "strategy trial," in which patients are treated with combinations of DMARDs versus monotherapy toward a target, generally a disease activity score – DAS [26] or DAS28 [27] – to indicate low disease activity or remission, with a protocol requiring adjustment of treatment at frequent visits.

   Eight "strategy trials" have been reported in RA [112–119] (Table 6), all of which documented significant advantages to intensification of therapies based on careful patient monitoring aimed at a target measure versus traditional therapy that was unchanged over longer periods. All eight trial results indicate that a strategy of aiming for low disease activity or remission appears more important than the agent used [120]. A "treat-to-target" strategy is emerging as the standard of care in RA [121]. Similarly, almost all patients with any inflammatory rheumatic disease are treated with combinations of medications, which cannot be studied optimally in clinical trials which restrict dosage and combinations.
7. *Surrogate markers and indices used in clinical trials may be suboptimal measures to detect changes in clinical status or predict important clinical outcomes.*
   The ultimate goal of treatment for a chronic disease is to prevent or postpone the most feared long-term consequences, such as death and disability, which generally result from poorly controlled dysregulation such as inflammation, leading to

Table 6 "Strategy" tight control clinical trials in rheumatoid arthritis

Study	Participants	Interventions	Outcomes
Pure intensive strategy versus usual care			
Grigor et al. [112]	$N=111$, DAS >2.4, disease duration <5 years	Intensive management: monthly assessment – if DAS >2.4, escalation of therapy according to step-up protocol	*Primary*: proportion of patients with a good response (defined as a DAS <2.4 and a fall in this score from baseline by >1.2)
TICORA study		Routine care: usual rheumatology follow-up	*Secondary*: proportion of patients in remission (DAS <1.6), ACR20/50/70, radiographic progression
2 sites 18-month open-label RCT in Glasgow, Scotland		Intra-articular triamcinolone in all swollen joints	
Fransen et al. [113]	$N=384$ meet 1987 ACR criteria	Conventional treatment	*Primary*: proportion of patients with DAS28 < 3.2 at week 24; *Secondary*: dose changes in individual DMARDs and changes in patient pain, global disease activity, and disability
Multicenter; 6-month cluster RCT at 24 sites; The Netherlands		DAS28 collected at selected visits	
Verstappen et al. [114]	$N=299$ participants meeting the 1987 ACR criteria, disease duration <1 year	Conventional strategy	*Primary*: remission for at least 3 months – no SJC, ≤ 3TJC, ESR ≤20, global VAS ≤20
CAMERA study		Intensive strategy group according to a computer decision program	*Secondary*: improvement in single measures; mean change in disease activity
2-year multicenter open-label strategy trial			
"*Hybrid*": *Initial parallel design treatment groups plus "intensive strategy"*			
Goekoop-Ruiterman et al. [115]	$N=508$ participants meeting the 1987 ACR criteria, ≥6 SJC and TJC, disease duration ≤2 years	Sequential monotherapy	*Primary*: functional capacity by HAQ and radiographic damage by modified Sharp/van der Heijde
BeSt study		Step-up combination MTX + SSZ + HCQ	*Secondary*: ACR20/50/70 and clinical remission defined as DAS44 < 1.6
1 (2–5)-year multicenter RCT in the Netherlands		Initial combination MTX + SSZ + Prednisone	
		Initial combination MTX + infliximab	

(continued)

Table 6 (continued)

Study	Participants	Interventions	Outcomes
Hetland et al. [116]	N=160 participants, disease duration <6 months	MTX+cyclosporine	*Primary*: ACR20 response at 2 years
CIMESTRA study		MTX+placebo	*Secondary*: remission, cumulative dose of betamethasone and radiographic progression
2-year multicenter placebo-controlled double-blind RCT in Denmark		Monthly assessments in both arms, betamethasone injection into all swollen joints; increase dose of MTX and/or cyclosporine by predefined protocol	
Saunders et al. [117]	N=96, DAS28>5.1, disease duration <5 years	"Step-up" SSZ, MTX, HCQ	*Primary*: mean decrease in DAS28 at 12 months
TICORAii		Parallel triple therapy with SSZ+MTX+HCQ	*Secondary*: EULAR good responses; # in remission: ACR20/50/70
12-month RCT at 3 sites in Glasgow		Intra-articular triamcinolone in all swollen joints	
Verschueren et al. [118]; 2 years at single site in Belgium	N=71 RA patients with unfavorable prognostic factors	Step-down group: modified COBRA	*Primary*: DMARD changes
		Step-up group: monotherapy with MTX, SSZ, HCQ, or AZA	*Secondary*: use of steroids, adverse events
Moreland et al. [119]	N=755 meet 1987 ACR criteria, >4 TJC or SJC, disease duration <3 years	Immediate MTX-etanercept	*Primary*: change in the DAS28 between week 48 and 102
TEAR study		Immediate MTX-SSZ-HCQ	*Secondary*: radiographic progression, ACR20/50/70, modified-HAQ
2-year multicenter RCT in USA		Step-up from MTX to MTX-etanercept	
		Step-up from MTX to MTX-SSZ-HCQ	

Abbreviations: *RCT*, randomized control trial, *MTX* methotrexate *SSZ*, sulfasalazine *HCQ* hydroxychloroquine, *AZA* azathioprine, *DAS28* disease activity score for 28-joint counts, *CDAI* Clinical Disease Activity Index, *HAQ* Health Assessment Questionnaire, *TJC* tender joint count, *SJC* swollen joint count, *ESR* erythrocyte sedimentation rate

cumulative organ damage. In a clinical trial over 1 year or even 5 years unless very large numbers of patients are enrolled, it is not pragmatically possible to assess long-term outcomes such as renal or cardiac damage in hypertension or joint destruction or work disability in RA. Furthermore, damage to organs usually is irreversible by interventions designed to control the dysregulation – generally inflammation; after damage is advanced, medical interventions may be of limited to no value (only surgery, dialysis, etc., are effective).

Therefore, interventions are properly studied to analyze reversible signs of disease, which are amenable to drug therapy, such as an elevated blood pressure in hypertension, reduced CD4 counts in HIV infection, or tender or swollen joints in RA. These "surrogate markers" are related to the long-term consequences of damage, e.g., reduced mortality rates associated with control of blood pressure [6, 7] or serum glucose [8]. However, in some instances, the correlation between surrogate markers and long-term outcomes is not robust at all. For example, there is little association between joint tenderness and radiographic damage to joints in RA [122]. Furthermore, the natural history of joint tenderness is to improve over a 5-year period, while patients may experience joint destruction with resultant deformity and limited functional capacity [123, 124]. Therefore, joint tenderness as a surrogate marker in a clinical trial may be limited in its capacity to represent future damage.

Identification of an appropriate surrogate marker has proven difficult in SLE. Indices for SLE, which are needed as no "gold standard" measure is available, have included the SLEDAI (Systemic Lupus Erythematosus Disease Activity Index) [34, 125], SLEDAI 2 K [126], BILAG (British Isles Lupus Assessment Group) index [35, 127], SLAM (Systemic Lupus Activity Measure) [128], ECLAM (European Consensus Lupus Activity Measurement) [129], and the SLICC/ACR (Systemic Lupus International Coordinating Clinics/American College of Rheumatology) damage index [130]. According to these measures, clinical trials of rituximab have shown no efficacy in SLE. By contrast, many clinicians find rituximab of value in routine clinical care of SLE [131], reminiscent of differences between clinical trial data and clinical experience with methotrexate in RA in the 1990s, noted above. One possible explanation is that the indices used to assess status and improvement in the reported clinical trials may be insufficiently sensitive to changes in SLE clinical status [132].

An example of the complexity of identifying an optimal measure for improvement in patients with SLE is seen in recent analyses of a clinical trial of abatacept in SLE [133]. The report of the clinical trial concluded that abatacept had no significant clinical efficacy in SLE. However, analyses of various clinical endpoints that have been used in other SLE clinical trials suggest that if different endpoints had been chosen, statistically significant advantages to abatacept versus placebo might have been found (Table 7) [133]. Therefore, the choice of a surrogate measure for long-term damage may greatly influence the results despite a control group.

8. *Rare adverse events cannot be identified in most trials.*
One particular limitation of clinical trials that cannot be surmounted, even with a representative sample, particularly in rare or unusual diseases such as many inflammatory rheumatic diseases, is the rare adverse event. For example, if a severe adverse event occurs in 1 in 10,000 patients, and only 1,000 are studied in clinical trials prior to approval of a medication, there is a reasonable chance that this possible important adverse event may not be observed at all in these trials. Therefore, it is probably always of value to collect post-registration surveillance data on at least 50–100,000 patients who take a given medication to monitor for unusual, but severe, adverse events. This goal can be accomplished in rheumatology if, say, 10,000 rheumatologists around the world monitored all their patients,

Table 7 Rates of complete response in patients with nephrotic levels of proteinuria (>339 mg/mmole (3 g/g)) at screening and/or baseline according to five sets of response criteria [133][a]

Criteria	Control treatment	Abatacept 10/10 treatment	Abatacept 30/10 treatment
BMS trial	1/54 (2 %)	1/49 (2 %)	2/56 (4 %)
ACR recommendations	1/54 (2 %)	3/49 (6 %)	7/56 (13 %)
LUNAR trial	2/53 (4 %)	8/48 (17 %)	13/56 (23 %)
ALMS trial	3/54 (6 %)	9/49 (18 %)	14/56 (25 %)
ACCESS trial	4/53 (8 %)	15/48 (31 %)	17/56 (30 %)

Abbreviations: *BMS* Bristol-Myers Squibb trial, *ACR* American College of Rheumatology, *LUNAR* Lupus Nephritis Assessment with Rituximab trial, *ALMS* Aspreva Lupus Management Study, *ACCESS* Abatacept and Cyclophosphamide Combination: Efficacy and Safety Study trial
[a]Patients in the abatacept treatment groups received 12 months of treatment at 10 mg/kg every 28 days (abatacept 10/10) or 12 months of treatment at 30 mg/kg every 28 days for 5 months followed by 10 mg/kg every 28 days for the remainder of the treatment period (abatacept 30/10). Values are the number of complete responders/number assessed (%)

including the 5–10 with rare diseases such as polymyositis, systemic sclerosis, and vasculitis, in identical long-term databases designed to pool the outcomes. The technology for this type of activity has been available for decades, but implementation to the rheumatology community (as well as general medical community) has been quite limited.

Intrinsic Limitations

Pragmatic limitations of clinical trials described above theoretically could be overcome by elimination of many logistical obstacles to an ideal trial. In other words, in theory, it might be possible (and desirable) to design a clinical trial that includes all patients with a given diagnosis, with no specific inclusion or exclusion criteria (other than those in whom the proposed study medication might be harmful), sufficient statistical power to observe trends that emerge from the study, indefinite continuation of the trial, and 20,000 subjects to detect rare adverse events. Nonetheless, limitations are seen to randomized controlled clinical trials that are simply intrinsic to the methodology, just as limitations exist to any scientific methodology, four of which are discussed below:

1. *The design of a clinical trial may greatly influence the results, despite inclusion of a control group.*
   The inclusion of a "control group," one of the defining characteristics in the basic design of a randomized controlled clinical trial, is commonly thought to eliminate bias in comparing results of one intervention to another or to a placebo. A control group certainly reduces bias once patients are entered into a trial, but does not eliminate all sources of bias. None the less, the design of the trial itself may strongly influence results in favor or against a particular conclusion.

Consider, for example, a simple clinical trial to compare a new medication versus placebo in a given condition. Two design options may be (*1*) to require "failure" with two previous standard treatments, so that patients have an opportunity to receive "standard of care" prior to enrollment in a clinical trial, or (*2*) to include only patients who have had no previous treatment for the condition.

Clinical research (and common sense) suggest that, in general, a medication is more likely to show efficacy when used as the first rather than as the third medication in a patient after two prior failures. A requirement for two prior failures selects for patients who are in general (although not always) more refractory to treatment. A new medication may show statistically significant differences in efficacy versus a placebo when used as the first therapy for a disease, but be only marginally better than a placebo in patients receiving the medication as their third therapy.

Another example might involve a clinical trial to compare outcomes in patients with a form of cancer who participate or do not participate in a support group. Consider two alternative designs: (*a*) offering the clinical trial to all patients at the time of diagnosis prior to any treatment; (*b*) offering the clinical trial only to patients who have persistent disease after standard treatment with surgery, radiation, and/or chemotherapy. Either design would appear quite reasonable, as patients who might be "cured" through standard treatment might be spared the trouble and expense of a support group, while "incurable" patients may benefit. However, these two designs might lead to different results. Patients beginning standard treatment would, by definition, have a higher likelihood of overall success, which might give an opportunity for a support group to add to this success. By contrast, patients who have failed standard treatment might be expected to have a lesser possibility of overall success, with a lesser possibility of additional value of a support group.

The design of a clinical trial obviously cannot preordain the results. Nonetheless, the design of a clinical trial can greatly "tilt" the probability that an intervention will or will not appear to be more efficacious than a placebo. A "control" group does not invariably eliminate biases, which are intrinsic to the design of any study.

2. *Clinical trial data are reported in groups and generally ignore individual variation*

As noted in the introductory comments, the prototype clinical trials were performed to analyze antibiotics in activity versus infectious bacteria. Bacteria are simple single-cell organisms, which present a target for antibiotics to eradicate from the body. A single optimal medication for *all* patients might be identified for treatment of a specific bacterium, particularly when the capacity of a medication to affect a target pathogen is tested in a laboratory "culture and sensitivities" analysis.

The treatment of complex multicellular and multiorgan human patients clearly is not as simple. Variation in responses among individuals to a medication would be *expected* in drugs designed to treat multicellular human organisms for such disorders as overproduction of gastric acid, control of blood pressure,

Table 8 Arthrotec compared to acetaminophen (ACTA) crossover clinical trial: patient ratings of each drug [134]

Patient ratings	Group I Arthrotec → acetaminophen *N* (%)	Group II acetaminophen → Arthrotec *N* (%)	Total *N* (%)
Arthrotec better or much better	52 (58 %)	48 (57 %)	100 (57 %)
No difference	18 (20 %)	21 (25 %)	39 (22 %)
Acetaminophen better or much better	20 (22 %)	15 (18 %)	35 (20 %)

management of pain, or reduction of depression. However, in general, a clinical trial is reported to identify the "best" therapy for *all* patients, rather than to identify *which* therapy might be most effective for *particular* individual patients.

Crossover clinical trials in which two agents are compared often document the phenomenon of individual variation in responses to two or more treatments. For example, in a crossover clinical trial of Arthrotec (diclofenac coated with misoprostol) compared to acetaminophen (ACTA trial), 57 % of individuals reported that Arthrotec was superior, 21 % that acetaminophen was superior, and 22 % found the two medications of equal efficacy (Table 8) [134]. An accurate interpretation of the data might be that Arthrotec is better for most individuals, but acetaminophen is better for some individual patients. However, the usual interpretation of such data is that Arthrotec is "superior" to acetaminophen in general.

This limitation may have significant consequences for therapies for individual patients. Many hospital formularies will select only a single medication from a given category, such as H2 blockers to reduce acid in peptic ulcer and reflux disease, tricyclic antidepressants, or NSAIDs. The reasoning is that it is cost-effective to have available only a single medication among several that all act according to a similar mechanism. However, each individual medication may be superior in some individual patients, due to different receptors, metabolism, and other idiosyncratic characteristics of the host. The interpretation that a single optimal medication exists for *all* patients with a disease is an incorrect assumption, probably based in large part on the origin of clinical trials in studies of antibiotic medications designed to interact primarily with simple bacterial cells, rather than complex human organisms.

3. *Interpretation of adverse events is not standardized and depends on assessment of risks and benefits which differ widely among individuals.*
   All interventions, including medications, physical therapy, exercise programs, etc., may be associated with some type of adverse event in certain individuals, ranging from renal damage to inconvenient travel to a support group. Consider, for example, in a comparison of two medications, that Medication A leads to remission in 95 % of patients with few adverse event effects, but 1 in 10,000

patients experiences renal failure, while Medication B leads to improvement in 50 % of patients, no remissions, and "nuisance" gastrointestinal side effects in 20 % of patients, but leads to no severe harm to internal organs. Which is the preferred medication? That depends in large part on how an individual patient assesses risks and benefits, which varies widely among individual patients and individuals in general. As an example to patients, the author often asks a patient to assess the risk/benefit of playing a lottery, pointing out that there is no single "correct" answer. A committee verdict concerning groups cannot provide optimal guidance to each individual patient.

In general, the community of health professionals accepts the interpretation of the authors of a clinical trial regarding risks and benefits of a therapy. However, in actual practice, certain patients may prefer the odds of one alternative or the other and can make an informed decision as to which is the optimal treatment. A clinical trial infers a "black and white" choice, while the actual results suggest "shades of gray." This interpretive component in analysis of results of a clinical trial may explain occasional contentious disagreement within FDA advisory groups concerning approval of certain new medications or procedures such as mammography in 40- to 50-year-old women. A positive or negative recommendation depends on analysis of risks versus benefits, interpretation of which varies greatly among patients (as well as "experts").

4. *The format of a clinical trial compromises the "placebo effect" in not informing patients that they may not receive the "best" therapy.*
   Considerable information has been reported over the last few decades concerning the "placebo" effect in any patient intervention [135]. After all, until the twentieth century, most medications were of little efficacy and yet health professionals were highly regarded as providing "curative" medications in many situations. This placebo effect is compromised considerably when a health professional invites a patient to participate in a "scientific experiment" to recognize the best therapy, rather than telling a patient that she/he will receive the "best therapy."

   Most clinical trials show substantial benefit to participants in both placebo and treatment groups, suggesting that there nonetheless exists a considerable "placebo effect" even within the clinical trial methodology. It may be argued that both arms of a clinical trial are diminished in their therapeutic efficacy by loss of possible placebo effect, but this loss is "controlled for." It seems clear, nonetheless, that some of the therapeutic "placebo" benefit which results from patients being told that they are being given an optimal therapy is lost in the circumstances of the clinical trial.

Summary and Conclusion

Clinical trials remain the optimal method to compare one therapy with another or a placebo independent of inevitable biases associated with choices of therapies [1, 82]. Nonetheless, clinical trials have limitations. In this chapter, selected randomized controlled clinical trials conducted in chronic rheumatic diseases, including

RA, SLE, polymyositis, and OA, as well as other chronic cardiovascular diseases, have been summarized to illustrate some of these limitations. Some limitations may be overcome by longer trials and meta-analyses. However, pragmatic and intrinsic limitations will always affect the clinical trial methodology to some extent. A greater awareness of these limitations would be of benefit to health professionals and the general public in interpreting results and implications of clinical trials for clinical care.

References

1. Feinstein AR. An additional basic science for clinical medicine: II. The limitations of randomized trials. Ann Intern Med. 1983;99:544–50.
2. Engel GL. The biopsychosocial model and the education of health professionals. Ann N Y Acad Sci. 1978;310:169–81.
3. Howick J. The philosophy of evidence-based medicine. Oxford: Wiley-Blackwell; 2011.
4. Streptomycin treatment of pulmonary tuberculosis. Br Med J. 1948;2(4582):769–82.
5. Hill AB. Suspended judgment: memories of the British streptomycin trial in tuberculosis. The first randomized clinical trial. Control Clin Trials. 1990;11:77–9.
6. Veterans Administration Cooperative Study on Antihypertensive Agent. Effects of treatment on morbidity in hypertension: results in patients with diastolic blood pressures averaging 115 through 129 mm Hg. JAMA. 1967;202:1028–34.
7. Veterans Administration Cooperative Study on Antihypertensive Agent. Effects of treatment on morbidity in hypertension: II. Results in patients with diastolic blood pressure averaging 90 through 114 mm Hg. JAMA. 1970;213:1143–50.
8. The effect of intensive treatment of diabetes on the development and progression of long-term complications in insulin-dependent diabetes mellitus. The Diabetes Control and Complications Trial Research Group. N Engl J Med. 1993;329(14):977–86.
9. Krause D, Schleusser B, Herborn G, Rau R. Response to methotrexate treatment is associated with reduced mortality in patients with severe rheumatoid arthritis. Arthritis Rheum. 2000;43:14–21.
10. Choi HK, Hernán MA, Seeger JD, Robins JM, Wolfe F. Methotrexate and mortality in patients with rheumatoid arthritis: a prospective study. Lancet. 2002;359:1173–7.
11. Wolfe F, Michaud K, Gefeller O, Choi HK. Predicting mortality in patients with rheumatoid arthritis. Arthritis Rheum. 2003;48:1530–42.
12. Jacobsson LTH, Turesson C, Nilsson JA, Petersson IF, Lindqvist E, Saxne T, et al. Treatment with TNF blockers and mortality risk in patients with rheumatoid arthritis. Ann Rheum Dis. 2007;66(5):670–5.
13. Pincus T, Gibofsky A, Weinblatt ME. Urgent care and tight control of rheumatoid arthritis as in diabetes and hypertension: better treatments but a shortage of rheumatologists. Arthritis Rheum. 2002;46(4):851–4.
14. Pincus T, Yazici Y, Sokka T. Complexities in assessment of rheumatoid arthritis: absence of a single gold standard measure. Rheum Dis Clin North Am. 2009;35(4):687–97.
15. Waaler E. On the occurrence of a factor in human serum activating the specific agglutination of sheep blood corpuscles. APMIS. 1940;17:172–8.
16. Rose HM, Ragan C, Pearce E, Lipman MO. Differential agglutination of normal and sensitized sheep erythrocytes by sera of patients with rheumatoid arthritis. Proc Soc Exp Biol Med. 1948;68:1–6.
17. Hargraves MM, Richmond H, Morton R. Presentation of two bone marrow elements: the "tart" cell and "L.E." cell. Proc Staff Meet Mayo Clin. 1948;23:25–8.

18. Nishimura K, Sugiyama D, Kogata Y, Tsuji G, Nakazawa T, Kawano S, et al. Meta-analysis: diagnostic accuracy of anti-cyclic citrullinated peptide antibody and rheumatoid factor for rheumatoid arthritis. Ann Intern Med. 2007;146(11):797–808.
19. Wolfe F, Michaud K. The clinical and research significance of the erythrocyte sedimentation rate. J Rheumatol. 1994;21:1227–37.
20. Wolfe F. Comparative usefulness of c-reactive protein and erythrocyte sedimentation rate in patients with rheumatoid arthritis. J Rheumatol. 1997;24:1477–85.
21. Sokka T, Pincus T. Erythrocyte sedimentation rate, C-reactive protein, or rheumatoid factor are normal at presentation in 35 %-45% of patients with rheumatoid arthritis seen between 1980 and 2004: analyses from Finland and the United States. J Rheumatol. 2009;36(7): 1387–90.
22. Munves EF, Schur PH. Antibodies to Sm and RNP: prognosticators of disease involvement. Arthritis Rheum. 1983;26:848–53.
23. Pincus T. A pragmatic approach to cost-effective use of laboratory tests and imaging procedures in patients with musculoskeletal symptoms. Prim Care. 1993;20:795–814.
24. Pincus T. Laboratory tests in rheumatic disorders. In: Klippel JH, Dieppe PA, editors. Rheumatology. 2nd ed. London: Mosby International; 1997. p. 10.1–8.
25. Goldsmith CH, Smythe HA, Helewa A. Interpretation and power of pooled index. J Rheumatol. 1993;20:575–8.
26. van der Heijde DM, van't Hof M, van Riel PL, van de Putte LB. Development of a disease activity score based on judgment in clinical practice by rheumatologists. J Rheumatol. 1993;20:579–81.
27. Prevoo MLL, van't Hof MA, Kuper HH, van Leeuwen MA, van de Putte LBA, van Riel PLCM. Modified disease activity scores that include twenty-eight-joint counts: development and validation in a prospective longitudinal study of patients with rheumatoid arthritis. Arthritis Rheum. 1995;38:44–8.
28. Aletaha D, Smolen J. The simplified disease activity index (SDAI) and the clinical disease activity index (CDAI): a review of their usefulness and validity in rheumatoid arthritis. Clin Exp Rheumatol. 2005;23:S100–8.
29. Pincus T, Strand V, Koch G, Amara I, Crawford B, Wolfe F, et al. An index of the three core data set patient questionnaire measures distinguishes efficacy of active treatment from placebo as effectively as the American College of Rheumatology 20 % response criteria (ACR20) or the disease activity score (DAS) in a rheumatoid arthritis clinical trial. Arthritis Rheum. 2003;48(3):625–30.
30. Pincus T, Bergman MJ, Yazici Y, Hines P, Raghupathi K, Maclean R. An index of only patient-reported outcome measures, routine assessment of patient index data 3 (RAPID3), in two abatacept clinical trials: similar results to disease activity score (DAS28) and other RAPID indices that include physician-reported measures. Rheumatology (Oxford). 2008; 47(3):345–9.
31. Pincus T, Swearingen CJ, Bergman M, Yazici Y. RAPID3 (routine assessment of patient index data 3), a rheumatoid arthritis index without formal joint counts for routine care: proposed severity categories compared to DAS and CDAI categories. J Rheumatol. 2008;35: 2136–47.
32. Petri M, Hellmann DB, Hochberg M. Validity and reliability of lupus activity measures in the routine clinic setting. J Rheumatol. 1992;19:53–9.
33. Bencivelli W, Vitali C, Isenberg DA, Smolen JS, Snaith ML, Sciuto M, et al. Disease activity in systemic lupus erythematosus: report of the Consensus Study Group of the European Workshop for Rheumatology Research III. Development of a computerised clinical chart and its application to the comparison of different indices of disease activity. The European Consensus Study Group for Disease Activity in SLE. Clin Exp Rheumatol. 1992;10(5): 549–54.
34. Hawker G, Gabriel S, Bombardier C, Goldsmith C, Caron D, Gladman D. A reliability study of SLEDAI: a disease activity index for systemic lupus erythematosus. J Rheumatol. 1993;20: 657–60.

35. Hay EM, Bacon PA, Gordon C, Isenberg DA, Maddison P, Snaith ML, et al. The BILAG index: a reliable and valid instrument for measuring clinical disease activity in systemic lupus erythematosus. Q J Med. 1993;86(7):447–58.
36. Gladman DD, Urowitz MB, Goldsmith CH, Fortin P, Ginzler E, Gordon C, et al. The reliability of the Systemic Lupus International Collaborating Clinics/American College of Rheumatology Damage Index in patients with systemic lupus erythematosus. Arthritis Rheum. 1997;40(5):809–13.
37. Mosca M, Bencivelli W, Vitali C, Carrai P, Neri R, Bombardieri S. The validity of the ECLAM index for the retrospective evaluation of disease activity in systemic lupus erythematosus. Lupus. 2000;9(6):445–50.
38. Swaak AJ, van den Brink HG, Smeenk RJ, Manger K, Kalden JR, Tosi S, et al. Systemic lupus erythematosus. Disease outcome in patients with a disease duration of at least 10 years: second evaluation. Lupus. 2001;10(1):51–8.
39. Lam GKW, Petri M. Assessment of systemic lupus erythematosus. Clin Exp Rheumatol. 2005;23:S120–32.
40. Luqmani RA, Bacon PA, Moots RJ, Janssen BA, Pall A, Emery P, et al. Birmingham Vasculitis Activity Score (BVAS) in systemic necrotizing vasculitis. Q J Med. 1994;87:671–8.
41. Bacon PA, Moots RJ, Exley E, Luqmani R, Rasmussen N. VITAL assessment of vasculitis – workshop report. Clin Exp Rheumatol. 1995;13:275–8.
42. Exley AR, Bacon PA, Luqmani RA, Kitas GD, Gordon C, Savage COS, et al. Development and initial validation of the Vasculitis Damage Index for the standardized clinical assessment of damage in the systemic vasculitides. Arthritis Rheum. 1997;40:371–80.
43. Whiting O'Keefe QE, Stone JH, Hellmann DB. Validity of a vasculitis activity index for systemic necrotizing vasculitis. Arthritis Rheum. 1999;42:2365–71.
44. Stone JH, Hoffman GS, Merkel PA, Min Y, Uhlfelder ML, Hellmann DB, et al. A disease-specific activity index for Wegener's granulomatosis: modification of the Birmingham Vasculitis Activity Score. Arthritis Rheum. 2001;44:912–20.
45. Seo P, Min Y, Holbrook JT, Hoffman GS, Merkel PA, Spiera R, et al. Damage caused by Wegener's granulomatosis and its treatment: prospective data from the Wegener's Granulomatosis Etanercept Trail (WGET). Arthritis Rheum. 2005;52:2168–78.
46. Clegg DO, Reda DJ, Weisman MH, Blackburn WD, Cush JJ, Cannon GW, et al. Comparison of sulfasalazine and placebo in the treatment of ankylosing spondylitis. A Department of Veterans Affairs Cooperative Study. Arthritis Rheum. 1996;39(12):2004–12.
47. Fleischer JAB, Feldman SR, Rapp SR, Reboussin DM, Exum ML, Clark AR, et al. Disease severity measures in a population of psoriasis patients: the symptoms of psoriasis correlate with self-administered psoriasis area severity index scores. J Invest Dermatol. 1996;107:26–9.
48. Kavanaugh A, Cassell S. The assessment of disease activity and outcomes in psoriatic arthritis. Clin Exp Rheumatol. 2005;23:S142–7.
49. Dougados M, Gueguen A, Nakache JP, Nguyen M, Mery C, Amor B. Evaluation of a functional index and an articular index in ankylosing spondylitis. J Rheumatol. 1988;15:302–7.
50. Calin A, Garrett S, Whitelock H, Kennedy LG, O'Hea J, Mallorie P, et al. A new approach to defining functional ability in ankylosing spondylitis: the development of the Bath Ankylosing Spondylitis Functional Index. J Rheumatol. 1994;21(12):2281–5.
51. Calin A, Nakache JP, Gueguen A, Zeidler H, Mielants H, Dougados M. Defining disease activity in ankylosing spondylitis: is a combination of variables (Bath Ankylosing Spondylitis Disease Activity Index) an appropriate instrument? Rheumatology (Oxford). 1999;38(9):878–82.
52. Calin A, MacKay K, Santos H, Brophy S. A new dimension to outcome: application of the Bath Ankylosing Spondylitis Radiology Index. J Rheumatol. 1999;26(4):988–92.
53. Zochling J, Braun J. Assessment of ankylosing spondylitis. Clin Exp Rheumatol. 2005;23:S133–41.
54. Pincus T, Segurado OG. Most visits of most patients with rheumatoid arthritis to most rheumatologists do not include a formal quantitative joint count. Ann Rheum Dis. 2006;65:820–2.

55. Anderson J, Caplan L, Yazdany J, Robbins ML, Neogi T, Michaud K, et al. Rheumatoid arthritis disease activity measures: American College of Rheumatology recommendations for use in clinical practice. Arthritis Care Res (Hoboken). 2012;64(5):640–7.
56. Castrejón I, McCollum L, Durusu Tanriover M, Pincus T. Importance of patient history and physical examination in rheumatoid arthritis compared to other chronic diseases: results of a physician survey. Arthritis Care Res. 2012;64(8):1250–5.
57. Pincus T, Swearingen CJ. The HAQ compared with the MDHAQ: "keep it simple, stupid" (KISS), with feasibility and clinical value as primary criteria for patient questionnaires in usual clinical care. Rheum Dis Clin North Am. 2009;35(4):787–98.
58. Pincus T, Skummer PT, Grisanti MT, Castrejón I, Yazici Y. MDHAQ/RAPID3 can provide a roadmap or agenda for all rheumatology visits when the entire MDHAQ is completed at all patient visits and reviewed by the doctor before the encounter. Bull NYU Hosp Jt Dis. 2012;70(3):177–86.
59. Pincus T, Oliver AM, Bergman MJ. How to collect an MDHAQ to provide rheumatology vital signs (function, pain, global status, and RAPID3 scores) in the infrastructure of rheumatology care, including some misconceptions regarding the MDHAQ. Rheum Dis Clin North Am. 2009;35(4):799–812.
60. OCEBM Levels of Evidence Working Group. The Oxford 2011 Levels of Evidence. http://www.cebm.net/index.aspx?o=5653, Oxford Centre for Evidence-Based Medicine. Oxford: Oxford Centre for Evidence-Based Medicine; 2011. Ref Type: Generic.
61. Smith GCS, Pell JP. Parachute use to prevent death and major trauma related to gravitational challenge: systematic review of randomised controlled trials. BMJ. 2003;327:1459–61.
62. Glasziou P, Chalmers I, Rawlins M, McCulloch P. When are randomised trials unnecessary? Picking signal from noise. BMJ. 2007;334(7589):349–51.
63. Aronson JK, Hauben M. Anecdotes that provide definitive evidence. BMJ. 2006;333(7581):1267–9.
64. Freiman JA, Chalmers TC, Smith Jr H, Kuebler RR. The importance of beta, the type II error and sample size in the design and interpretation of the randomized control trial: survey of 71 "negative" trials. N Engl J Med. 1978;299:690–4.
65. Sackett DL, Gent M. Controversy in counting and attributing events in clinical trials. N Engl J Med. 1979;301:1410–2.
66. Sackett DL. The competing objectives of randomized trials. N Engl J Med. 1980;303:1059–60.
67. Huskisson EC. Important factors in the success and failure of clinical trials (closing remarks). Agents Actions Suppl. 1980;7:323–4.
68. Freireich EJ. The randomized clinical trial as an obstacle to clinical research. In: Varco RL, Delaney JP, editors. Controversy in surgery. 2nd ed. Philadelphia: W.B. Saunders; 1983. p. 5–12.
69. Diamond GA, Forrester JS. Clinical trials and statistical verdicts: probable grounds for appeal. Ann Intern Med. 1983;98:385–94.
70. Chalmers TC, Celano P, Sacks HS, Smith Jr H. Bias in treatment assignment in controlled clinical trials. N Engl J Med. 1983;309:1358–61.
71. Bombardier C, Tugwell P. Controversies in the analysis of longterm clinical trials of slow acting drugs (editorial). J Rheumatol. 1985;12:403–5.
72. Guyatt G, Sackett D, Taylor DW, Chong J, Roberts R, Pugsley S. Determining optimal therapy – randomized trials in individual patients. N Engl J Med. 1986;314:889–92.
73. Gotzsche PC. Methodology and overt and hidden bias in reports of 196 double-blind trials of nonsteroidal antiinflammatory drugs in rheumatoid arthritis. Control Clin Trials. 1989;10:31–56.
74. Sanz I, Dang H, Takei M, Talal N, Capra JD. VH sequence of a human anti-Sm autoantibody. Evidence that autoantibodies can be un-mutated copies of germline genes. J Immunol. 1989;142:883–7.
75. Klippel JH. Comment: winning the battle, losing the war? Another editorial about RA. J Rheumatol. 1990;17:1118–22.

76. Felson DT, Anderson JJ, Meenan RF. Time for changes in the design, analysis, and reporting of rheumatoid arthritis clinical trials. Arthritis Rheum. 1990;33:140–9.
77. Hawley DJ, Wolfe F. Are the results of controlled clinical trials and observational studies of second line therapy in rheumatoid arthritis valid and generalizable as measures of rheumatoid arthritis outcome: analysis of 122 studies. J Rheumatol. 1991;18:1008–14.
78. Rothwell PM. Can overall results of clinical trials be applied to all patients? Lancet. 1995;345:1616–9.
79. Cleophas TJ, Zwinderman AH. Limitations of randomized clinical trials. Proposed alternative designs. Clin Chem Lab Med. 2000;38(12):1217–23.
80. Grossman J, Mackenzie FJ. The randomized controlled trial: gold standard, or merely standard? Perspect Biol Med. 2005;48(4):516–34.
81. Ho PM, Peterson PN, Masoudi FA. Evaluating the evidence: is there a rigid hierarchy? Circulation. 2008;118(16):1675–84.
82. Pincus T. Rheumatoid arthritis: disappointing long-term outcomes despite successful short-term clinical trials. J Clin Epidemiol. 1988;41:1037–41.
83. Pincus T, Wolfe F. Response to letter: gold therapy for rheumatoid arthritis: challenges to traditional paradigms. Ann Intern Med. 1992;117:169–70.
84. Pincus T. Limitations of randomized controlled clinical trials to recognize possible advantages of combination therapies in rheumatic diseases. Semin Arthritis Rheum. 1993;23 Suppl 1:2–10.
85. Pincus T, Stein M. What is the best source of useful data on the treatment of rheumatoid arthritis: clinical trials, clinical observations, or clinical protocols? J Rheumatol. 1995;22: 1611–7.
86. Pincus T, Stein CM. Why randomized controlled clinical trials do not depict accurately long-term outcomes in rheumatoid arthritis: some explanations and suggestions for future studies. Clin Exp Rheumatol. 1997;15 Suppl 17:S27–38.
87. Pincus T, Sokka T. Clinical trials in rheumatic diseases: designs and limitations. Rheum Dis Clin North Am. 2004;30:701–4.
88. Pincus T, Sokka T. Complexities in the quantitative assessment of patients with rheumatic diseases in clinical trials and clinical care. Clin Exp Rheumatol. 2005;23:S1–9.
89. Chalmers TC, Block JB, Lee S. Controlled studies in clinical cancer research. N Engl J Med. 1972;287:75–8.
90. Williams HJ, Ward JR, Reading JC, Brooks RH, Clegg DO, Skosey JL, et al. Comparison of auranofin, methotrexate, and the combination of both in the treatment of rheumatoid arthritis: a controlled clinical trial. Arthritis Rheum. 1992;35:259–69.
91. Felson DT, Anderson JJ, Meenan RF. The comparative efficacy and toxicity of second-line drugs in rheumatoid arthritis: results of two metaanalyses. Arthritis Rheum. 1990;33:1449–61.
92. Pincus T, Marcum SB, Callahan LF. Long-term drug therapy for rheumatoid arthritis in seven rheumatology private practices: II. Second-line drugs and prednisone. J Rheumatol. 1992;19: 1885–94.
93. Donahue KE, Gartlehner G, Jonas DE, Lux LJ, Thieda P, Jonas BL, et al. Systematic review: comparative effectiveness and harms of disease-modifying medications for rheumatoid arthritis. Ann Intern Med. 2008;148(2):124–34.
94. Sokka T, Kautiainen H, Toloza S, Makinen H, Verstappen SM, Hetland ML, et al. QUEST-RA: quantitative clinical assessment of patients with rheumatoid arthritis seen in standard rheumatology care in 15 countries. Ann Rheum Dis. 2007;66:1491–6.
95. Bunch TW, Worthington JW, Combs JJ, Ilstrup DM, Engel AG. Azathioprine with prednisone for polymyositis: a controlled, clinical trial. Ann Intern Med. 1980;92:365–9.
96. Bunch TW. Prednisone and azathioprine for polymyositis: long-term followup. Arthritis Rheum. 1981;24:45–8.
97. Austin III HA, Klippel JH, Balow JE, le Riche NGH, Steinberg AD, Plotz PH, et al. Therapy of lupus nephritis: controlled trial of prednisone and cytotoxic drugs. N Engl J Med. 1986; 314:614–9.
98. Sokka T, Pincus T. Eligibility of patients in routine care for major clinical trials of anti-tumor necrosis factor alpha agents in rheumatoid arthritis. Arthritis Rheum. 2003;48(2):313–8.

99. Sokka T, Pincus T. An early rheumatoid arthritis treatment evaluation registry (ERATER) in the United States. Clin Exp Rheumatol. 2005;23:S178–81.
100. Gogus F, Yazici Y, Yazici H. Inclusion criteria as widely used for rheumatoid arthritis clinical trials: patient eligibility in a Turkish cohort. Clin Exp Rheumatol. 2005;23(5):681–4.
101. Pincus T, Marcum SB, Callahan LF, Adams RF, Barber J, Barth WF, et al. Long-term drug therapy for rheumatoid arthritis in seven rheumatology private practices: I. Nonsteroidal anti-inflammatory drugs. J Rheumatol. 1992;19:1874–84.
102. Donadio Jr JV, Holley KE, Wagoner RD, Ferguson RH, McDuffie FC. Further observations on the treatment of lupus nephritis with prednisone and combined prednisone and azathioprine. Arthritis Rheum. 1974;17:573–81.
103. Hahn BH, Kantor OS, Osterland CK. Azathioprine plus prednisone compared with prednisone alone in the treatment of systemic lupus erythematosus: report of a prospective controlled trial in 24 patients. Ann Intern Med. 1975;83:597–605.
104. Sztejnbok M, Stewart A, Diamond H, Kaplan D. Azathioprine in the treatment of systemic lupus erythematosus. Arthritis Rheum. 1971;14:639–45.
105. Cade R, Spooner G, Schlein E, Pickering M, DeQuesada A, Holcomb A, et al. Comparison of azathioprine, prednisone, and heparin alone or combined in treating lupus nephritis. Nephron. 1973;10:37–56.
106. Felson DT, Anderson J. Evidence for the superiority of immunosuppressive drugs and prednisone over prednisone alone in lupus nephritis: results of a pooled analysis. N Engl J Med. 1984;311:1528–33.
107. A randomized trial of propranolol in patients with acute myocardial infarction. I. Mortality results. JAMA. 1982;247(12):1707–14.
108. Ruberman W, Weinblatt E, Goldberg JD, Chaudhary BS. Psychosocial influences on mortality after myocardial infarction. N Engl J Med. 1984;311:552–9.
109. The Coronary Drug Project Research Group. Influence of adherence to treatment and response of cholesterol on mortality in the coronary drug project. N Engl J Med. 1980;303:1038–41.
110. Boers M. Add-on or step-up trials for new drug development in rheumatoid arthritis: a new standard? Arthritis Rheum. 2003;48:1481–3.
111. Smolen JS, Aletaha D, Bijlsma JW, Breedveld FC, Boumpas D, Burmester G, et al. Treating rheumatoid arthritis to target: recommendations of an international task force. Ann Rheum Dis. 2010;69(4):631–7.
112. Grigor C, Capell H, Stirling A, McMahon AD, Lock P, Vallance R, et al. Effect of a treatment strategy of tight control for rheumatoid arthritis (the TICORA study): a single-blind randomised controlled trial. Lancet. 2004;364:263–9.
113. Fransen J, Moens HB, Speyer I, van Riel PL. Effectiveness of systematic monitoring of rheumatoid arthritis disease activity in daily practice: a multicentre, cluster randomised controlled trial. Ann Rheum Dis. 2005;64:1294–8.
114. Verstappen SM, Jacobs JW, van der Veen MJ, Heurkens AH, Schenk Y, Ter Borg EJ, et al. Intensive treatment with methotrexate in early rheumatoid arthritis: aiming for remission. Computer Assisted Management in Early Rheumatoid Arthritis (CAMERA, an open-label strategy trial). Ann Rheum Dis. 2007;66(11):1443–9.
115. Goekoop-Ruiterman YP, de Vries-Bouwstra JK, Allaart CF, van Zeben D, Kerstens PJ, Hazes JM, et al. Clinical and radiographic outcomes of four different treatment strategies in patients with early rheumatoid arthritis (the BeSt study): a randomized, controlled trial. Arthritis Rheum. 2005;52:3381–90.
116. Hetland ML, Stengaard-Pedersen K, Junker P, Lottenburger T, Hansen I, Andersen LS, et al. Aggressive combination therapy with intra-articular glucocorticoid injections and conventional disease-modifying anti-rheumatic drugs in early rheumatoid arthritis: second-year clinical and radiographic results from the CIMESTRA study. Ann Rheum Dis. 2008;67: 815–22.
117. Saunders SA, Capell HA, Stirling A, Vallance R, Kincaid W, McMahon AD, et al. Triple therapy in early active rheumatoid arthritis: a randomized, single-blind, controlled trial comparing step-up and parallel treatment strategies. Arthritis Rheum. 2008;58(5):1310–7.

118. Verschueren P, Esselens G, Westhovens R. Daily practice effectiveness of a step-down treatment in comparison with a tight step-up for early rheumatoid arthritis. Rheumatology (Oxford). 2008;47(1):59–64.
119. Moreland LW, O'Dell JR, Paulus HE, Curtis JR, Bathon JM, St Clair EW, et al. A randomized comparative effectiveness study of oral triple therapy versus etanercept plus methotrexate in early aggressive rheumatoid arthritis: the treatment of Early Aggressive Rheumatoid Arthritis Trial. Arthritis Rheum. 2012;64(9):2824–35.
120. Sokka T, Pincus T. Rheumatoid arthritis: strategy more important than agent. Lancet. 2009;374(9688):430–2.
121. Turchetti G, Smolen JS, Kavanaugh A, Braun J, Pincus T. Treat-to-target in rheumatoid arthritis: clinical and pharmacoeconomic considerations. Clin Exp Rheumatol. 2012;30(4 Suppl 73):S1–169. Ref Type: Journal (Full).
122. Fuchs HA, Callahan LF, Kaye JJ, Brooks RH, Nance EP, Pincus T. Radiographic and joint count findings of the hand in rheumatoid arthritis: related and unrelated findings. Arthritis Rheum. 1988;31:44–51.
123. Callahan LF, Pincus T, Huston III JW, Brooks RH, Nance Jr EP, Kaye JJ. Measures of activity and damage in rheumatoid arthritis: depiction of changes and prediction of mortality over five years. Arthritis Care Res. 1997;10:381–94.
124. Mulherin D, Fitzgerald O, Bresnihan B. Clinical improvement and radiological deterioration in rheumatoid arthritis: evidence that pathogenesis of synovial inflammation and articular erosion may differ. Br J Rheumatol. 1996;35:1263–8.
125. Bombardier C, Gladman DD, Urowitz MB, Caron D, Chang CH. Derivation of the SLEDAI A disease activity index for lupus patients. The Committee on Prognosis Studies in SLE. Arthritis Rheum. 1992;35(6):630–40.
126. Gladman DD, Ibanez D, Urowitz MB. Systemic lupus erythematosus disease activity index 2000. J Rheumatol. 2002;29(2):288–91.
127. Isenberg DA, Rahman A, Allen E, Farewell V, Akil M, Bruce IN, et al. BILAG 2004. Development and initial validation of an updated version of the British Isles Lupus Assessment Group's disease activity index for patients with systemic lupus erythematosus. Rheumatology (Oxford). 2005;44(7):902–6.
128. Liang MH, Socher SA, Larson MG, Schur PH. Reliability and validity of six systems for the clinical assessment of disease activity in systemic lupus erythematosus. Arthritis Rheum. 1989;32:1107–18.
129. Vitali C, Bencivelli W, Isenberg DA, Smolen JS, Snaith ML, Sciuto M, et al. Disease activity in systemic lupus erythematosus: report of the Consensus Study Group of the European Workshop for Rheumatology Research II. Identification of the variables indicative of disease activity and their use in the development of an activity score. The European Consensus Study Group for Disease Activity in SLE. Clin Exp Rheumatol. 1992;10(5):541–7.
130. Gladman D, Ginzler E, Goldsmith C, Fortin P, Liang M, Urowitz M, et al. The development and initial validation of the Systemic Lupus International Collaborating Clinics/American College of Rheumatology Damage Index for systemic lupus erythematosus. Arthritis Rheum. 1996;39:363–9.
131. Gunnarsson I, Jonsdottir T. Rituximab treatment in lupus nephritis–where do we stand? Lupus. 2013;22(4):381–9.
132. Petri M. Disease activity assessment in SLE: do we have the right instruments? Ann Rheum Dis. 2007;66 Suppl 3:iii61–4.
133. Wofsy D, Hillson JL, Diamond B. Abatacept for lupus nephritis: alternative definitions of complete response support conflicting conclusions. Arthritis Rheum. 2012;64(11):3660–5.
134. Pincus T, Koch GG, Sokka T, Lefkowith J, Wolfe F, Jordan JM, et al. A randomized, double-blind, crossover clinical trial of diclofenac plus misoprostol versus acetaminophen in patients with osteoarthritis of the hip or knee. Arthritis Rheum. 2001;44:1587–98.
135. Kaptchuk TJ. Powerful placebo: the dark side of the randomised controlled trial. Lancet. 1998;351:1722–5.

Methodological Issues Relevant to Observational Studies, Registries, and Administrative Health Databases in Rheumatology

Marie Hudson and Samy Suissa

Randomized controlled trials (RCTs) remain the gold standard for evidence-based therapy. However, RCTs are expensive to conduct and thus often provide data on limited numbers of highly selected patients followed for short durations of time. Indeed, in a systematic review of 29 RCTs of antitumor necrosis factor (TNF) drugs in rheumatoid arthritis, over 40 % of the studies followed subjects for less than 14 weeks [1]. Thus, the well-accepted limitations of RCTs include lack of generalizability, insufficiently long follow-up to answer many questions relating to long-term drug safety, and sample sizes too small to study particular rare events. In response to this, several drug and disease registries have been established to provide long-term follow-up on patients in routine clinical care. In addition, administrative databases have the additional advantage of large study populations, thus offering the potential to identify rare events. Observational (i.e., nonexperimental) studies of registry data and administrative databases using pharmacoepidemiological approaches have thus become useful sources of information concerning the effectiveness and safety of treatments in rheumatology.

On the other hand, observational studies involving complex time-varying medication use with multiple drugs and time-dependent risks are subject to method-

M. Hudson, MD, MPH (✉)
Division of Rheumatology and Centre for Clinical Epidemiology, Department of Medicine, Lady Davis Institute for Medical Research, Jewish General Hospital, McGill University, 3755 Côte-Sainte-Catherine Road, Montreal, QC H3T 1E2, Canada
e-mail: marie.hudson@mcgill.ca

S. Suissa, PhD
Centre for Clinical Epidemiology, Lady Davis Institute for Medical Research, Jewish General Hospital, McGill University, 3755 Côte-Sainte-Catherine Road, Montreal, QC H3T 1E2, Canada
e-mail: samy.suissa@mcgill.ca

H. Yazici et al. (eds.), *Understanding Evidence-Based Rheumatology*,
DOI 10.1007/978-3-319-08374-2_9

Table 1 Summary of strengths and limitations of RCTs and observational studies

	RCTs	Observational studies
Strengths	Randomization	Large sample sizes and greater statistical power
	Blinding	Greater external validity (more representative population)
Limitations	External validity is limited (usually highly selected population)	Case definition/validation
	Short duration (limiting assessment of long-term efficacy and safety)	Selection bias, information bias, and confounding
	Relatively small samples and low statistical power (limiting ability to detect rare harms)	Informative patient dropout and missing data
	Occasionally not ethical (e.g., randomizing to a harmful exposure such as smoking)	In the case of administrative databases, secondary use of data that lack patient-level data (e.g., measures of disease activity, laboratory tests)
	Recruitment challenging in rare diseases	

ological challenges that, unless recognized and addressed, can lead to confusing results. Indeed, in the past several years, observational studies related to the safety of new drugs used for rheumatic diseases have been published with apparent discrepant results. For example, initial reports on the association between anti-TNF drugs and the risk of serious infection suggested a range of estimates, from no increased risk to a greater than twofold risk. However, these apparent discrepant results were subsequently shown to be reconcilable. Indeed, additional studies designed to examine these differences revealed that the risk of infection appeared to be time-dependent, with an early increase in risk that normalized over time [2]. The differences were found to have arisen from differences in study design and analytical approaches. This emphasizes the importance of robust methodology to ensure the validity of observational studies using pharmacoepidemiology approaches.

Recently, two consensus documents have identified methodologic issues of particular relevance to observational studies of registry and administrative health databases in rheumatology that, if improperly addressed, threaten the validity of their results, namely, confounding by indication, channeling bias, immortal time bias, and depletion of susceptible bias [3, 4]. In addition, they provide guidance on a number of additional methodological, analytical, and reporting points that are designed to enhance study quality.

The aim of this chapter is to compare the strengths and limitations of RCTs and observational study designs (Table 1), to review selected methodological biases in observational studies, to discuss some approaches to avoid or reduce these biases, and to provide examples using selected published studies that have compared results before and after adjusting for possible confounding or bias to illustrate the magnitude of the methodological challenges.

Comparison of RCTs and Observational Study Designs

Evidence-based medicine is the application of the most valid scientific evidence to the care of patients. The strength of evidence is graded in large part based on study design, with randomized clinical trials (RCTs) receiving a higher grade than observational studies. Indeed, randomization and blinding are key attributes of RCTs that deal with the major problems due to confounding and other potential sources of bias inherent in observational studies.

However, RCTs are subject to some important limitations. First, RCTs may lack external validity. Indeed, to be clinically useful, the results of a study "must be relevant to a definable group of patients in a particular clinical setting"[5]. Common issues that potentially affect external validity of RCTs include the setting (e.g., recruitment from primary or academic care centers), eligibility criteria (e.g., magnitude of disease activity), exclusion criteria (e.g., patients with various comorbidities), characteristics of the study subjects (e.g., sociodemographic characteristics such as sex, ethnicity, and education), fixed treatment regimens and intense follow-up. Many examples of lack of generalizability in rheumatology are available. Several papers have been published showing that RA patients in routine care would not be eligible for major clinical trials of anti-TNF drugs, based on strict eligibility and exclusion criteria [6–8]. Geographic setting has also been recognized as a potential factor affecting generalizability. In 2011, belimumab was the first therapy in more than 50 years to be approved by the FDA for the treatment of systemic lupus erythematosus (SLE). At least half of the trial research done for belimumab was conducted outside North America and benefits were found to be consistently lower for subjects in the USA and Canada [9]. Factors contributing to such geographic differences were postulated to include variations in the underlying patient characteristics and variation in study execution. The increasing numbers of trials being conducted globally makes this threat to generalizability of growing concern. Finally, the exclusion of patients with comorbidity is particularly of concern in the context of drug safety rather than effectiveness, as these are the very same patients who may be susceptible to adverse events of the study drug.

Second, RCTs are expensive to undertake and for that reason are often of relatively short duration and underpowered to detect rare outcomes. This limits the ability of demonstrating long-term effectiveness or safety. Open-label extension (OLE) studies are often performed following the successful completion of an RCT and are reported commonly in the rheumatology literature [10]. Although the purpose of OLE studies includes collecting valuable long-term efficacy and safety data, OLE are not as robust as RCTs and should be viewed with considerable circumspection. At this point, the RCT has essentially turned into an observational study. Indeed, to begin with, the characteristics of the study participants who continue in an OLE study may differ significantly from the individuals who dropped out of the RCT. In addition, bias may also be introduced in the assessment of outcomes because of unblinding. Hence, OLE studies may underestimate side effects or harms because those who continue on treatment are those less likely to have dropped out or had side effects during the course of the RCT or overestimate treatment effects because assessments are no longer blinded. In addition, the lack of a comparator group limits the ability to draw robust conclusions from OLE studies. Indeed, the effect of treatment knowledge on behavior may be profound and lead to an inability to distinguish temporal trends from treatment-related effects. In a recent OLE study of strontium ranelate for the treatment of postmenopausal osteoporosis, the 10-year population consisted of only 7 % (237/3,352) of the original trial population [11]. Although the baseline characteristics of the OLE study group were representative of the original population, the possibility of confounding bias cannot be ruled out. The authors also acknowledged that the absence of a comparator group was an important limitation. Finally, it should be noted that if an original RCT was underpowered to detect rare harms, the likelihood of observing these rare harms in OLE remains low. Indeed, OLE of bisphosphonates for the treatment of postmenopausal osteoporosis failed to identify the increased risk of atypical femoral fractures associated with these drugs [12].

RCTs are not always feasible. In studies of harm in particular, it would not be ethical to randomize subjects to harmful exposures (e.g., smoking) and most RCTs are underpowered to detect rare harms.

Finally, RCTs for rare diseases can be particularly challenging logistically because of the difficulty in recruiting sufficient numbers of subjects. In such small RCTs, it may be particularly difficult to distinguish true negative results from false negative results due to low power. Systemic sclerosis is a relatively rare rheumatic disease and this has contributed to the fact that there have been few RCTs in this disease. One of the few RCTs in systemic sclerosis randomized a total of 71 early diffuse subjects to methotrexate or placebo [13]. The study found that methotrexate was associated with a nonsignificant ($p > 0.05$) improvement in two primary outcomes (modified Rodnan skin score and UCLA skin score) and a statistically significant benefit in physician global assessments of disease activity ($p = 0.04$), a third primary outcome, compared to placebo. The authors concluded that there was insufficient evidence to reject the null hypothesis of no treatment effect. Unfortunately, the study was labelled a "negative" trial, when in fact the study had been powered to find an optimistically large effect (35 % difference in skin scores over 1 year) and was therefore clearly underpowered to detect smaller but clinically relevant treatment effects. Indeed, a reanalysis of the data using Bayesian models, which make efficient use of all available data and present results that are more clinically relevant than that which is possible with a p-value from an RCT of a rare disease, found that there was 96 % probability that at least two of three primary outcomes were better on methotrexate compared to placebo [14]. The results of the initial RCT notwithstanding, methotrexate has continued to be commonly used in systemic sclerosis in routine clinical practice [15].

The limitations of RCTs highlight the fact that data from methodologically rigorous observational studies can be extremely valuable. Indeed, with improved methodology to minimize confounding and other biases, as well as newer statistical methods, estimates of treatment effects in observational studies are, for the most part, similar to those from those in RCTs [16–18]. In addition, by expanding the setting to more representative populations, observational studies of treatment effects in routine clinical settings, in particular among subjects who would not have been eligible for RCTs, are useful sources of data. For example, anti-TNF drugs have been shown to be effective in routine clinical practice for patients who would not have been eligible for RCTs albeit with more modest results [19, 20]. These important findings suggest that the current use of biologics in routine clinical practice may be suboptimal and alternative, more cost-effective ways of using these potent but expensive and potentially toxic drugs should be explored. Nevertheless, observational studies of the intended effects of a drug to assess effectiveness remain a challenge as they are subject to greater degree of confounding by indication.

Table 2 Summary of biases in observational studies

	Definition	Examples	Clues for identification of bias	Possible solutions
Selection bias	Selection or exclusion criteria for entering the study associated with both the drug exposure and the outcome	Depletion of susceptibles	Is the risk of the outcome a function of time, higher early after the initiation of drug exposure?	Equal cohort entry point for all drug exposure groups
				New-user designs
Information bias	Also known as measurement or classification bias; this bias results from the inaccurate determination of exposure or outcome	Immortal time bias	Is information about exposure classified in the same way for cases and comparisons?	Survival analysis with time-dependent exposures
Confounding	Lack of comparability between drug groups under comparison. The observed association between an exposure and an outcome may be accounted by a third factor, when that factor is associated with both the exposure and outcome but is not in the causal pathway between the exposure and the outcome	Confounding by indication or confounding by disease severity	Could the outcome attributed to the drug also be an outcome of more severe disease?	Restriction, matching, stratification
				Multivariate regression techniques
				Propensity score modeling
		Channeling bias	Could the treatment have been preferentially prescribed to patients with special preexisting morbidity or because of ineffective current therapy?	Stratification

Time-Related and Other Biases in Observational Studies

In routine clinical practice, exposure to drug therapy is not randomized, but rather dependent on a multitude of patient and physician characteristics. Thus, analysis of clinical data captured in registries and administrative datasets is generally subject to confounding bias and several other sources of bias. The biases are generally classified as selection, information, or confounding bias with different mechanisms described leading to these (Table 2) [21]. In the field of rheumatology, confounding by indication, channeling bias, immortal time bias, and depletion of susceptibles are among the more common mechanisms of bias that have threatened the validity of observational studies of registry and administrative health data.

Confounding by Indication

Confounding by indication may occur in observational studies if patients with more severe disease are preferentially prescribed selected, presumably more intensive, treatments (e.g., different drugs, regimes or doses) [22]. In such situations, differences in outcomes of treatment groups may be due to differences in baseline disease severity rather than treatment itself. Such confounding may affect results in different ways, including attenuating the true effect of treatment (i.e., making it harder to show the effect of treatment because those treated have more severe disease) or suggesting increased harms associated with treatment. In rheumatoid arthritis, for example, patients selected to receive anti-TNF drugs likely have more active disease than those who are not given these drugs. Yet, there is evidence to suggest that the risk of lymphoma in rheumatoid arthritis is particularly associated with disease activity [23]. Thus, increased rates of lymphoma associated with anti-TNF therapy could reflect, at least in part, confounding by indication, whereby patients with the highest risk of lymphoma preferentially receive anti-TNF drugs. The problem of confounding by indication is compounded by the fact that treatment decisions may be affected not only by differences in baseline disease severity but by the natural course of the disease and by treatment response, which can both be subject to considerable interindividual variation.

Various statistical techniques can be used to minimize the effect of confounding by indication in observational studies, including multivariate regression analyses, traditional propensity scores, high-dimensional propensity scores, and instrumental variables to adjust for both baseline and time-dependent confounders. In recent years, studies have also been reported using inverse-probability-weighted (also called inverse-propensity-weighted) marginal structural models [24–27]. Simply put, this type of analysis attempts to balance potential confounders among treated and untreated subjects by reweighing observations according to the inverse of the probability of receiving their observed drug exposure. The approach is similar to analysis via propensity matching estimators, applied over time to account for changing values of the confounders [28]. By reweighing, rather than matching subjects, one is able to make use of all of the subject level data available for the analysis and account for their changes over time. Another advantage of weighting is that fewer assumptions need to be made about the underlying probability models [24]. Finally, missing data due to subject dropout can be accounted for in a straightforward manner by incorporating the estimated probability of study completion in the weight for each subject [25]. Thus, marginal structural models attempt to correct for bias due to confounding (both due to the observational nature of the data and time-varying confounding) and bias due to subject dropout and to estimate the causal effect of treatment.

An example of confounding by indication and statistical adjustment for this comes from a study using the Norfolk Arthritis Register to investigate the benefit of disease-modifying antirheumatic drugs (DMARD) treatment on the long-term functional outcomes of patients with inflammatory polyarthritis [29]. The investigators acknowledged that, in the setting of an observational cohort study, the effect of treatment on outcomes could be confounded by differences both in baseline and time-dependent disease characteristics. They therefore used marginal structural models to adjust for time-dependent confounding. They reported on 642 subjects who had completed a Health Assessment Questionnaire (HAQ) both at baseline and at the 10-year assessment. Of these, 54 % had been treated with DMARDs by 10 years. As expected, patients who did not require DMARDs during 10 years of follow-up had better baseline HAQ scores (median 0.50, IQR 0.13; 0.88) and smaller mean change in HAQ over the follow-up period (0.13; 95 % CI 0.05, 0.21) than those who were treated (baseline median HAQ 1.00; IQR 0.50, 1.50 and mean change over 10 years of 0.24; 95 % CI 0.14, 0.33). When adjusted only for baseline differences in HAQ scores, those ever treated with DMARDs had a significantly greater deterioration in function over 10 years than those never treated (adjusted mean difference in change in HAQ 0.30; 95 % CI 0.18, 0.42). However, after adjustment for the time-dependent confounders using a weighted structural marginal model, there was no significant difference in the change in HAQ between those ever treated and those not treated (−0.01; 95 % CI −0.20, 0.19). In other words, after allowing for the fact that treatment was more likely to be given to those with severe inflammatory polyarthritis, treatment appeared to move patients onto a trajectory that they would have followed if they had had milder disease not requiring treatment. Although the possibility of residual confounding cannot be excluded even using this type of sophisticated statistical approach, the magnitude of confounding by indication appears to be greatly mitigated by it.

Channeling Bias

Channeling bias is a form of confounding by indication that involves not only disease status but also individual patient profiles and medication use tailored to this. In other words, patients at high risk for a given complication may be preferentially prescribed or switched to a certain treatment because an alternative treatment is known to be associated with that particular complication. Thus, one subtle difference between confounding by indication and channeling bias is that in the former case the confounding results from a patient's indication for a certain treatment, whereas in the latter case, it results from a contraindication to that treatment. Another is that channeling bias generally also involves switching of treatment from an older to a newer agent.

In a population-based safety study examining the association between leflunomide and interstitial lung disease (ILD) using a large claims database, we found that in the overall analysis, leflunomide (rate ratio 1.9), but not methotrexate (rate ratio 1.4), was associated with the risk of ILD [30]. We found that patients with a history of ILD were almost twice as likely to have received leflunomide compared to methotrexate (adjusted odds ratio 1.9; 95 % CI 1.5, 2.3) as a first DMARD. In a stratified analysis, we showed that in patients without prior exposure to methotrexate and without a history of ILD, methotrexate (rate ratio 3.1) but not leflunomide (rate ratio 1.2) was associated with ILD, whereas in the subgroup of patients with either a prior exposure to methotrexate or a history of ILD, methotrexate was highly *protective* against ILD (rate ratio 0.4) and leflunomide was associated with a significant increase (rate ratio 2.6) in the risk of ILD. We concluded that this stratified analysis provided strong evidence that patients with a history of ILD may have been preferentially prescribed leflunomide rather than methotrexate on the assumption that, in contrast to methotrexate, no lung toxicity was known to be associated with leflunomide. Thus, channeling bias must be considered in studies of harm and proper stratified analysis of the data is necessary to determine whether this bias may have influenced the results.

Immortal Time Bias

A study investigated whether the use of antimalarials in patients with systemic lupus erythematosus (SLE) could be associated with cancer incidence [31]. The authors used a cohort of 235 SLE patients followed for up to 31 years, of which 13 patients developed cancer during follow-up. The comparison of time to cancer incidence was based on comparing the 156 patients who had "ever" received antimalarials during follow-up with the 79 who did not. The Cox proportional hazards model was used to estimate the adjusted hazard ratio of 0.15 (95 % CI 0.02, 0.99). This result implied that the incidence of cancer of all types could be significantly reduced by 85 % in SLE patients treated with antimalarials.

However, this analysis was subject to a bias created by looking at "ever" exposure to antimalarials during follow-up. Immortal time refers to a time period during cohort follow-up when, *by design*, subjects cannot die or have the outcome event under study [32, 33]. Thus, exposed patients are necessarily "immortal" (in this case cancer-free) during the time span between cohort entry and the first prescription for an antimalarial. On the other hand, the comparison patients who did not receive antimalarials had no such cancer-free period as they could have developed cancer anytime during follow-up. Thus, the comparison of the time to cancer incidence between these two groups provided an advantage to exposed patients because they were guaranteed, by design, a cancer-free period. To the extent that this immortal time period is in fact unexposed but misclassified as exposed, the immortal time bias is a form of information bias. This type of bias will result in lowering the rate ratio (i.e., closer to the null if the effect is harmful (>1) or away from the null if the effect is nil or protective (<1)).

A time-dependent Cox proportional hazard model or similar approach to data analysis that classifies the person-time from cohort entry until the first prescription as unexposed and the subsequent person-time as exposed is a simple approach to avoid an immortal time bias. We replicated the abovementioned study in a population-based cohort of 23,810 rheumatoid arthritis patients, identified from provincial healthcare databases between 1980 and 2003 [34]. We identified all cancer cases occurring during follow-up and obtained information on the timing of antimalarial agents, as well as all relevant concomitant medications. The analysis was based on an approach that considered the time-dependent nature of the antimalarial prescriptions and classified the time prior to the first one correctly as unexposed. As a result, the adjusted rate ratio of cancer incidence with antimalarial use was 1.1 (95 % CI 0.9, 1.3). This is quite different from the protective effect reported using the approach subject to immortal time bias described above.

Other examples of immortal time bias are found in the rheumatology literature. In a study from the LUMINA cohort, the use of hydroxychloroquine was reported to reduce the incidence of renal damage by 88 % (hazard ratio 0.12; 95 % CI 0.02, 0.97) [35]. However, exposure to hydroxychloroquine was measured as "any use during the follow-up period" (i.e., ever/never used). In so doing, unexposed person-time from cohort entry to the start of actual exposure was misclassified as exposed. This "immortal" time period during which the outcome under study could not have occurred conferred an undue advantage to the exposed group. As a result, the protective effect of hydroxychloroquine was overestimated [36]. Another similar example involving hydroxychloroquine comes from the ARAMIS cohort of rheumatoid arthritis patients. In that study, 4 years or more of exposure was associated with a very significant 77 % reduction in the incidence of diabetes (hazard ratio 0.23; 95 % CI 0.11, 0.50) [37]. Immortal time bias was introduced by the inherent requirement of 4 years with no diabetes to determine the exposure, whereas the nonexposed reference patients were permitted, by the analysis, to develop diabetes as of day 1 of cohort entry.

Depletion of Susceptibles

The time-varying hazard functions of several medications commonly used in rheumatology have been described, for example, the higher risk of infection present with early exposure to TNF antagonists [38–40] and the higher risk of myocardial infarction or acute renal failure associated with early exposure to rofecoxib [41, 42] and other NSAIDs [42]. If a study sample is underrepresented by those individuals most susceptible to an event possibly because of early attrition due to the development of a complication and overrepresented by low-risk individuals who tolerate the drug, a depletion of susceptible bias can result and will tend to underestimate the magnitude of harm associated with a treatment.

A depletion of susceptible bias can result from study design or analysis. In a study using a large, population-based administrative database designed to examine the risk of myocardial infarction associated with COX-2 inhibitors, only those individuals who were given *at least two successive prescriptions* of the drugs of interest were included (with the purported intent of excluding "sporadic" users of NSAIDs) [43]. The authors found no increase in the risk of myocardial infarction associated with the use of rofecoxib compared to controls. It is possible that excluding subjects who received only one rofecoxib prescription may have excluded patients among the most susceptible to the increased risk in myocardial infarction that has been since confirmed with rofecoxib and that this may have contributed to an underestimation of the true risk.

Misspecification of the "at-risk" period may also result in a depletion of susceptible bias. Dixon et al. provided an excellent example using the British Biologic Register [38]. This group had previously reported no increase in the risk of serious infection associated with TNF antagonists in rheumatoid arthritis [44]. However, they subsequently reanalyzed their data and found that the magnitude of the risk of infection varied depending on different definitions of the "at-risk" period. For example, when the at-risk period was defined as "receiving treatment," there was no significant risk of infection associated with anti-TNF therapy (adjusted incidence rate ratio 1.22; 95 % CI 0.88, 1.69). However, there was a strong trend towards increased risk when the at-risk period was defined as "ever receiving treatment" (adjusted incidence rate ratio 1.35; 95 % CI 0.99, 1.85). They concluded that these result were consistent with a "depletion of susceptible" effect, whereby in an analysis with follow-up limited to the period of exposure, those at greater risk of infections are excluded from the analysis early and those who continue to receive treatment are really a healthier group at an overall lower risk. Care in defining the risk window and the use of sensitivity analyses to investigate alternative definitions of exposure can help to address this potential bias.

Finally, the depletion of susceptible phenomenon can have a major impact in prevalent cohort studies, in other words studies that include *prevalent* users of a drug, because of the exclusion of subjects in the early high-risk period and the over-representation of lower-risk subjects who survived this early high-risk period. The "new-user" design has been proposed as solution to overcome this problem [45].

The Quagmire of Biologics and Malignancies

The relative strengths and limitations of RCTs and observational studies, and the challenges in practicing evidence-based medicine are highlighted by the controversy surrounding the association between biologics and malignancies in RA. A thorough review by Chakravarty et al. found that RA was not associated with a significantly increased *overall* risk of malignancies compared to the general population [46]. On the other hand, a subsequent meta-analysis of 21 observational studies by Smitten et al. found a small but significant increase in overall risk (standardized incidence ratio (SIR) 1.05, 95 % CI 1.01, 1.09) [47]. More importantly, though, this meta-analysis, demonstrated that such overall findings obscure the more informative fact that RA may be associated with an increase in some and a decrease in other site-specific malignancies. Indeed, in this meta-analysis, there was an increase in the risk of lymphoma (SIR 2.08, 95 % CI 1.80–2.39) and lung cancer (SIR 1.63, 95 % CI 1.43–1.987), but a decrease in the risk of colorectal (SIR 0.77; 95 % CI 0.65–0.90) and breast cancer (SIR 0.84; 95 % CI 0.79, 0.90) [47].

This study underscores the fact that the relationship between RA and malignancies is complex. There are multiple theoretical pathways by which RA and malignancies may be associated [48]. Two such pathways are the disease per se and the drugs used to treat the disease. As far as the disease is concerned, autoimmune dysfunction and chronic inflammation have been proposed as mechanisms whereby the risk of certain malignancies, in particular lymphoproliferative cancers, may be increased in RA. In particular, higher disease severity in RA has been associated with a greater risk of lymphoma [23]. On the other hand, drugs used to treat RA modulate the immune system and may, also in part, be responsible for the increased risk of malignancy [49]. In particular, cytokine pathways, including tumor necrosis factor (TNF), play an important role in tumor surveillance. Thus, blocking this pathway with anti-TNF drugs could theoretically contribute to an increased risk of malignancy. Moreover, lacking a randomized trial, it may be difficult to tease apart the effects of the disease and the drugs to the extent that stronger immunosuppression is used in more severe disease, so that any observational study would be subject to intractable confounding by disease severity. Finally, to add to the complexity, the question of how the possible risks of malignancy resulting from the disease or the drugs relate, whether additively, synergistically, or perhaps negatively with, for example, the reduction of the chronic inflammation by the drugs mitigating the risk associated with the disease itself, remains unresolved [50].

Insofar as the evidence is concerned, none of the individual RCTs of anti-TNF drugs in RA showed a significantly increased risk of lymphoma or cancer. However, a 2006 meta-analysis of nine trials (*N* 5,014) of ≥12 weeks duration (range 12–54 weeks) with infliximab or adalimumab in RA patients showed a three-fold increase in the overall risk of cancer relative to placebo (pooled odds ratio 3.3; 95 % CI 1.2–9.1) [51]. The absolute rates of events were, however, fairly low, with 29 malignancies reported in 3,192 patients on treatment (0.9 %) compared to 3 in 1,428 (0.2 %) in those on placebo. A follow-up report placed the relative risk at 2.02 (95 % CI 0.95, 4.29) when additional trial data were added [52]. On the other hand, a meta-analysis of etanercept trial data in patients with rheumatic diseases (18 rheumatoid arthritis, 2 psoriatic arthritis and 2 ankylosing spondylitis trials with 6,798 person-years of exposure) showed no increased risk with this drug [53] although the exact number of malignancies in the treated and control patients was not reported. Finally, the results of an FDA-requested analysis was published in response to the meta-analysis of infliximab and adalimumab data and reported no increase in the risk of malignancy in patients with RA treated with infliximab and adalimumab when compared to general population rates available from the Surveillance, Epidemiology, and End Results (SEER) database and with etanercept when compared to placebo [54].

More recently, an individual patient data meta-analysis of 74 RCTs of etanercept, infliximab, and adalimumab identified 130 (0.84 %) of 15,418 individuals randomized to anti-TNF therapy diagnosed with cancer, compared to 48 (0.64 %) of 7,486 individuals randomized to comparators [55]. The overall relative risk of all-site cancer (excluding non-melanoma skin cancers) associated with the three anti-TNF drugs was 0.99 (95 %CI 0.61, 1.68). However, there were indications of differences in control group cancer risk between the three drugs and some indication of an increased cancer risk with infliximab, although this latter observation was severely limited by the small numbers of events (two or less in the infliximab comparators). In addition, the numbers of site-specific cancers, in particular lymphomas, were too small to permit robust statistical modeling of site-specific cancer risks. Thus, the authors concluded that despite a reassuring overall short-term risk, they could neither refute nor verify that *individual* anti-TNF drugs could affect the short-term risk of cancer and that there might be important site-specific differences. In addition, the authors acknowledged that the short duration of the trials included in their analyses precluded as assessment of long-term cancer risks associated with anti-TNF drugs. They thus concluded that "[a]lthough this individual patient data meta-analysis represents the best available evidence to date regarding short-term risks, analyses of long-term risks as well as further explorations of the risk for site-specific cancers…require larger study populations and longer follow-up. The ongoing long-term follow-up via registries is important in this respect."

Observational studies of RA patients treated with anti-TNF drugs have not, to date, shown a substantial increase in the overall risk of cancer (excluding skin cancers) or lymphoma [56–60]. A recent meta-analysis of RA registries and prospective observational studies reported a pooled risk estimate of 0.95 (95 % CI 0.85, 1.05) in the risk of all-site malignancy in subjects exposed to anti-TNF therapy [61]. Of note, the risk for individual anti-TNF agents has not been reported to be different either, although this analysis has also been limited by small numbers, and in one study that assessed drug-specific risks by time since treatment start, differences by drug and time of exposure were observed, with subjects exposed to adalimumab (RR 1.91; 95 % CI 1.11, 3.31), but not etanercept or infliximab, found to be at higher risk of overall cancer in the first year but not thereafter [62]. The meta-analysis specifically excluded studies using administrative databases to reduce heterogeneity. Nonetheless, a recent study using two US and one Canadian administrative database showed no significantly increased risk of either solid (HR 0.91, 95 % CI 0.65, 1.26) or hematological (HR 1.37; 95 % CI 0.71, 2.65) malignancies in subjects exposed to anti-TNF drugs [63].

Despite the accumulating evidence from both RCTs and observational studies suggesting that the risk of malignancy is not substantially increased with anti-TNF drugs in RA, concerns persist. The evidence remains sparse regarding many important questions, including whether the association between anti-TNF drugs and malignancies is a class effect or whether there might be individual drug effects, whether there are differences between overall versus site-specific cancers, and whether risk varies over time. Indeed, absence of evidence cannot be construed as evidence of absence. The fact that current treatment guidelines on these questions are still largely based on consensus recommendations speaks to the fact that the evidence to date remains incomplete [64]. In addition to the inherent limitations of RCTs and observational studies already discussed above, future RCTs will no doubt exclude patients with a history of malignancy or with comorbidities associated with higher risk of malignancy and subjects entered into observational studies will be screened for malignancies prior to exposure, thereby reducing the likelihood of finding what are already rare events. In addition, with signals relating to infliximab and adalimumab, both monoclonal antibodies, but not etanercept, a receptor fusion protein, there may be a perception that monoclonal antibodies are associated with a greater risk of malignancy and channeling bias based on a patient's perceived risk of malignancy may result. Finally, finding an appropriate comparator group for RA subjects exposed to anti-TNF drugs who are likely to be under greater cancer surveillance will be particularly challenging. We believe that the answers to these questions will hinge not so much on one or another study design, but rather on the incremental accumulation of evidence from methodologically rigorously conducted studies using a variety of designs and statistical analyses.

Standards for Reporting of Registry and Administrative Database Research in Rheumatology

The setting of the study has implications on access to medication, eligibility criteria, and drug penetration and may introduce additional problems of confounding beyond the control of the investigators. For example, guidelines effective in many jurisdictions limit the prescription of biologic drugs to patients with more severe disease and/or failure of one or more traditional DMARD. The challenge here is to identify an appropriate comparison group. Indeed, the selection of the comparison cohort remains one of the most important challenges in observational setting [65] and has the potential to influence the interpretation of study results. An illustration comes from a comparison of the results of the British [44] and German [66] biologic registries. Despite fairly similar absolute risks of serious infections in patients treated with anti-TNF drugs in those two studies (ranging from 51.3 to 64 per 1,000 person-years, with overlapping confidence intervals), the estimates in the British study suggested no increased risk of serious infections in patients treated with anti-TNF drugs, whereas the German study suggested a doubling in risk. This may have resulted from the fact that the estimates of risk in the respective controls were very different, with the British controls having a two-fold increase in risk of serious infections compared to the German controls (41.1; 95 % CI 31.4, 53.5, per 1,000 person-years compared to 23; 95 % CI 13, 39, per 1,000 person-years, respectively).

In addition, temporal trends may also influence the characteristics of the treated patients. For example, biologic drugs were initially used as drugs of last resort in patients with long-standing refractory rheumatoid arthritis. As clinical practice has evolved, rheumatoid arthritis patients with less severe disease are now commonly treated much earlier with these drugs. Data from the Swedish ARTIS biologic registry illustrates this well (Table 3) [67]. These data show that the clinical characteristics of patients newly started on biologics has changed considerably over time,

Table 3 Temporal trends in clinical profiles of rheumatoid arthritis subjects starting biologic drugs

	1999	2002	2005	2008
Median disease duration, years	9.8	8.2	7.5	7.0
Tender joint count*	10.6	8.7	8.3	7.7
Swollen joint count*	11.9	9.5	8.4	7.5
C-reactive protein (mg/L)*	46.4	34.9	25.4	18.4
DAS-28*	6.0	5.5	5.2	5.0
Health Assessment Questionnaire*	1.7	1.4	1.2	1.2

DAS-28 28-joint Disease Activity Score
**p* for trend <0.05

with many markers of disease activity indicating that patients with milder disease are being increasingly treated with biologics earlier. Observational data sources are increasingly being used to pursue comparative effectiveness studies in rheumatic diseases (discussed below) [68, 69]. However, for the reasons indicated above, great caution will have to be exercised when comparing established and more recently introduced biologics. Better effectiveness and safety profiles of newer drugs could reflect, at least in part, differences in clinical characteristics of the patients exposed to established and newer drugs.

Several important sets of reporting guidelines on research methods and findings of observational studies have been published [70, 71]. This has resulted in greatly enhancing the quality of observational health research and strengthening results of studies. Papers providing reporting guidelines with specific applications for studies of biologic registers and administrative health data in rheumatic disease research have also been published [3, 4, 72]. In addition to what has been previously discussed, issues of case definition (in particular osteoarthritis and rheumatoid arthritis) and comorbid diseases (e.g., cardiovascular disease, infections, cancer, osteoporosis, fractures, and renal disease) relevant to rheumatic diseases are addressed. Finally, they emphasize the importance of detailed reporting of setting and characteristics of exposed and comparator groups, as well as analyzing results under various specifications of statistical models to assess the sensitivity of the results to model assumptions.

New Use of Registry and Administrative Health Data: Comparative Effectiveness Studies

With the increasing number of new targeted therapies to treat rheumatoid arthritis, registry and administrative heath data have found a new role, namely, to allow comparative effectiveness studies in the absence of head-to-head trials [68, 69]. An example comes from the British Biologics Register in which, in rheumatoid arthritis patients having failed a first anti-TNF drug, the effectiveness of rituximab was compared to a second anti-TNF drug as second-line treatment. In total, 1,328 patients were included in the analysis of treatment response, and 937 patients were included in the analysis of Health Assessment Questionnaire (HAQ) scores. Six months after switching, 54.8 % of patients who switched to rituximab were responders according to the EULAR criteria compared to 47.3 % of those who switched to a second anti-TNF. A total of 38.4 % of rituximab patients achieved a clinically important improvement in HAQ score compared to 29.6 % in anti-TNF patients. After adjustment using propensity scores, patients who switched to rituximab were significantly more likely to achieve EULAR response (odds ratio 1.31; 95 % CI 1.02, 1.69) compared to those who switched to an alternative anti-TNF. Rituximab patients were also significantly more likely to achieve improvements in HAQ score (odds ratio 1.49; 95 % CI 1.07, 2.08). Restriction has also been proposed as a useful tool to adjust for confounding by indication in studies of comparative effectiveness using administrative databases [73].

Defining treatment effectiveness using large registries and administrative databases without measures of disease status can be more challenging. Nevertheless, time to discontinuation may be an accepted measure, and more sophisticated definitions incorporating biologic dose escalation or switching, adjunct drug use (DMARDs, oral and parenteral glucocorticoids, NSAIDs), and composite measures of disease severity have been used [74–77]. In addition, comparative effectiveness studies will also be relevant for other rheumatic diseases where new and expensive targeted therapies have been or are being developed, including systemic lupus erythematosus and gout. Guidelines to minimize bias in comparative effectiveness studies of registries have been formulated [78–80].

Conclusion

Observational studies of registry and administrative health data have their unique advantages and disadvantages compared to RCTs [81]. In addition to what has been discussed above, challenges of longitudinal studies of registry data also include patient dropout, loss to follow-up, and missing data, and challenges of administrative health database studies include defining exposure (e.g., drug dispensed may not equate to drug taken, affecting measures of medication compliance) and residual confounding from unavailable patient data (e.g., smoking status, body mass index, disease severity, etc.). Pharmacoepidemiological studies also are susceptible to several time-related biases that can generally be avoided with proper study design and careful data analysis. Nevertheless, studies from large, unselected samples with prolonged follow-up are a highly useful source of data because of the generalizability of their results and the power to detect rare events. Standards for conducting and reporting studies of registry and administrative health data have been proposed and have the potential to enhance the validity of observational studies in rheumatology. In addition, a better understanding of study design and data analysis and new statistical techniques have contributed to ensuring that analysis of registry data and administrative databases is robust. Finally, registry and administrative health databases have provided a new opportunity to undertake useful comparative effectiveness research, especially given that head-to-head comparison of expensive, targeted therapies remains unlikely.

References

1. Chen YF, Jobanputra P, Barton P, Jowett S, Bryan S, Clark W, Fry-Smith A, Burls A. A systematic review of the effectiveness of adalimumab, etanercept and infliximab for the treatment of rheumatoid arthritis in adults and an economic evaluation of their cost-effectiveness. Health Technol Assess. 2006;10(42):iii–iv, xi–xiii, 1–229.
2. Askling J, Dixon W. The safety of anti-tumour necrosis factor therapy in rheumatoid arthritis. Curr Opin Rheumatol. 2008;20:138–44.
3. Dixon WG, Carmona L, Finckh A, Hetland ML, Kvien TK, Landewe R, Listing J, Nicola PJ, Tarp U, Zink A, Askling J. EULAR points to consider when establishing, analysing and reporting safety data of biologics registers in rheumatology. Ann Rheum Dis. 2010;69(9): 1596–602.
4. Bernatsky S, Lix L, O'Donnell S, Lacaille D. Consensus statements for the use of administrative health data in rheumatic disease research and surveillance. J Rheumatol. 2013;40(1):66–73.
5. Rothwell PM. External validity of randomised controlled trials: "to whom do the results of this trial apply?". Lancet. 2005;365(9453):82–93.
6. Sokka T, Pincus T. Eligibility of patients in routine care for major clinical trials of anti-tumor necrosis factor alpha agents in rheumatoid arthritis. Arthritis Rheum. 2003;48(2):313–8.
7. Yazici Y, Erkan D. Eligibility of rheumatoid arthritis patients seen in clinical practice for rheumatoid arthritis clinical trials: comment on the article by Sokka and Pincus. Arthritis Rheum. 2003;48(12):3611; author reply 3613–5.
8. Greenberg JD, Kishimoto M, Strand V, Cohen SB, Olenginski TP, Harrington T, Kafka SP, Reed G, Kremer JM. Tumor necrosis factor antagonist responsiveness in a United States rheumatoid arthritis cohort. Am J Med. 2008;121(6):532–8.
9. Kandala NB, Connock M, Grove A, Sutcliffe P, Mohiuddin S, Hartley L, Court R, Cummins E, Gordon C, Clarke A. Belimumab: a technological advance for systemic lupus erythematosus patients? Report of a systematic review and meta-analysis. BMJ Open. 2013;3(7):e002852.
10. Taylor WJ, Weatherall M. What are open-label extension studies for? J Rheumatol. 2006; 33(4):642–3.
11. Reginster JY, Kaufman JM, Goemaere S, Devogelaer JP, Benhamou CL, Felsenberg D, Diaz-Curiel M, Brandi ML, Badurski J, Wark J, Balogh A, Bruyere O, Roux C. Maintenance of antifracture efficacy over 10 years with strontium ranelate in postmenopausal osteoporosis. Osteoporos Int. 2012;23(3):1115–22.
12. Black DM, Kelly MP, Genant HK, Palermo L, Eastell R, Bucci-Rechtweg C, Cauley J, Leung PC, Boonen S, Santora A, de Papp A, Bauer DC. Bisphosphonates and fractures of the subtrochanteric or diaphyseal femur. N Engl J Med. 2010;362(19):1761–71.
13. Pope JE, Bellamy N, Seibold JR, Baron M, Ellman M, Carette S, Smith CD, Chalmers IM, Hong P, O'Hanlon D, Kaminska E, Markland J, Sibley J, Catoggio L, Furst DE. A randomized, controlled trial of methotrexate versus placebo in early diffuse scleroderma. Arthritis Rheum. 2001;44(6):1351–8.
14. Johnson SR, Feldman BM, Pope JE, Tomlinson GA. Shifting our thinking about uncommon disease trials: the case of methotrexate in scleroderma. J Rheumatol. 2009;36(2):323–9.
15. Pope JE, Ouimet JM, Krizova A. Scleroderma treatment differs between experts and general rheumatologists. Arthritis Rheum. 2006;55(1):138–45.
16. Benson K, Hartz AJ. A comparison of observational studies and randomized, controlled trials. N Engl J Med. 2000;342(25):1878–86.

17. Concato J, Shah N, Horwitz RI. Randomized, controlled trials, observational studies, and the hierarchy of research designs. N Engl J Med. 2000;342(25):1887–92.
18. Ioannidis JP, Haidich AB, Pappa M, Pantazis N, Kokori SI, Tektonidou MG, Contopoulos-Ioannidis DG, Lau J. Comparison of evidence of treatment effects in randomized and nonrandomized studies. JAMA. 2001;286(7):821–30.
19. Kievit W, Fransen J, Oerlemans AJ, Kuper HH, van der Laar MA, de Rooij DJ, De Gendt CM, Ronday KH, Jansen TL, van Oijen PC, Brus HL, Adang EM, van Riel PL. The efficacy of anti-TNF in rheumatoid arthritis, a comparison between randomised controlled trials and clinical practice. Ann Rheum Dis. 2007;66(11):1473–8.
20. Wolfe F, Michaud K. The loss of health status in rheumatoid arthritis and the effect of biologic therapy: a longitudinal observational study. Arthritis Res Ther. 2010;12(2):R35.
21. Delgado-Rodriguez M, Llorca J. Bias. J Epidemiol Community Health. 2004;58(8):635–41.
22. Landewe RB. The benefits of early treatment in rheumatoid arthritis: confounding by indication, and the issue of timing. Arthritis Rheum. 2003;48(1):1–5.
23. Baecklund E, Ekbom A, Sparen P, Feltelius N, Klareskog L. Disease activity and risk of lymphoma in patients with rheumatoid arthritis: nested case-control study. BMJ. 1998;317(7152): 180–1.
24. Hernán M, Brumback B, Robins J. Marginal structural models to estimate the joint causal effect of nonrandomized treatments. J Am Stat Assoc. 2001;96(454):440–8.
25. Hernan MA, Brumback BA, Robins JM. Estimating the causal effect of zidovudine on CD4 count with a marginal structural model for repeated measures. Stat Med. 2002; 21(12): 1689–709.
26. Choi HK, Hernan MA, Seeger JD, Robins JM, Wolfe F. Methotrexate and mortality in patients with rheumatoid arthritis: a prospective study. Lancet. 2002;359(9313):1173–7.
27. Herrick AL, Lunt M, Whidby N, Ennis H, Silman A, McHugh N, Denton CP. Observational study of treatment outcome in early diffuse cutaneous systemic sclerosis. J Rheumatol. 2010;37(1):116–24.
28. Rubin DB. Estimating causal effects from large data sets using propensity scores. Ann Intern Med. 1997;127(8 Pt 2):757–63.
29. Farragher TM, Lunt M, Plant D, Bunn DK, Barton A, Symmons DP. Benefit of early treatment in inflammatory polyarthritis patients with anti-cyclic citrullinated peptide antibodies versus those without antibodies. Arthritis Care Res (Hoboken). 2010;62(5):664–75.
30. Suissa S, Hudson M, Ernst P. Leflunomide use and the risk of interstitial lung disease in rheumatoid arthritis. Arthritis Rheum. 2006;54(5):1435–9.
31. Ruiz-Irastorza G, Ugarte A, Egurbide M, Garmendia M, Pijoan J, Martinez-Berriotxoa A, Aguirre C. Antimalarials may influence the risk of malignancy in systemic lupus erythematosus. Ann Rheum Dis. 2007;66(6):815–7.
32. Suissa S. Immortal time bias in pharmocepidemiology. Am J Epidemiol. 2008;167(4):492–9.
33. Suissa S. Immortal time bias in observational studies of drug effects. Pharmacoepidemiol Drug Saf. 2007;16(3):241–9.
34. Bernatsky S, Clarke A, Suissa S. Antimalarial drugs and malignancy: no evidence of a protective effect in rheumatoid arthritis. Ann Rheum Dis. 2008;67(2):277–8.
35. Pons-Estel GJ, Alarcon GS, McGwin Jr G, Danila MI, Zhang J, Bastian HM, Reveille JD, Vila LM. Protective effect of hydroxychloroquine on renal damage in patients with lupus nephritis: LXV, data from a multiethnic US cohort. Arthritis Rheum. 2009;61(6):830–9.
36. Vinet E, Bernatsky S, Suissa S. Have some beneficial effects of hydroxychloroquine been overestimated? Potential biases in observational studies of drug effects: comment on the article by Pons-Estel et al. Arthritis Rheum. 2009;61(11):1614–5; author reply 1615–6.
37. Wasko MC, Hubert HB, Lingala VB, Elliott JR, Luggen ME, Fries JF, Ward MM. Hydroxychloroquine and risk of diabetes in patients with rheumatoid arthritis. JAMA. 2007; 298(2):187–93.
38. Dixon WG, Symmons DP, Lunt M, Watson KD, Hyrich KL, Silman AJ. Serious infection following anti-tumor necrosis factor alpha therapy in patients with rheumatoid arthritis: lessons from interpreting data from observational studies. Arthritis Rheum. 2007;56(9):2896–904.

39. Askling J, Fored CM, Brandt L, Baecklund E, Bertilsson L, Feltelius N, Coster L, Geborek P, Jacobsson LT, Lindblad S, Lysholm J, Rantapaa-Dahlqvist S, Saxne T, van Vollenhoven RF, Klareskog L. Time-dependent increase in risk of hospitalisation with infection among Swedish RA patients treated with TNF antagonists. Ann Rheum Dis. 2007;66(10):1339–44.
40. Curtis JR, Xi J, Patkar N, Xie A, Saag KG, Martin C. Drug-specific and time-dependent risks of bacterial infection among patients with rheumatoid arthritis who were exposed to tumor necrosis factor alpha antagonists. Arthritis Rheum. 2007;56(12):4226–7.
41. Levesque LE, Brophy JM, Zhang B. Time variations in the risk of myocardial infarction among elderly users of COX-2 inhibitors. CMAJ. 2006;174(11):1563–9.
42. Schneider V, Levesque LE, Zhang B, Hutchinson T, Brophy JM. Association of selective and conventional nonsteroidal antiinflammatory drugs with acute renal failure: A population-based, nested case-control analysis. Am J Epidemiol. 2006;164(9):881–9.
43. Mamdani M, Rochon P, Juurlink DN, Anderson GM, Kopp A, Naglie G, Austin PC, Laupacis A. Effect of selective cyclooxygenase 2 inhibitors and naproxen on short-term risk of acute myocardial infarction in the elderly. Arch Intern Med. 2003;163(4):481–6.
44. Dixon WG, Watson K, Lunt M, Hyrich KL, Silman AJ, Symmons DP. Rates of serious infection, including site-specific and bacterial intracellular infection, in rheumatoid arthritis patients receiving anti-tumor necrosis factor therapy: results from the British Society for Rheumatology Biologics Register. Arthritis Rheum. 2006;54(8):2368–76.
45. Ray WA. Evaluating medication effects outside of clinical trials: new-user designs. Am J Epidemiol. 2003;158(9):915–20.
46. Chakravarty EF, Genovese MC. Associations between rheumatoid arthritis and malignancy. Rheum Dis Clin North Am. 2004;30(2):271–84, vi.
47. Smitten AL, Simon TA, Hochberg MC, Suissa S. A meta-analysis of the incidence of malignancy in adult patients with rheumatoid arthritis. Arthritis Res Ther. 2008;10(2):R45.
48. Michaud K, Wolfe F. Comorbidities in rheumatoid arthritis. Best Pract Res Clin Rheumatol. 2007;21(5):885–906.
49. Radis CD, Kahl LE, Baker GL, Wasko MC, Cash JM, Gallatin A, Stolzer BL, Agarwal AK, Medsger Jr TA, Kwoh CK. Effects of cyclophosphamide on the development of malignancy and on long-term survival of patients with rheumatoid arthritis. A 20-year followup study. Arthritis Rheum. 1995;38(8):1120–7.
50. Symmons DP, Silman AJ. Anti-tumor necrosis factor alpha therapy and the risk of lymphoma in rheumatoid arthritis: no clear answer. Arthritis Rheum. 2004;50(6):1703–6.
51. Bongartz T, Sutton AJ, Sweeting MJ, Buchan I, Matteson EL, Montori V. Anti-TNF antibody therapy in rheumatoid arthritis and the risk of serious infections and malignancies: systematic review and meta-analysis of rare harmful effects in randomized controlled trials. JAMA. 2006;295(19):2275–85.
52. Costenbader KH, Glass R, Cui J, Shadick N. Risk of serious infections and malignancies with anti-TNF antibody therapy in rheumatoid arthritis. JAMA. 2006;296(18):2201; author reply 2203–4.
53. Fleischmann R, Baumgartner SW, Weisman MH, Liu T, White B, Peloso P. Long term safety of etanercept in elderly subjects with rheumatic diseases. Ann Rheum Dis. 2006;65(3): 379–84.
54. Okada SK, Siegel JN. Risk of serious infections and malignancies with anti-TNF antibody therapy in rheumatoid arthritis. JAMA. 2006;296(18):2201–2; author reply 2203–4.
55. Askling J, Fahrbach K, Nordstrom B, Ross S, Schmid CH, Symmons D. Cancer risk with tumor necrosis factor alpha (TNF) inhibitors: meta-analysis of randomized controlled trials of adalimumab, etanercept, and infliximab using patient level data. Pharmacoepidemiol Drug Saf. 2011;20(2):119–30.
56. Geborek P, Bladstrom A, Turesson C, Gulfe A, Petersson IF, Saxne T, Olsson H, Jacobsson LT. Tumour necrosis factor blockers do not increase overall tumour risk in patients with rheumatoid arthritis, but may be associated with an increased risk of lymphomas. Ann Rheum Dis. 2005;64(5):699–703.

57. Wolfe F, Michaud K. Biologic treatment of rheumatoid arthritis and the risk of malignancy: analyses from a large US observational study. Arthritis Rheum. 2007;56(9):2886–95.
58. Wolfe F, Michaud K. The effect of methotrexate and anti-tumor necrosis factor therapy on the risk of lymphoma in rheumatoid arthritis in 19,562 patients during 89,710 person-years of observation. Arthritis Rheum. 2007;56(5):1433–9.
59. Askling J, Fored CM, Baecklund E, Brandt L, Backlin C, Ekbom A, Sundstrom C, Bertilsson L, Coster L, Geborek P, Jacobsson LT, Lindblad S, Lysholm J, Rantapaa-Dahlqvist S, Saxne T, Klareskog L, Feltelius N. Haematopoietic malignancies in rheumatoid arthritis: lymphoma risk and characteristics after exposure to tumour necrosis factor antagonists. Ann Rheum Dis. 2005;64(10):1414–20.
60. Askling J, Fored CM, Brandt L, Baecklund E, Bertilsson L, Feltelius N, Coster L, Geborek P, Jacobsson LT, Lindblad S, Lysholm J, Rantapaa-Dahlqvist S, Saxne T, Klareskog L. Risks of solid cancers in patients with rheumatoid arthritis and after treatment with tumour necrosis factor antagonists. Ann Rheum Dis. 2005;64(10):1421–6.
61. Mariette X, Matucci-Cerinic M, Pavelka K, Taylor P, van Vollenhoven R, Heatley R, Walsh C, Lawson R, Reynolds A, Emery P. Malignancies associated with tumour necrosis factor inhibitors in registries and prospective observational studies: a systematic review and meta-analysis. Ann Rheum Dis. 2011;70(11):1895–904.
62. Askling J, van Vollenhoven RF, Granath F, Raaschou P, Fored CM, Baecklund E, Dackhammar C, Feltelius N, Coster L, Geborek P, Jacobsson LT, Lindblad S, Rantapaa-Dahlqvist S, Saxne T, Klareskog L. Cancer risk in patients with rheumatoid arthritis treated with anti-tumor necrosis factor alpha therapies: does the risk change with the time since start of treatment? Arthritis Rheum. 2009;60(11):3180–9.
63. Setoguchi S, Solomon DH, Weinblatt ME, Katz JN, Avorn J, Glynn RJ, Cook EF, Carney G, Schneeweiss S. Tumor necrosis factor alpha antagonist use and cancer in patients with rheumatoid arthritis. Arthritis Rheum. 2006;54(9):2757–64.
64. Bombardier C, Hazlewood GS, Akhavan P, Schieir O, Dooley A, Haraoui B, Khraishi M, Leclercq SA, Legare J, Mosher DP, Pencharz J, Pope JE, Thomson J, Thorne C, Zummer M, Gardam MA, Askling J, Bykerk V. Canadian Rheumatology Association recommendations for the pharmacological management of rheumatoid arthritis with traditional and biologic disease-modifying antirheumatic drugs: part II safety. J Rheumatol. 2012;39(8):1583–602.
65. Kelsey J, Whittemore A, Evans A, Thompson W. Methods in observational epidemiology. 2nd ed. New York: Oxford University Press; 1996.
66. Listing J, Strangfield A, Kary S, Rau R, von Hinueber U, Stoyanova-Scholz M, Gromnica-Ihle E, Antoni C, Herzer P, Kekow J, Schneider M, Zink A. Infections in patients with rheumatoid arthritis treated with biologic agents. Arthritis Rheum. 2005;52(11):3403–12.
67. Simard JF, Arkema EV, Sundstrom A, Geborek P, Saxne T, Baecklund E, Coster L, Dackhammar C, Jacobsson L, Feltelius N, Lindblad S, Rantapaa-Dahlqvist S, Klareskog L, van Vollenhoven RF, Neovius M, Askling J. Ten years with biologics: to whom do data on effectiveness and safety apply? Rheumatology (Oxford). 2011;50(1):204–13.
68. Kim SY, Solomon DH. Use of administrative claims data for comparative effectiveness research of rheumatoid arthritis treatments. Arthritis Res Ther. 2011;13(5):129.
69. Yun H, Curtis JR. New methods for determining comparative effectiveness in rheumatoid arthritis. Curr Opin Rheumatol. 2013;25(3):325–33.
70. von Elm E, Altman DG, Egger M, Pocock SJ, Gotzsche PC, Vandenbroucke JP. The Strengthening the Reporting of Observational Studies in Epidemiology (STROBE) statement: guidelines for reporting observational studies. Lancet. 2007;370(9596):1453–7.
71. EQUATOR Network. Enhancing the Quality and Transparency of health Research. http://www.equator-network.org/resource-centre/library-of-health-research-reporting/reporting-guidelines/observational-studies/.
72. Wolfe F, Lassere M, van der Heijde D, Stucki G, Suarez-Almazor M, Pincus T, Eberhardt K, Kvien TK, Symmons D, Silman A, van Riel P, Tugwell P, Boers M. Preliminary core set of

domains and reporting requirements for longitudinal observational studies in rheumatology. J Rheumatol. 1999;26(2):484–9.

73. Psaty BM, Siscovick DS. Minimizing bias due to confounding by indication in comparative effectiveness research: the importance of restriction. JAMA. 2010;304(8):897–8.
74. Wolfe F, Michaud K, Stephenson B, Doyle J. Toward a definition and method of assessment of treatment failure and treatment effectiveness: the case of leflunomide versus methotrexate. J Rheumatol. 2003;30(8):1725–32.
75. Curtis JR, Baddley JW, Yang S, Patkar N, Chen L, Delzell E, Mikuls TR, Saag KG, Singh J, Safford M, Cannon GW. Derivation and preliminary validation of an administrative claims-based algorithm for the effectiveness of medications for rheumatoid arthritis. Arthritis Res Ther. 2011;13(5):R155.
76. Curtis JR, Chastek B, Becker L, Harrison DJ, Collier D, Yun H, Joseph GJ. Further evaluation of a claims-based algorithm to determine the effectiveness of biologics for rheumatoid arthritis using commercial claims data. Arthritis Res Ther. 2013;15(2):404.
77. Vinet E, Kuriya B, Widdifield J, Bernatsky S. Rheumatoid arthritis disease severity indices in administrative databases: a systematic review. J Rheumatol. 2011;38(11):2318–25.
78. Hennessy S. When should we believe nonrandomized studies of comparative effectiveness? Clin Pharmacol Ther. 2011;90(6):764–6.
79. Gabriel SE, Normand SL. Getting the methods right–the foundation of patient-centered outcomes research. N Engl J Med. 2012;367(9):787–90.
80. Patient-Centered Outcomes Research Institute. Research Methodology. http://www.pcori.org/research-we-support/methodology/.
81. Elkayam O, Pavelka K. Biologic registries in rheumatology: lessons learned and expectations for the future. Autoimmun Rev. 2013;12(2):329–36.

Systematic Reviews and Meta-analyses in Rheumatology

Theo Stijnen and Gulen Hatemi

Introduction

Meta-analysis is the method of combining data from independent studies to address a specific, well-defined question using appropriate statistical methods. The choice of statistical methods depends on several factors such as how similar the results of individual studies were or the characteristics of the subjects included in those studies and the sample sizes of each study. The selection of studies that will be included in the meta-analysis and extraction of appropriate data from these studies is based on systematic review. The systematic review, in turn, should rely on a thorough systematic literature search and be reproducible in order to minimize bias. For reliable results from the meta-analysis, the systematic review has to have clearly defined, predetermined objectives and methodology. In addition to testing the null hypothesis according to treatment effect and integrating the effect sizes derived from the collected studies, systematic reviews and meta-analyses help determine the shortcomings of the available data and may suggest further trials to answer the study question.

T. Stijnen, MSc, PhD (✉)
Department of Medical Statistics and Bioinformatics, Leiden University Medical Center, P.O. Box 9600, 2300RC Leiden, The Netherlands
e-mail: T.Stijnen@lumc.nl

G. Hatemi, MD
Division of Rheumatology, Department of Internal Medicine, Istanbul University, Cerrahpasa Medical School, Cerrahpasa Tip Fakultesi, Kocamustafapasa, Istanbul, 34365, Turkey
e-mail: gulenhatemi@yahoo.com

H. Yazici et al. (eds.), *Understanding Evidence-Based Rheumatology*,
DOI 10.1007/978-3-319-08374-2_10

Meta-analyses can be used to answer several types of questions in rheumatology. One of the most common uses has been collating studies aiming to determine the efficacy or safety of certain treatment modalities, in comparison to either placebo or another treatment modality. Determining the efficacy of a certain drug where studies have shown controversial results such as sulfasalazine for ankylosing spondylitis or using network meta-analysis methods for comparing the efficacy of certain drugs such as TNF-alpha inhibitors, where head-to-head trials are rarely conducted, are examples for meta-analyses evaluating efficacy [1, 2]. Determining the efficacy over a more specific end point, such as renal involvement in SLE, would be another use of meta-analyses [3, 4]. This method would also be helpful for conditions that are less frequent manifestations of a disease and usually not evaluated on their own. An example is to evaluate the efficacy of etanercept for uveitis in AS by bringing together data from several etanercept trials in AS [5]. Safety issues such as the risk of a specific adverse event, for example, tuberculosis among patients receiving these agents, can also be addressed. Another use of meta-analysis is in determining the diagnostic performance and accuracy of a certain test or method, such as QuantiFERON for screening for latent tuberculosis or comparison of different imaging modalities for determining joint erosions in rheumatoid arthritis [6, 7]. Bringing together genome-wide association studies or genetic polymorphism studies and studies on the cost-effectiveness of certain interventions has been other areas where meta-analyses have been used [8–10]. Finally, a common use of systematic reviews in rheumatology has been the development of recommendations. Examples of this would be EULAR recommendations, which have been developed covering several areas in rheumatology, by combining the evidence obtained by systematic reviews and the opinions of experts of that area [11, 12].

Meta-analyses are considered to have the highest level in the evidence hierarchy [13]. However, caution is required. Conducting and interpreting meta-analyses can be a challenging process due to potential biases. It is important for experts of the field to be involved in the meta-analysis which is not solely extracting numbers from studies. Expert help is needed for formulating the selection criteria for studies that will be included in a meta-analysis. The outcomes that are analysed will have an important impact on the results. In this chapter, we will try to summarize the methods used in conducting a systematic review and the statistical methods which are used to bring together data extracted from individual studies.

Systematic Literature Review

A complete and precise systematic literature search is the backbone of a good meta-analysis. The first step is to define the study question well and then to formulate it into a searchable question. The quality of meta-analyses and systematic reviews depends on a well-conducted systematic literature search.

Just like any trial, a systematic literature review should try to answer a specific question, have predefined inclusion and exclusion criteria and be reproducible.

Formulation of the Research Question

Formulating the clinical question into a research question is important since the selection criteria for the articles to be included and excluded, identifying the types of study designs to be included, determining the search strategy and the type of data that will be extracted from each study all depend on this step.

The components of a formulated research question are abbreviated as PICO. "P" stands for patient or population. When talking about patients, it is important to specify the criteria used to identify those patients. A simple example would be rheumatoid arthritis. Results of a systematic review including RA patients diagnosed by 1984 criteria may be different from one including patients diagnosed by 2010 criteria. Other features such as demographic characteristics may also be important according to the study question. For example, a meta-analysis on the efficacy of colchicine on mucocutaneous lesions in Behcet's syndrome should evaluate men and women separately, since individual trials have shown that treatment response may vary according to gender in these patients. More detailed specifications may be necessary depending on the question. For example, on a meta-analysis of biologic agents in methotrexate-resistant RA patients, it would be wise to prespecify the methotrexate dose and duration that should have been used before classifying the patient as methotrexate resistant. Comorbid conditions may also be important.

The "I" stands for the intervention and "C" stands for the comparator. Here the dose, duration, timing, mode or route of application and the concomitant medications need to be specified. For example, in a review of TNF-alpha antagonists, whether concomitant methotrexate was used or not may substantially affect the results. Specifying the comparator is also crucial since, for example, including "standard therapy" as comparator may result in substantial heterogeneity across studies, as standard therapy may vary in different settings. Another important issue is duration, especially when evaluating adverse events. One aspect is that the possibility of having an adverse event would increase as time passes. Thus, it would be unfair to compare the adverse events in studies with different durations. Another issue related to duration of intervention is the use of patient years. This approach would underestimate adverse events that occur mostly at the beginning of therapy, such as activation of latent tuberculosis with TNF-alpha inhibitors, since they will be diluted as the study duration increases.

The "O" stands for outcome, and this may be the most challenging part of formulating the research question. Validated and good outcome measures are available for some rheumatologic conditions such as rheumatoid arthritis. However, this is not the case for many other rheumatologic conditions. One of the important points in choosing outcomes is to decide whether you want to use a dichotomous versus a continuous outcome. If a dichotomous outcome is chosen, then inclusion of manuscripts with different cut-off points for the positivity may be a problem. If continuous outcomes are chosen, it is important to evaluate whether the difference that is detected is clinically meaningful. Having standard cut-off points for positivity is also an important issue in systematic reviews of diagnostic methods.

The homogeneity across trials for the components of PICO is even more important if a network meta-analysis method is being used for comparing different treatment modalities.

Development of Search Strategy

In addition to the components of PICO, the search strategy also takes into account the types of study designs which will be preferred. For example, if the question is related to treatment, then one would search for randomized controlled trials. On the other hand if the question is about the incidence or prevalence of a certain condition, then cohort studies, surveys or cross-sectional studies would be preferred. Finally, if the etiology of a certain condition is tried to be determined, then case-control studies or cohort studies could be selected.

Determining the databases which will be used is another important point and depends on the type of research question. For example, in rheumatology, if the study question involves allied health or nursing, it would be wise to include "Cumulative Index to Nursing and Allied Health" (CINAHL) in the databases that will be searched. Selection of key terms is another important step in the development of a search strategy. These should enable a thorough search in order not to miss any relevant studies.

Selection of Studies on the Basis of Inclusion/ Exclusion Criteria

The literature search is performed according to the search strategy, using the pre-determined key terms and limits in the databases. The studies are usually first screened by reading the title and abstract, and studies which are not relevant are excluded. The excluded articles and the reasons for exclusion should also be noted at this step. The full texts of the remaining articles are scrutinized to determine whether they fulfil the inclusion criteria. Hand search of the references of these articles may also be helpful to determine articles that were not retrieved with the original literature search.

It should be remembered that there may be studies that have not been published or published only in local journals which are not covered by the databases. The fact that these articles tend to be those reporting negative results may cause bias in the meta-analysis. One study that formally looked at this has shown that published studies yield larger estimates of intervention efficacy compared to unpublished ones, including meeting abstracts (OR 1.15; 95 % CI 1.04–1.28) [14].

Judgment of Methodological Quality of Selected Studies and Assessing Studies for the Risk of Bias

The quality of the studies that are included is important, because the validity of the meta-analysis depends on the reliability of the information coming from the studies which have been analysed. Several systems have been proposed for evaluating the quality of studies. JADAD or Downs and Black are examples of such scoring systems [15, 16]. However, there may also be some disadvantages of using such systems. Due to the differences in these scoring systems, a study may get different scores depending on the system that has been used [17]. Each item used in these systems may not be equally important in every systematic literature search, depending on the research question. Thus, between two trials getting the same score, one may be more prone to bias compared to the other, depending on the outcome that we are looking for. Moreover, the results of such scoring systems may be difficult for the reader to interpret.

Cochrane reviews use another method to overcome this. Each trial is indicated to have low risk, high risk or unclear risk of bias in random sequence generation, allocation concealment, masking of participants and personnel, masking of outcome assessment, incomplete outcome data, selective reporting and other biases [18]. Just like the systematic literature search, the assessment of the risk of bias should be evaluated by two independent authors, since this evaluation can somewhat be subjective.

After determining the study qualities, with which ever method you choose, the impact of this on the results must be analysed. Depending on the research question, studies with shortcomings that may have impact over the results of the meta-analysis may be excluded. Alternatively, a sensitivity analysis may be performed to determine whether these studies should be excluded or not. Analysis of subgroups and meta-regression can also be used.

Data Extraction (Table 1)

The data which is extracted from studies include data on the PICO of that study, publication year and duration of the study, study design and factors related to the quality or risk of bias. About the participants, the number, age, sex and diagnosis; the criteria used for diagnosis; and other factors related to the study question such as the ethnicity, disease duration and predisposing factors to the condition that is being assessed should be noted. For the intervention and comparator, data on details such as the dose, frequency, mode, duration and timing of intervention may be extracted. Regarding the outcomes, it is important to note how the outcome is defined, the unit of measurement as well as upper and lower limits of normal for laboratory parameters and the time from baseline that the outcome is evaluated. If the outcome is dichotomous, then noting the number of patients having that

Table 1 Data extraction

Parameters that are commonly extracted from studies
Characteristics of the manuscript
Author
Publication year
Study duration
Study design
Factors related to risk of bias
Participant characteristics
Number
Age
Sex
Diagnosis/criteria used for diagnosis
Ethnicity
Disease duration
Predisposing factors to the condition that is being assessed
Characteristics of the intervention and comparator
Dose
Frequency
Mode
Duration
Timing
Characteristics of the outcomes
How the outcome is defined
The unit of measurement
Upper and lower limits of normal for laboratory parameters
Time from baseline that the outcome is evaluated
Others
How the missing data is handled
Outcomes of specific subgroups

outcome and the total number of patients in each group would be sufficient. If the outcome is continuous, then in addition to the mean value, a measure of variability such as the standard deviation, standard error and/or the confidence intervals should be tabulated. While some of these data are readily presented in studies, some of them may have to be calculated using the data at hand. Finally, there may be data specific for each research question that needs to be extracted such as how the missing data is handled or outcomes of specific subgroups.

The data extraction should also ideally be performed by two independent observers. Just like the clinical report forms (CRF) that one would use in clinical trials, it is important to have standard forms for data extraction in order to make the process homogenous and keep track of missing data.

Summarizing the Data and (if Possible) Pooling (Meta-analysis)

It is not uncommon for a systematic review to yield articles which show substantial heterogeneity in methodology and results which make it impossible to pool the data and perform a meta-analysis. If this is the case, usually results of the individual trials are summarized with emphasis on their characteristics and potential biases.

If it is reasonable to pool and combine the data from individual studies statistically, then meta-analysis can be performed. The type of data, in terms of being continuous or dichotomous, and its heterogeneity are factors that need to be considered when deciding which statistical methods will be used for the meta-analysis. These will be further discussed in the following sections.

Reporting the Results

The PRISMA statement provides a guideline for reporting systematic reviews and meta-analyses to achieve a standard in manuscripts [19]. It is very important to report the number of studies which are identified by the literature search in each of the databases or other sources, number of articles that had been screened and excluded after reading the title and the abstract as well as the articles that are excluded after reading the full text and the reasons for excluding them.

The possible factors that may affect the outcome of the studies, assessed by quality or risk of bias assessment and results of the sensitivity analysis, should also be reported.

The reliability of the result of the meta-analysis is evaluated by the GRADE approach in Cochrane reviews. Here the reliability of the results is graded in four levels from very low to high, depending on whether the evidence is coming from studies with the preferred study design, the presence of factors decreasing the quality of evidence such as limitations in the design of included studies, inconsistency of results, indirectness of evidence, imprecision and publication bias and the presence of factors which increase the quality of evidence, such as large magnitude of effect or dose–response gradient, which are mainly used for evaluating observational studies. It is important to provide some form of evaluation of the reliability of the results to help the readers to be able to interpret the results correctly.

Choice of the Effect Parameter

Once the article data are extracted, the first step in the meta-analysis is the choice of the effect parameter. There are several possibilities. If the outcome variable is continuous, for instance the decrease in a depression score during treatment, then a straightforward choice would be the difference between the mean decrease in the experimental treatment group and that in the control group. When the absolute difference between the means is difficult to compare between the studies, for instance if depression is rated by different instruments across studies, usually the

Table 2 Extracted data

Study	Patients with aTNF response/total no. of patients	
	ADA positive	ADA negative
1	0/10	24/24
2	1/5	22/25
3	9/21	76/100
4	4/13	2/2
5	3/13	13/16
6	4/18	17/17
7	1/11	20/27
8	8/22	20/29
9	3/23	56/62
10	0/7	10/13
11	4/7	23/24
12	1/10	37/41
13	2/6	20/23

standardised difference is chosen, which is the difference between the group means divided by (mostly) the pooled standard deviation at baseline. This means that the difference between the groups is expressed in the number of standard deviations. When the standard deviation or standard error with the sample size is known for each treatment group, the 95 % confidence intervals (CI) can be calculated. It is customary to present the 95 % CIs of all studies in a figure called the forest plot. This plot provides a first impression of the evidence in favour of an effect of the experimental treatment relative to the control treatment.

In case of a dichotomous outcome variable, like for instance, the patient does or does not respond to a treatment, the data for each study can be represented in a 2×2 table. Then the treatment effect can be characterised by either the odds ratio (OR), the risk ratio (RR, also called the relative risk) or the risk difference (RD). As an example, we take a meta-analysis reported by Gârces et al. [20]. They investigated the effect of anti-drug antibodies (ADA) on drug response (positive or negative) to antitumour necrosis factor (aTNF) biological therapies. In Table 2, the extracted data are given. There are 13 studies, and for each of them, the number of responding patients and the total number of patients are given for the ADA-positive and ADA-negative group separately.

Given the choice of the effect measure (RD, OR or RR), a 95 % CI is calculated with the usual formulas, and these are presented in the forest plot. In practice, one of the three possible effect measures is taken, but here we show for illustration all three forest plots (Fig. 1). The confidence intervals are made in the usual way, taking estimate $\pm 1.96 \times$ standard error.

These figures have been made with the meta-analysis package of Stata [21]. The program employs the usual approximate formulas for the confidence intervals, which can be somewhat inaccurate if the number of responding or non-responding patients is small. This is the case here for some of the studies, and the confidence intervals of these studies are therefore rather inaccurate, as is illustrated by some studies having a confidence interval for the RD that exceeds the value −1, which is impossible since

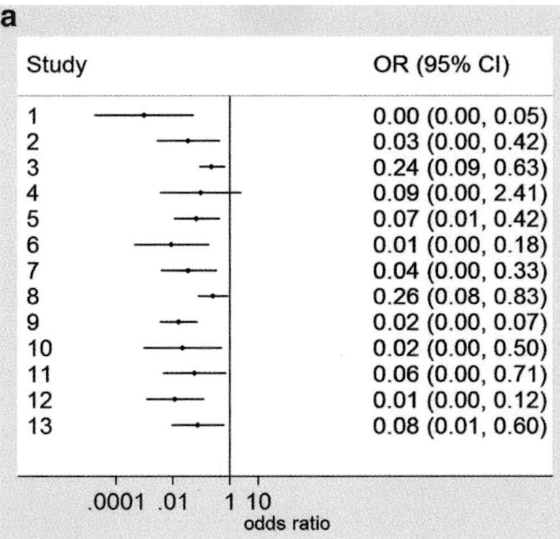

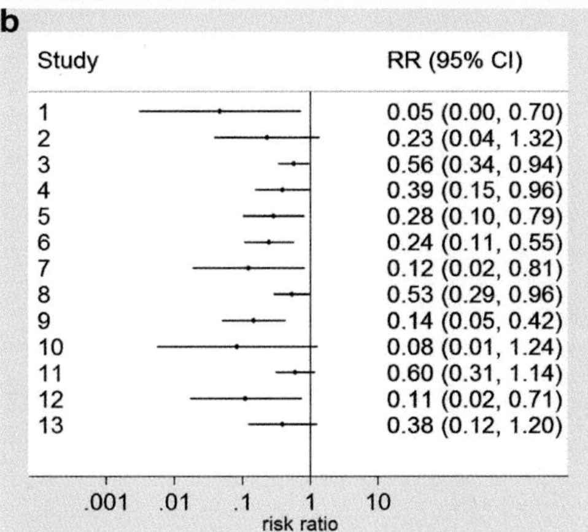

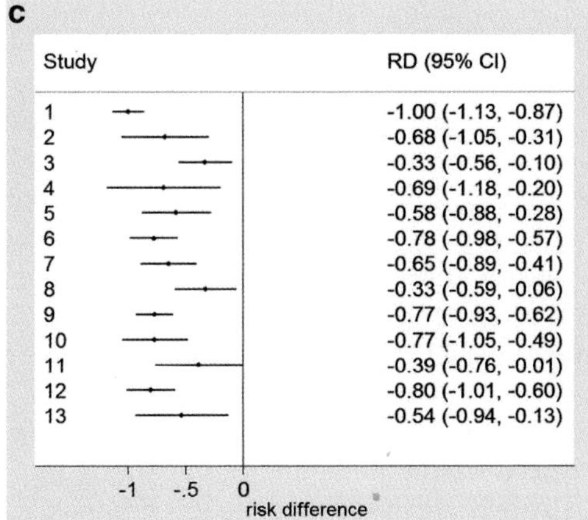

Fig. 1 (**a–c**) Forest plots for the meta-analysis data of Table 2, for three different effect measures

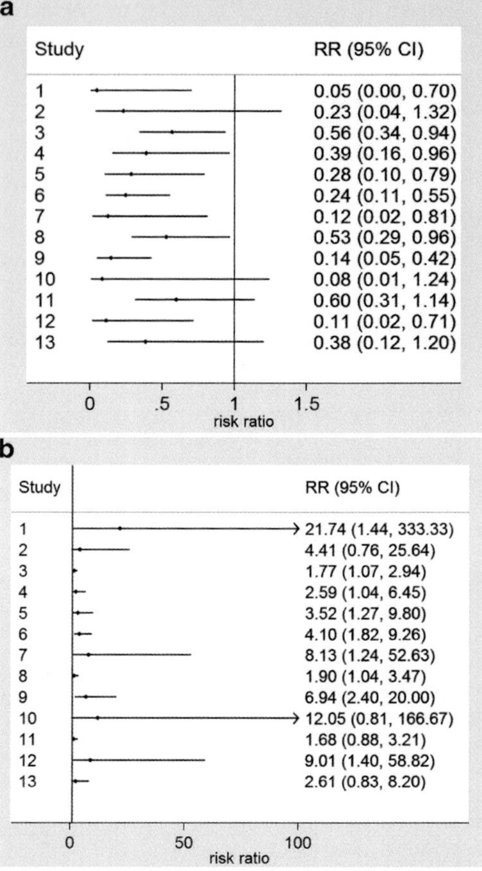

Fig. 2 (**a**, **b**) Forest plots for the RRs of the meta-analysis data of Table 2. (**a**) RR of response in ADA-positive versus ADA-negative group and (**b**) RR of response in ADA-negative versus ADA-positive group

a difference between two proportions cannot exceed 1 in absolute value. Some programs are able to calculate better confidence intervals in the case of small numbers.

Notice that the ratio measures are represented on a logarithmic scale, which is customarily done for ratio measures. The advantage of the logarithmic scale is that the CIs are symmetric and that the figure does not essentially change visually if the numerator and denominator are interchanged. As an illustration in Fig. 2, we have given the forest plots for the RR on the non-logarithmic scale. Figure 2a gives the RR of the ADA-positive group relative to the ADA-negative group, while Fig. 2b shows the RR of the ADA-negative relative to the ADA-positive group.

Notice that the confidence intervals are very asymmetric and the figures look much less attractive than Fig. 1b. Some of the confidence intervals in Fig. 2b do not even fit within the figure. Furthermore, Fig. 2a, b look very different, while essentially they are the same since it is arbitrary what to take as the numerator or denominator of the risk ratio.

In the rest of this chapter, we take the RR as the effect measure. All methods discussed are equally applicable to other choices for the effect measure.

Meta-analysis

The forest plot in Fig. 1b is very nice in the sense that it gives a complete description of all the available data. In this case, the overall conclusion, at least qualitatively, is clear. On the average, there is definitely an effect of ADA positivity on the response to anti-TNF treatment. However, the conclusion is not always this clear in meta-analyses. In addition, we would like to answer more specific questions such as: What is the overall (average) effect across studies? What is the corresponding confidence interval? Is the overall effect statistically significant? Is there variability in the effects across studies, and if so, how large is it? The meta-analysis answers these types of questions as well. Sometimes the meta-analysis is also called "pooling the data", but this does not mean that all data are simply thrown together, in one 2×2 table. To carry out a meta-analysis, all that is needed is the estimated effect and its standard error per study. The method of analysis is independent of the specific choice of the effect measure.

Fixed-Effect Meta-analysis

The starting point is the availability of the effect estimate and its standard error for each study. It is important to realise that the observed effect in a study is not the true value of the effect in that study, but only its estimate. The true effect of a study would only be known if the study had an infinitely large sample size. Due to sampling variability, the observed effect deviates from the true effect. The studies are called homogeneous if it is reasonable to assume that all true effects are equal across studies. In that case, since there is one common effect to all the studies, the meta-analysis is called a fixed-effect analysis. The first question is how to make an estimate of the value of the common treatment effect? It is tempting to just take the simple mean of all observed effects. However, larger studies are more informative than smaller studies, as is reflected in smaller standard errors. Thus, we should better calculate a *weighted* mean instead of a simple mean, such that the larger studies have a larger weight. Statistical theory says that the optimal weights are equal to the inverse squared standard errors. So, if a study has a two times smaller standard error than another study, then the first study should count four times as heavy as the second. Weighting by the inverse squared standard errors is often very similar to weighting by the total sample sizes. For ratio measures, the calculations are done on the logarithmic scale and translated to the original scale afterwards. In Fig. 3, the resulting overall estimate of the RR in our example is given as 0.39. It means that the probability to respond for ADA-positive patients is 0.39 times the probability to respond for ADA-negative patients, or, in other words, the probability to respond is reduced by 61 % in ADA-positive patients compared to ADA-negative patients.

The last column in Fig. 3 gives the logarithmic standard errors. These were used to calculate the weights as 1 over the squared standard error. By dividing these weights by the sum of all the weights, one gets the weight percentages of each study. For instance, the largest study, number 3, determines 25 % of the overall estimate of the RR.

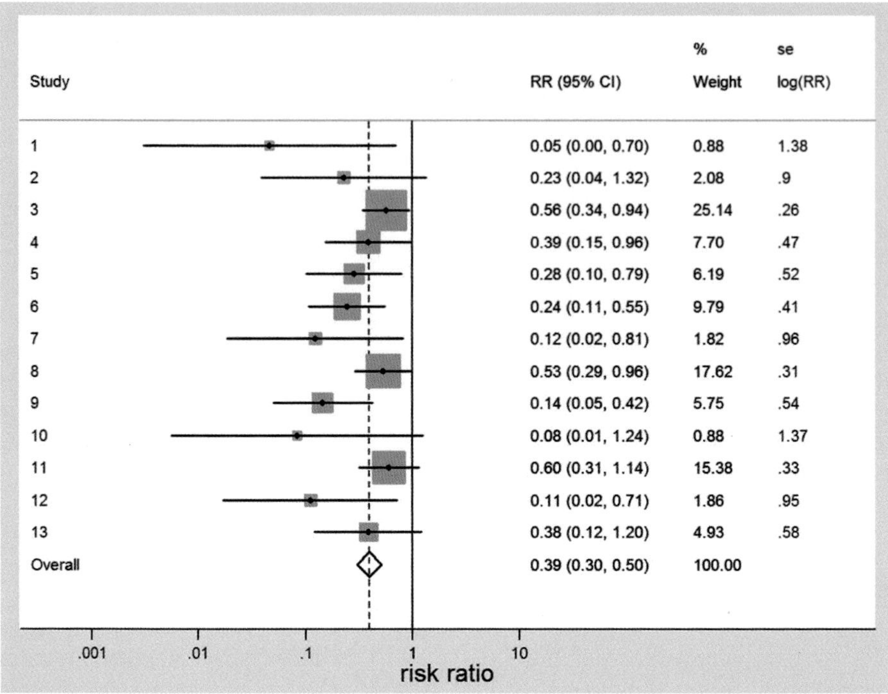

Fig. 3 Forest plots and results of a fixed-effects meta-analysis for the risk ratios of the data of Table 2

Furthermore, it is seen that the two smallest studies hardly influence the overall estimate, since they count each for less than 1 %. The grey boxes in the figure are meant to draw the attention to the more influential studies: The sizes of the boxes are proportional to the weights.

How precise is the overall estimate? That is characterised by its 95 % confidence interval as given in the figure. There is a simple formula for the standard error of the overall effect on the logarithmic scale: It is equal to 1 over the square root of the sum of all the weights. This standard error is used to calculate the 95 % CI in the usual way on the logarithmic scale, and then the anti-logarithm is taken. In our example, the confidence interval runs from 0.30 to 0.50, which is a quite narrow confidence interval, showing the power of meta-analysis. The conclusion of the meta-analysis is that, under the assumption of homogeneity, the best estimate of the risk ratio is 0.39 and that it is 95 % certain that the unknown true value of the RR lies between 0.30 and 0.50.

From the forest plot, it is clear that the 95 % CI of the overall effect is far away from the value RR = 1, indicating that the overall effect is statistically very significantly smaller than one. A formal test is carried out by calculating the Z-value as the logarithm of the overall effect divided by its standard error and referring the Z-value to the standard normal distribution. In this example, we get $Z = 7.28$ with $P < 0.00001$.

Heterogeneity

The above conclusion is only justified if the assumption of one common effect across all studies is plausible. In our example, it is unclear from the forest plot whether the variability that we see is only due to within study sampling variability. A part of the variability may also be due to the differences in true effects across studies. Which part of the variability in the forest plot is due to heterogeneity in true effects? That is expressed by the I-squared measure. In our example, $I^2 = 29$ %, indicating that there might be a non-negligible between-studies heterogeneity. The I^2 value means that 29 % of the variability in the forest plot is due to real heterogeneity across studies, while the remaining 71 % is due to random sampling variation. It is also possible to test the null hypothesis of homogeneity by Cochrane's Q test. In our example, the *P*-value is 0.15, indicating that there is no statistically significant heterogeneity. However, the power of this test is notably low, so this does not mean that we can exclude heterogeneity and conclude homogeneity. One could even argue that a priori at least some heterogeneity is very likely, since there are always smaller or larger differences between studies. Studies can differ in numerous aspects, such as in gender and age distribution, severity and stages of the disease, duration of follow-up, differences in concomitant treatments, etc. Thus, it might be more realistic to use a meta-analysis method that allows possible heterogeneity across studies. This is what a random-effects meta-analysis does. Among biostatisticians, there is a broad consensus that a random-effects meta-analysis is the preferred method of analysis. Moreover, if the between-studies variation turns out to be small, the random-effects method returns the same results as a fixed-effects analysis.

Random-Effects Meta-Analysis

This method accounts for possible heterogeneity in the true effects of the studies. The studies in the meta-analysis are conceived to be a sample from a large imaginary population of studies. The true effects of these studies vary according to some distribution in this imaginary population. The variability of this distribution is characterised by its standard deviation, say σ, or its square σ^2, the variance. The mean of the distribution, say θ, is the main parameter of interest, of which we want to have an estimate and confidence interval. θ is often called the overall effect and σ (σ^2) is called the between-studies standard deviation (variance).

In the random-effects approach, the estimate of the overall effect θ is again calculated as a weighted mean of the observed effects. In the fixed-effect method, the weights were equal to $1/\text{se}^2$, with se being the standard error of the observed effect of a study. In the presence of heterogeneity, statistical theory says that the optimal weights are equal to $1/(\text{se}^2 + \sigma^2)$. So first, we need an estimate of σ^2. There are two main methods to estimate σ. The first is the well-known method of DerSimonian and Laird [22], which is easily calculated by hand and therefore is mostly used. The other one is the maximum likelihood method, which is considered

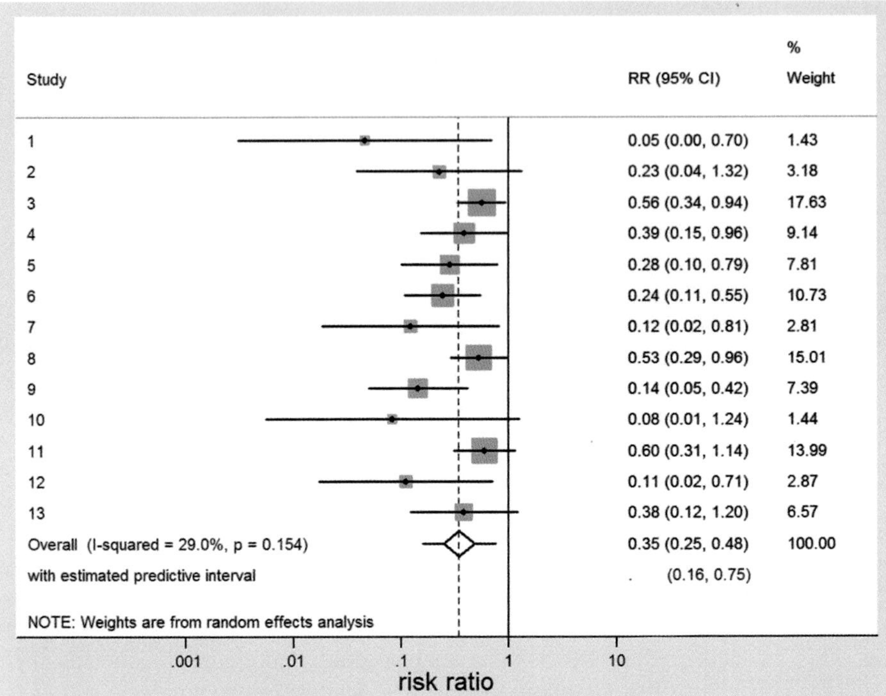

Fig. 4 Result of standard DerSimonian–Laird random-effects method for the data of Table 2

to be a somewhat better method but for which a computer is needed. Once the estimate of σ is available, all calculations proceed exactly the same as for the fixed-effects method. Notice that if the estimate of the between-studies variation is zero, the random-effects analysis produces results identical to the fixed analysis. The result of the random-effects meta-analysis for our example is given in Fig. 4.

The estimate of the overall RR from the random-effects analysis is 0.35 with a 95 % CI running from 0.25 to 0.48. The overall estimate is different from the fixed-effect analysis because now the studies have other weights, in fact $1/(\text{se}^2+\sigma^2)$ instead of $1/\text{se}^2$. Smaller studies get more and larger studies less weight compared to the fixed-effects method. The larger the between-studies variance σ^2, the more equal the weights become across studies. In the extreme case where σ is very large compared to all se's, all studies count evenly. In this example, the overall effects of the fixed and random meta-analysis are very similar, but in other cases, there can be a substantial difference. Notice that the confidence interval is somewhat wider than for the fixed-effect analysis. That is because in a random-effects meta-analysis always the standard error of the overall effect estimate is larger than in a fixed-effect analysis. In the example, the logarithmic standard error is 0.15 for the random-effects method against 0.13 for the fixed-effect method. This explains why in practice mostly the *P*-value from the fixed-effect method is smaller than from the random-effects method.

The random-effects method gives an estimate of the between-studies standard deviation of the true effects (on the logarithmic scale). In the example, the estimate is equal to 0.31. This estimate can be used to give a concrete description of the heterogeneity in true RRs across studies. If the distribution of true RRs on the logarithmic scale is assumed to be approximately normal, then, very roughly, 95 % of the true RRs will lie between $\ln(0.35) \pm 2 \times 0.31 = (-1.67, -0.45)$. Therefore, approximately 95 % of the true RRs should reside between $\exp(-1.67) = 0.19$ and $\exp(-0.45) = 0.64$. In Fig. 4a, a more sophisticated and accurate interval is given by Stata, (0.16, 0.75). In the figure, it is called predictive interval. If a new study would be done, then with 95 % certainty the true RR of that study would fall in this prediction interval.

Publication Bias and the Funnel Plot

Even more than in individual studies, bias is lurking around the corner in meta-analyses. Of course a meta-analysis can only give valid results if all individual studies are unbiased. However, besides that, in a meta-analysis, there is always a risk of bias caused by possibly missing studies. Maybe more relevant studies have been done which are not published for some reason. If the missing studies are randomly missing, then the studies in the meta-analysis still constitute a random sample, and there is no danger of bias. However, there is a big chance that the missing studies are selectively missing (see chapter "The randomized controlled trial: methodological perspectives"). For instance, studies with a nonsignificant result, or studies with an unexpected outcome, are more difficult to publish, especially if they are small. To get an impression whether there might be publication bias, a funnel plot can be drawn. This is a graph where the observed effects are on the horizontal axis while a measure of precision of the observed effect, (mostly the standard error) is on the vertical axis. The funnel plot should be approximately symmetric around the overall effect, since each individual study has an equal chance to show an effect above rather than below the mean effect. Thus, if there is a clear trend in funnel plot, that might be an indication that there are missing studies causing bias. Figure 5 shows the funnel plot for our example.

The figure is clearly not symmetric around the overall effect, and a clear trend is seen. There are formal tests of symmetry in a funnel plot, the most well-known being the tests of Egger [23] and Begg [24], which both give $P < 0.001$ and confirm the trend seen in the figure. This strongly suggests that there are a number of smaller studies missing that had a less unfavourable effect or even a favourable effect of ADA positivity on treatment response. If this is true, then the overall RR of 0.35 would be biased downwards and a better estimate should be nearer to one. Before drawing the conclusion that there is publication bias, one should try to exclude other explanations of the observed pattern in the funnel plot. For instance, it might be that larger studies are different from smaller studies in some aspects related to the effect of ADA positivity on treatment response.

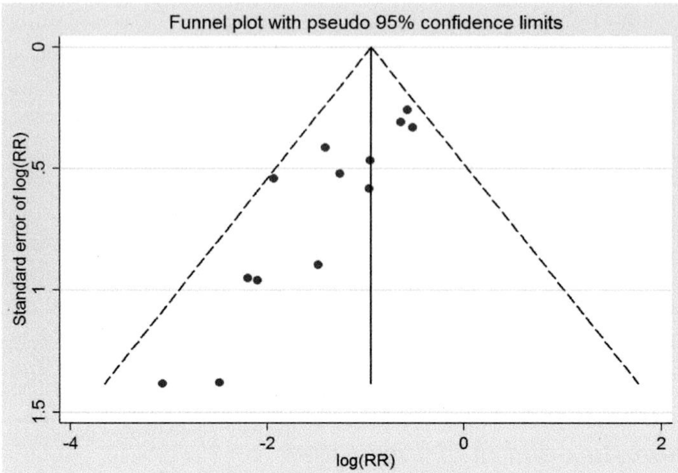

Fig. 5 Funnel plot for the data of Table 2. The vertical line corresponds with the overall effect. Studies within the *dotted lines* have an RR not significantly different from the overall RR

Concluding Remarks on the Statistical Methods for Meta-analyses

We have discussed general meta-analysis methods that can be applied when an observed effect and its standard error are available per study. These methods are appropriate irrespective of the chosen effect measure.

As always true for statistics, there are some underlying assumptions to the methods. One of the assumptions is that the observed effects have an approximate normal distribution. In general, the logarithm of a risk ratio is nicely approximately normal, except when the number of events (or nonevents) is small in a group. That was typically the case for a number of studies in our example. In such cases, there are often alternative methods available performing better [25].

In this chapter, only the most basic meta-analysis methods were discussed. There are many possible extensions and generalisations available. The reader is referred, for instance, to two useful Statistics in Medicine tutorials [25, 26]. One of the extensions is multivariate meta-analysis [25, 26], a technique to analyse several outcomes simultaneously. Another extension is meta-regression [26]. This technique might be used to investigate the relation between the size of the effect and study characteristics. For instance, in our example, the trend seen in Fig. 5 may be explained by larger studies that had been more recently conducted than the smaller studies. Then a meta-regression with the year of publication as explanatory variable could be performed. Another extension is network meta-analysis. An example of a simple network is where one is interested in the comparison between two treatments, A and B. Suppose that besides the articles reporting on the direct comparison between A and B, there are also other articles found in the literature on the comparison of A and B with another treatment, C. It is clear that the latter articles also carry (indirect) information on the A with B comparison, via the A versus C and B versus C comparisons. The goal of a network meta-analysis is to combine all direct and indirect information available in the literature on treatment comparisons. See, for instance, Singh et al. [27] for an example of network meta-analysis in rheumatology. There are also many special methods for specific applications, such as meta-analysis of diagnostic tests [28] and meta-analysis of survival data [29].

References

1. Ferraz MB, Tugwell P, Goldsmith CH, Atra E. Meta-analysis of sulfasalazine in ankylosing spondylitis. J Rheumatol. 1990;17(11):1482–6.
2. Shu T, Chen GH, Rong L, Feng F, Yang B, Chen R, Wang J. Indirect comparison of anti-TNF-α agents for active ankylosing spondylitis: mixed treatment comparison of randomized controlled trials. Clin Exp Rheumatol. 2013;31(5):717–22.
3. Henderson LK, Masson P, Craig JC, Roberts MA, Flanc RS, Strippoli GF, Webster AC. Induction and maintenance treatment of proliferative lupus nephritis: a meta-analysis of randomized controlled trials. Am J Kidney Dis. 2013;61(1):74–87.
4. Dooley MA, Houssiau F, Aranow C, D'Cruz DP, Askanase A, Roth DA, Zhong ZJ, Cooper S, Freimuth WW, Ginzler EM, BLISS-52 and −76 Study Groups. Effect of belimumab treatment on renal outcomes: results from the phase 3 belimumab clinical trials in patients with SLE. Lupus. 2013;22(1):63–72.
5. Sieper J, Koenig A, Baumgartner S, Wishneski C, Foehl J, Vlahos B, Freundlich B. Analysis of uveitis rates across all etanercept ankylosing spondylitis clinical trials. Ann Rheum Dis. 2010;69(1):226–9.
6. Pai M, Zwerling A, Menzies D. Systematic review: T-cell-based assays for the diagnosis of latent tuberculosis infection: an update. Ann Intern Med. 2008;149(3):177–84.
7. Baillet A, Gaujoux-Viala C, Mouterde G, Pham T, Tebib J, Saraux A, Fautrel B, Cantagrel A, Le Loët X, Gaudin P. Comparison of the efficacy of sonography, magnetic resonance imaging and conventional radiography for the detection of bone erosions in rheumatoid arthritis patients: a systematic review and meta-analysis. Rheumatology (Oxford). 2011;50(6): 1137–47.
8. Rodriguez-Fontenla C, Calaza M, Evangelou E, Valdes AM, Arden N, Blanco FJ, Carr A, Chapman K, Deloukas P, Doherty M, Esko T, Garces CM, Gomez-Reino JJ, Helgadottir H, Hofman A, Jonsdottir I, Kerkhof HJ, Kloppenburg M, McCaskie A, Ntzani EE, Ollier WE, Oreiro N, Panoutsopoulou K, Ralston SH, Ramos YF, Riancho JA, Rivadeneira F, Slagboom PE, Styrkarsdottir U, Thorsteinsdottir U, Thorleifsson G, Tsezou A, Uitterlinden AG, Wallis GA, Wilkinson JM, Zhai G, Zhu Y, the arcOGEN consortium, Felson DT, Ioannidis JP, Loughlin J, Metspalu A, Meulenbelt I, Stefansson K, van Meurs JB, Zeggini E, Spector TD, Gonzalez A. Assessment of osteoarthritis candidate genes in a meta-analysis of 9 genome-wide association studies. Arthritis Rheum. 2013. doi:10.1002/art.38300. [Epub ahead of print] PubMed PMID: 24338622.
9. López-Mejías R, Genre F, García-Bermúdez M, Corrales A, González-Juanatey C, Llorca J, Miranda-Filloy JA, Rueda-Gotor J, Blanco R, Castañeda S, Martín J, González-Gay MA. The ZC3HC1 rs11556924 polymorphism is associated with increased carotid intima-media thickness in patients with rheumatoid arthritis. Arthritis Res Ther. 2013;15(5):R152.
10. Jansen JP, Gaugris S, Choy EH, Ostor A, Nash JT, Stam W. Cost effectiveness of etoricoxib versus celecoxib and non-selective NSAIDS in the treatment of ankylosing spondylitis. Pharmacoeconomics. 2010;28(4):323–44.

11. Hatemi G, Silman A, Bang D, Bodaghi B, Chamberlain AM, Gul A, Houman MH, Kötter I, Olivieri I, Salvarani C, Sfikakis PP, Siva A, Stanford MR, Stübiger N, Yurdakul S, Yazici H. Management of Behçet disease: a systematic literature review for the European League Against Rheumatism evidence-based recommendations for the management of Behçet disease. Ann Rheum Dis. 2009;68(10):1528–34.
12. Hatemi G, Silman A, Bang D, Bodaghi B, Chamberlain AM, Gul A, Houman MH, Kötter I, Olivieri I, Salvarani C, Sfikakis PP, Siva A, Stanford MR, Stübiger N, Yurdakul S, Yazici H, EULAR Expert Committee. EULAR recommendations for the management of Behçet disease. Ann Rheum Dis. 2008;67(12):1656–62.
13. Guyatt GH, Haynes RB, Jaeschke RZ, Cook DJ, Green L, Naylor CD, Wilson MC, Richardson WS. Users' Guides to the Medical Literature: XXV. Evidence-based medicine: principles for applying the Users' Guides to patient care Evidence-Based Medicine Working Group. JAMA. 2000;284(10):1290–6.
14. McAuley L, Pham B, Tugwell P, Moher D. Does the inclusion of grey literature influence estimates of intervention effectiveness reported in meta-analyses? Lancet. 2000;356(9237): 1228–31.
15. Jadad AR, Carroll D, Moore A, McQuay H. Developing a database of published reports of randomised clinical trials in pain research. Pain. 1996;66(2–3):239–46.
16. Downs SH, Black N. The feasibility of creating a checklist for the assessment of the methodological quality both of randomised and non-randomised studies of health care interventions. J Epidemiol Community Health. 1998;52(6):377–84.
17. Moher D, Jadad AR, Tugwell P. Assessing the quality of randomized controlled trials. Current issues and future directions. Int J Technol Assess Health Care. 1996;12(2):195–208.
18. Higgins JPT, Green S, editors. Cochrane handbook for systematic reviews of interventions version 5.1.0 [updated March 2011]. The Cochrane Collaboration. 2011. Available from: www.cochrane-handbook.org.
19. Moher D, Liberati A, Tetzlaff J, Altman DG, The PRISMA Group. Preferred reporting items for systematic reviews and meta- analyses: the PRISMA statement. PLoS Med. 2009;6(6): e1000097.
20. Gârces S, Demengeot J, Benito-Garcia E. The immunogenicity of anti-TNF therapy in immune-mediated inflammatory diseases: a systematic review of the literature with a meta-analysis. Ann Rheum Dis. 2013;72:1947–55.
21. Sterne JAC, editor. Meta-analysis in Stata: an updated collection from the Stata journal. College Station: Stata Press; 2009.
22. DerSimonian R, Laird N. Meta-analysis in clinical trials. Control Clin Trials. 1986;7:177–88.
23. Egger MG, Davey Smith G, Schneider M, Minder C. Bias in meta-analysis detected by a simple, graphical test. BMJ. 1997;315:629–34.
24. Begg CB, Mazumdar M. Operating characteristics of a rank correlation test for publication bias. Biometrics. 1994;50:1088–101.
25. Stijnen T, Hamza TH, Özdemir P. Random effects meta-analysis of event outcome in the framework of the generalized linear mixed model with applications in sparse data. Stat Med. 2010;29:3046–67.
26. van Houwelingen JC, Arends LR, Stijnen T. Advanced methods in meta-analysis: multivariate approach and meta-regression. Stat Med. 2002;21:589–624.
27. Singh JA, Wells GA, Christensen R, Tanjong Ghogomu E, Maxwell L, Macdonald JK, Filippini G, Skoetz N, Francis D, Lopes LC, Guyatt GH, Schmitt J, La Mantia L, Weberschock T, Roos JF, Siebert H, Hershan S, Lunn MP, Tugwell P, Buchbinder R. Adverse effects of biologics: a network meta-analysis and Cochrane overview. The Cochrane Collaboration. Published by John Wiley & Sons, Ltd. 2013. Available from: www.update-software.com/bcp/wileypdf/en/cd008794.pdf.
28. Arends LR, Hamza TH, van Houwelingen JC, Heijenbrok-Kal MH, Hunink MG, Stijnen T. Bivariate random effects meta-analysis of ROC curves. Med Decis Making. 2008;8:621–38.
29. Parmar MKB, Torri V, Stewart L. Extracting summary statistics to perform meta-analyses of the published literature for survival endpoints. Stat Med. 1999;17:2815–34.

Ethical Issues in Study Design and Reporting

Hasan Yazici, Emmanuel Lesaffre, and Yusuf Yazici

We plan to deviate somewhat in this chapter from the usual accounts of ethical issues in medicine. We are mainly concerned here with ethical issues as they relate to study design and reporting. Secondly, we propose that ethical transgressions as they relate to medicine can be classified into two main categories. We like to call the first category pudendal and the second cerebral. Table 1 gives a brief, but incomplete list of what we mean.

The distinguishing characteristic of the pudendal form is that there is actually no real debate in the medical community that they represent ethical transgressions and this awareness is shared with the public. This is much akin to the US Supreme Court justice P. Stewart's well known definition of pornography "But I know it when I see it…" [1]. On the other hand those which we like to call cerebral are perhaps more subtle. Not only the lay public is rather unaware of most, but we are afraid that a substantial portion of our colleagues in the medical community do not readily recognize them as transgressions and/or fully appreciate their importance. Furthermore, and with some wishful thinking, we reason that, as every seasoned hunter knows, one must always aim a bit higher to hit a target. So overcoming a cerebral problem might help us in overcoming the pudendal as well.

H. Yazici, MD (✉)
Division of Rheumatology, Department of Medicine, Cerrahpasa Medical Faculty, University of Istanbul, Istanbul, Turkey

E. Lesaffre, Dr, Sc
Department of Biostatistics, Erasmus MC, Rotterdam, The Netherlands

L-Biostat, KU Leuven, Leuven, Belgium

Y. Yazici, MD
Division of Rheumatology, NYU Hospital for Joint Diseases, New York University, New York, USA

H. Yazici et al. (eds.), *Understanding Evidence-Based Rheumatology*,
DOI 10.1007/978-3-319-08374-2_11

Table 1 Some Pudendal and the Cerebral Forms of Ethical Transgression

Pudendal	Cerebral
Direct bribery to promote drugs and medical equipment	Conducting/participating in unnecessary drug trials for the main purpose of promotion
Indirect bribery in the form of gifts, lavish meals and meeting facilities	Adjusting control groups in the direction of confirming the study hypothesis, i.e. exclusion of effective comparators in drug studies
Straightforward plagiarism or falsification of data	Many forms of statistical misconduct in data analysis and presentation, including resorting to pseudoscience in the latter
Disregarding patient autonomy in drug trials mainly in the form of conducting them among the less privileged by their geography and/or social status	Preparing practically incomprehensible informed consent forms which only please the corporate lawyer

1. Ethical Issues in Study Design

To remind ourselves briefly, clinical studies can either be observational or interventional. In turn, either type can be retrospective (usually observational), prospective (most frequently interventional) or cross-sectional (always observational).

The main ethical issue in study design, and this surely extends into the reporting phase, centers around whether the investigators tailor their work solely in the direction of the results they wish to observe and promote. Leaving aside the pudendal examples of painting the experimental mice in the direction of what they want to see as in the famous and notorious Summerlin example [2], there are many, at first sight seemingly acceptable, ways of proving oneself right.

Informed Consent

In any study involving humans the informed consent is the basis of our morality and legitimacy. Good accounts of its history, application and legal dimension are available [3]. Here we plan to emphasize several specific issues which we believe are of current and important concern in practice and research.

There is the prevailing opinion that the informed consent forms have become unduly long [4]. We agree, but unfortunately are unaware of formal data. The consent forms we have to ask our patients to sign are mainly prepared by the pharmaceutical companies or central grant giving bodies by an army of lawyers or bureaucrats for whom the main concern is, we strongly suspect, to avert any potential law suits.

Another issue is related to continuation studies which are popular especially in drug industry sponsored trials of their products. The usual scenario is that a certain drug turns out to be effective in a, let us say 12 months, study against placebo and/or the conventional treatment. At the end of this time the investigators and/or the sponsors decide to continue with the study often in an open or sometimes in a blind design. The common arguments for this continuation are to assess the beneficial effects over a longer time period, to assess any potential side effects, again over a longer time period; and to continue prescribing effective medication still again for a longer time period to patients who participated in the study. The downside, however is that perhaps no important additional data are collected from these continuation studies and at least some of these studies are mainly *seeding* studies for promotional purposes [5, 6]. Frequently it is neglected to include the second informed consent that deals with the extension arm of the study, in the trial report. The important issue here is whether the document explicitly warns patients that there is a chance that they agree to continue taking a drug which was just proven to be inferior to the new remedy. This scenario does not surely comply with the dictum of equipoise and patient autonomy. Some years ago we had explicitly brought this up as related to a well-known trial in rheumatology and the rather unfortunate investigator/ sponsor reply was that this should not cause any concern because "Patients and investigators were always free to stop participation in the trial" [7, 8].

The exact wording of the informed consent form is of special importance in safety trials. In this line and to the best of our knowledge there are at least two currently ongoing trials of assessing the cardiovascular safety of celecoxib, the well-known Cox 2 inhibitor, versus conventional non steroidal anti-inflammatory drugs (NSAIDs). One is in the USA: the Prospective Randomized Evaluation Of Celecoxib Integrated Safety vs Ibuprofen Or Naproxen (PRECISION)) and the other one in Europe: The Standard Care Versus Celecoxib Outcome Trial (SCOT). The rational as well as the methodology of these trials have been published in peer reviewed journals [9, 10]. Both are non-inferiority trials with the primary outcomes being the occurrence of fatal or non-fatal myocardial infarction, or stroke during the study period. This design is based on the hypothesis that there will not be meaningfully more of these outcome events among the celecoxib as compared to the traditional NSAID users. A legitimate question is then how one gets an informed consent for such a trial? Or more simply how does one tell the patient:

'You will be taking the medication A (the traditional NSAID) which is associated with a small extra risk of heart attack and/or a stroke. Here is this medication B (celecoxib), which is not only more easy on your stomach but does not cause meaningfully more heart attacks or stroke as compared to medication A. The main reason you are being enrolled in this trial is to formally test that the medication B does not substantially increase your chance of having more heart attacks or stroke as compared to medication A.'

No osteoarthritis patient *has* to take celecoxib or an NSAID, and may very well seek and get pain relief with weight loss, physical therapy, or simple analgesics like paracetamol. How is it then morally possible to expose a patient to a drug the use of which is associated with, however small, but potentially increased risk of cardiovascular events or stroke? Moreover how can this potential increase be worded in the informed consent document that thousands of patients have to sign before they take part in these studies? This exact issue was brought up some years ago with no satisfactory answer from the primary investigator [11].

More transparency is an impending need in informed consent forms as we have previously proposed [12]. The exact wording of these forms is currently only available (apart from the sponsors and the federal agencies) to the investigators, study participants and institutional review boards. When finally the related article appears, the readers, the journals and very importantly the reviewers, have no way of judging whether there had been any breach of patient autonomy. Our proposal is that a copy of all informed consent forms (and subsequent alterations) should be in the public domain. Any consideration of trade secrets or printed page limitations are not realistic since these forms are anyhow seen by the patients. A potential journal page allocation concern, on the other hand, cannot be of practical consequence in this digital age, either.

Our suggestion for transparency would discourage the industry and the investigators from embarking on promotional trials [13], i.e. Were the potential trial patients actually told this agent had been shown to be an effective medicine to start with? Finally our proposal would also possibly help to prevent the well known pudendal forms of ethical transgressions in drug research in underdeveloped regions of the globe.

Control Groups

A common way of proving oneself right is not giving due importance to the specificity of the observations made. That is, in many studies, often observational, the researchers focus on underpinning their prior beliefs, thereby neglecting the possibility that the initial reflections may be wrong. The litmus test for the specificity of what is observed is, of course, the control group.

The main reason for the inclusion of a control group, or groups, in any study is to assess specificity. If you are studying disease A and you hypothesize that an asset X is characteristically present among patients with disease A it is fairly obvious that you have also to look for the presence of X among healthy people and patients with diseases other than A. Smaller the frequency of the asset X in these groups (your control groups) more specific X becomes for disease A. The other (but often neglected) reason for having a control group is whether there is a need to assess the validity of a new measuring device. Suppose a laboratory method has been used to assess hypercoagulability in disease A and found it increased. Then, when our aim is to assess hypercoagulability this time in disease B, we might again include a group of patients with disease A. The behavior of the diagnostic test in the control group will then greatly help us to interpret our findings when we study disease B.

Above we plead to include a control group in almost every study, but the question is how the control group should be chosen. Too often the control group consists of healthy people only. The solo healthy control group design is quite inadequate in that this design does not tell us anything about the specificity of the observations we make for the disease we are studying. At the end of the study we might indeed observe differences between the disease being studied and the healthy controls in any parameter we have studied. However this does not mean the differences we observe are specific to that disease. In order to say that, we have to study other diseases (the diseased controls) and *not* observe these same changes. This specificity is crucial not only for diagnostic tests but, almost equally important, for our understanding of disease mechanisms. In a survey of publications about Behçet's syndrome among 282 full articles reporting original research in 15 high impact factor general medicine and subspecialty journals we saw that 9.3 % had not included a control group while a 58 % had included only healthy controls. In addition, this survey revealed a strikingly low frequency, 6/37 (12.8 %), of diseased controls in genetic association studies [14]. It is noteworthy that the authoritative STREGA (Strengthening the Reporting of Genetic Association Studies) which is an extension of the STROBE (Strengthening the Reporting of Observational Studies in Epidemiology) position paper does not include the inclusion of diseased controls as an important issue [15].

Let us see now briefly consider how what we discuss relates to the important issue of the discovery of the association of pyrin (MEFV) mutations and Familial Mediterranean Fever (FMF). This association was first described by two independent research consortiums in 1997, using positional cloning [16, 17]. It is to be noted that around one half of all patients with FMF do not have a family history of the same disease. So from the very start we did not know how the described association applied to non familial FMF patients. Furthermore, as is true for the vast majority of association studies, there were no diseased controls. Another issue was that these described pyrin mutations could be present in the heterozygote form in a condition which, in the majority of cases had a recessive pattern of inheritance. Up until recently these caveats were basically ignored and most of the articles about FMF began with a sentence to the effect that FMF was a disease caused by pyrin mutations. These assertive sentences did not even acknowledge that there might be other additional causes(s) of FMF, obviously including mutations in other genes working in tandem, as well.

Since 1997, we, however, understood that these pyrin mutations can also be increased in many other diseases ranging from Behçet's syndrome to endometriosis [18, 45], also being associated with disease severity in the former.

There is little doubt that pyrin is a very important molecule in the inflammatory cascade. However, we also know that the presence of pyrin mutations is not specific for FMF, let alone be causative. To complicate the issue further we also now acknowledge that the genetics of FMF is much more involved than we once we thought [20]. Some years ago when one of us (HY) had proposed the lack of diseased controls in the original MEFV work had hindered the advancement of FMF research for over a decade [21] one reviewer had commented "Had the initial FMF-pyrin work included diseased controls, for example patients with other auto or otherwise inflammatory conditions, the students of FMF would have been where they are now quite a number of years ago. We would respond that had the two FMF consortia used a Behçet's or Crohn's disease control group, they might still be searching for the gene now". This praise of non-specificity by the reviewer was most curious.

The mere presence of diseased controls in a study design does not guarantee that the specificity issue is adequately addressed. The ultimate guideline in selecting the control groups is , as much as possible, to assess the specificity of our observations for that clinical condition we are studying. So if our aim is to search for the specificity of a laboratory biomarker in one disease we should also search for it in a) among healthy people; b) among patients with diseases with clinical manifestations that are similar to the disease we are studying; and c) in other diseases which are not clinically similar but in which we strongly suspect our new laboratory biomarker will turn out to be positive. We should also not forget that our search for specificity does not end even after we include these 3 types of control groups. Very often we still have to check both the sensitivity and the specificity of the new biomarker among the young and the old, among the severe and the less severe and among patients from different ethnic or social backgrounds.

When we design a study to search for the specificity for a specific serological marker of inflammation (A) for patients with rheumatoid arthritis, it gives us limited information to utilize a group of patients with osteoarthritis as a diseased control group. A much more informative group would be patients with another disease which runs with systemic inflammation, like systemic lupus erythematosus (SLE) or ankylosing spondylitis. In this example, the business of selecting osteoarthritis as a control group for rheumatoid arthritis is called an under matching of the control group [22]. This undermatching exists where it is, or should be, obvious to the investigator that the specificity of the asset that is studied will turn out to be excellent, merely by the virtue of the fact that the clinical and the laboratory features of the diseased control group selected is inherently quite different from those of the disease under study. Since osteoarthritis is basically a non-inflammatory disease it would be most unlikely to observe an inflammatory marker to be present in osteoarthritis. Therefore, your under matching of the control group would cause you to erroneously consider what you had observed in RA was pretty specific for RA. An over matching of the control group, on the other hand, exists where it will, by definition, be difficult for the investigator to determine the specificity of a parameter for a disease A by the virtue of the fact that the selected control group will inherently have many features in common with the disease A. Let us assume that based on several individual case reports we suspect that patients with Behçet's syndrome (BS), in general, have enlarged prostate glands. Reasoning that almost every patient that attends a urology clinic has his prostate examined we consider that this would be a diseased control group very easy to study. Hence, we take the whole urology outpatient population for one full week as our diseased control group and examine every patient for his prostate size. This is surely overmatching the control group in that most patients who go to a urology clinic have enlarged prostates to start with.

Similarly, in randomized controlled trials of new remedies the way we choose our control group may influence considerably the results of the study. Particularly, undermatching of the traditional medication for efficacy is an important problem. This happens not uncommonly when you compare the efficacy of a new drug in group of patients using as the comparator another group of patients who you know as those who had not responded well to the traditional remedy. For example in the first randomized controlled trial of cyclosporine in BS from Japan [23] patients with resistant eye disease were randomized into receiving cyclosporine or colchicine. It is well known that all patients with BS receive colchicine from the start in Japan. So, in this particular example, the authors should have known that the eye disease in the group randomized to colchicine would not respond to this drug in any event since they had already used it before the trial had started with no effect on their eye disease. To randomize a portion of the patients to the same drug on which they had progressed to develop resistant disease is an obvious example of under matching.

An interesting example of undermatching can involve not only the control, but also the active arms of a randomized controlled trial. In this case we can say that all the groups were under matched to the hypothesis being tested. In a recent double blind randomized international trial of a new Syk inhibitor in rheumatoid arthritis, the authors reported the new medication was superior to placebo among patients who were non responsive to the traditional agent, methotrexate [24]. The design was a 3 arm study. All patients were using methotrexate at baseline at a dose ranging from 7.5-25.mg/week. One group received the new drug at a higher dose, the second group at a lower dose while the third group received placebo. At the end of the study the patients in both the low and the high dose groups did better than those who received placebo. Curiously, however, this good response was observed only among the patients from Eastern Europe and Latin America and not among those from the United States. We suggested that this might have been due to the fact that patients from Eastern Europe and Latin America had been on a lower dose of methotrexate before being called as "inadequate responders" to be enrolled in the trial as compared to US patients. In other words this proposed effect of the new agent may have disappeared if the patients had received the established effective dose of the traditional remedy before enrolling in the trial.

Under matching the control group may serve to prove a desirable outcome, as can be seen in the Actemra versus Methotrexate double-Blind Investigative Trial In monotherapy (AMBITION study) [25]. The aim of this trial was to compare the efficacy of monotherapy with tocilizumab or methotrexate in methotrexate naïve patients with rheumatoid arthritis. The primary outcomes were ACR responses. At the end of the trial, tocilizumab monotherapy was superior to monotherapy with MTX. This was a very interesting result not found, up to that time, with any other biologic in the same setting. In fact, a biologic monotherapy was generally similar in efficacy as MTX monotherapy while the combination of a biologic plus MTX was superior to either agent used alone when studied among MTX naïve patients with RA. Thus this trial in effect implied that tocilizumab was rather different in efficacy from other biologics. However, on a closer look one realized that about 35 % of patients had been on MTX prior to being enrolled in the trial and their MTX treatment had been discontinued prior to enrollment for reasons other than "inefficacy or adverse events". But, why would anyone stop MTX if efficacious without adverse events? Also, it is rather bizarre to enroll patients to MTX, a drug they had taken before, and compare this to a group of patients starting a brand new drug and to conclude that the new drug is better than MTX. The efficacy of monotherapy in the AMBITION study could not be confirmed in the FUNCTION study looking at the same ACR responses, presented as an abstract in 2013 [26]. In this properly done MTX naïve trial, the ACR scores between monotherapy MTX and tocilizumab were not different, re-enforcing the paradigm that monotherapy with a biologic has similar efficacy to MTX and combination is better when tested among MTX naïve patients.

Power Calculations

This is another important issue in study design. We need power calculations basically to control the probability of a Type II error (denoted as β), which is simply missing a real difference between the two arms of a study, due to an inadequate sample size. To avoid this, calculations are made in the study design to select a minimum number of study subjects necessary to limit this error to say 0.20. The information needed for a sample size calculation are [27]:

1) the anticipated clinically important difference between the effect of the primary outcome in the experimental treatment versus the control treatment. For continuous outcomes this is sometimes expressed as the effect size, which is the difference in treatment means of the primary outcome divided by the standard deviation of that outcome.
2) The selected probability of Type I error (denoted as α)
3) The aimed power, which is the probability of detecting the aimed clinical difference and is equal to $1\text{-}\beta$.

An underpowered study raises ethical concerns, especially for interventional studies. It is simply not justified to expose any subject (patients, but also animals) to an intervention if the likelihood of demonstrating a beneficial effect is slight. This being the case it is strange that sample size determinations are quite uncommon in investigative rheumatology. In the methodological audit of Behçet 's syndrome publications [14] only 3.0 % of 280 original articles had any power calculations. Included among these original articles were 6 drug trials, which usually have the highest frequency of including a power calculation. Still, only 1/6 of these trials had a power calculation.

Equipoise

The concept of equipoise is an important principle in study design. In the context of a drug study equipoise simply means that prior to the study the investigators assume an equal chance of efficacy for the active and the control arms of the study. Equipoise, or mainly its lack in many randomized clinical trials, was the subject matter of an important debate a decade ago [28, 29].

Fries and Krishnan [28] argued that the main reason that practically only randomized clinical trials with positive results are published was not mainly due to publication bias as commonly assumed, but was the result of a design bias. By the time a new drug reaches Phase III in drug development, equipoise in the randomized controlled trial may not hold true anymore. In brief, from the accumulated evidence from Phases I and II the investigators are quite often fairly certain that the drug under study should work. Felson and Glantz, on the other hand, disagreed [29] and maintained that publication bias, rather than the lack of equipoise, was the main reason that only trials with positive results got published.

We have the impression that the concept of equipoise, which usually is not adhered to in drug industry sponsored trials, is present more in publicly funded trials or in trials where the comparator is not a placebo but what is available as the best active drug.

As expected the debate about equipoise in controlled clinical trials continues and there is special concern that equipoise is can be jeopardized in trials with an adaptive design [30] in which the a priori assumption about the possible efficacy of the drug being tested changes during the course of the trial.

Popper's Falsification

The main discussion about the *cerebral* ethics as it relates to study design is centered on the investigators adhering to the general principle of falsification as the main business of any scientific investigation. According to Popper [31] a hypothesis can only be accepted (temporarily) when a rigorous attempt to falsify it turns out to be unsuccessful. In brief, Popper's philosophy tells investigators that the hypothesis they have formulated (through experience, knowledge, hard work and, on occasion, genius) can only be accepted when it has undergone an agonizing, deductive, and above all honest self-falsification. From this perspective any breach of self-falsification may be considered as an ethical transgression. To quote Feynman "For example, if you're doing an experiment, you should report everything that you think might make it invalid--not only what you think is right about it: other causes that could possibly explain your results; and things you thought of that you've eliminated by some other experiment, and how they worked--to make sure the other fellow can tell they have been eliminated."[32].

There surely have been severe criticisms of Popper's hypothesis driven self – falsification centered approach to scientific method [33, 34]. Namely, it has been argued that science does not progress through deductive self- falsification. To the contrary, it is the inductive reasoning based on accumulated knowledge and designing experiments to prove our hypothesis that keeps up the scientific progress. The Bayesian approach to knowledge accumulation is surely in this line (see chapter "A review of statistical approaches for the analysis of data in rheumatology"). Finally, the critics of Popper explicitly bring up the point that no investigator actually wants to disprove himself.

It has to be underlined that adherence to Popper's falsification principle to science, based on deductive principles, does not negate the validity and the usefulness of the Bayesian inductive approach. They surely complement each other in formulating/rejecting hypotheses and in collecting/interpreting data. It might be said that the scientists need the inductive (Bayesian) approach to formulate/expand their hypotheses and test to the limits of probability, the data they collect. However they also need the Popperian approach of deductive reasoning to be self-critical of their hypotheses through their interpretation of and the deduction from the data they collect.

II. Ethical Issues in Reporting

The various issues thus far discussed in the context of study design were mainly cerebral per our classification. The reader will note the issues will become somewhat more pudendal as we go into reporting. Even the famous Supreme Court decision we quoted in the opening lines will not much help us to tell the cerebral from the pudendal in many of these instances.

Authorship

One common debated issue, one that can even end research careers of both the novice and occasionally the master, is that of authorship in a scientific article. Unlike most of the ethical transgressions discussed, authorship entails an ethical debate mainly among the members of the scientific community. There is no question that a bonus authorship is an important issue but the impact of this transgression on the societal good is relatively less as compared to fudged data or trying to hide away from the public eye overt biases in the methodology and/or the results of a scientific study.

The International Committee of Medical Journal Editors advises that the authorship be based on [35]:

> *"1. Substantial contributions to the conception or design of the work; or the acquisition, analysis, or interpretation of data for the work; AND 2. Drafting the work or revising it critically for important intellectual content; AND 3. Final approval of the version to be published; AND 4. Agreement to be accountable for all aspects of the work in ensuring that questions related to the accuracy or integrity of any part of the work are appropriately investigated and resolved.*
>
> *In addition to being accountable for the parts of the work he or she has done, an author should be able to identify which co-authors are responsible for specific other parts of the work. In addition, authors should have confidence in the integrity of the contributions of their coauthors.*
>
> *All those designated as authors should meet all four criteria for authorship, and all who meet the four criteria should be identified as authors. Those who do not meet all four criteria should be acknowledged—see Section II.A.3 below. These authorship criteria are intended to preserve the status of authorship for those who deserve credit and can take responsibility for the work. The criteria are not intended for use as a means to disqualify colleagues from authorship who otherwise meet authorship criteria by denying them the opportunity to meet criterion #s 2 or 3. Therefore, all individuals who meet the first criterion should have the opportunity to participate in the review, drafting, and final approval of the manuscript."*

We have taken this long passage from the current official advice on purpose to demonstrate how debatable the issue of authorship is even among the *cognoscenti*, like the journal editors. The fight in academic circles, a consequence of the *publish or perish* motto, may stem from either the master abusing his/her seniority (insisting to be included in the authorship because he/she has given the idea or found the money or has contributed few minutes of his/her time in rewording the draft) or from the novice who has done all the scud work. Clearly, the rights of the novice should be protected in the first place. Therefore the deletion of the word "therefore" from the last paragraph from the quoted text would be in order.

Even after this alteration we suggest the ultimate guidelines for authorship in any scientific manuscript should and could not be made uniform for all purposes and instances. Conflicts can only be resolved on an individual, *case law* basis. Apart from the above discussed master-novice conflict in authorship, there are mainly three additional authorship issues, namely: guest, gift and ghost authorship.

The ethical transgression associated with the first two forms of authorship cannot be taken lightly. Guest authors are those with no substantial contribution study but are included in the authorship, even as first authors, benefiting from their prominence for promotional purposes. Gift authors are included just to please some colleagues. This exercise is surely pitiful as well.

Ghost authorship stands somewhat different from the other two. No doubt it is usually frowned upon [36]. This is most justified when a drug company hires a commercial firm to prepare almost the final form of a manuscript commonly and cleverly designed to put the company's product in the best possible light, and again usually with a long list of guest or gift authors. On the other hand, we consider it ethical if investigators provide their data, along with their interpretation to a professional firm to prepare a manuscript fully acknowledged in the final paper. Unfortunately what we have just described is also considered as ghost authorship and we argue this is unjustified.

Data Presentation

There are many ways by which the readership may be ill informed and on many occasions one considers this might, unfortunately, be intentional. The more common scenarios are trying to show the drug of interest is more efficacious than it really is, trying to show a drug is safer than it really is, and the display of mesmerizing science or statistical foot play of many forms.

The comparative efficacy of any one medication over another can be expressed in many different ways and if a reader is not aware of a few essential subtleties he/she may be easily misinformed. Assume it is reported that a new drug decreases after one year of treatment, the formation of new erosions among patients with rheumatoid arthritis in 50 % more among the patients as compared to what is observed among the rheumatoid arthritis patients receiving the old remedy. This difference can be pretty impressive at first sight; however it can equally be deceiving if we look at this 50 % difference in absolute terms. Assuming this was a randomized controlled trial of two groups of 100 patients with rheumatoid arthritis and two patients in each group had erosions to start with. If additional two patients in the old and one patient in the new drug group develop erosions at the end of one year this would give us 4 patients with erosions in the old drug and 3 patients with erosions in the new drug groups. This does represent 50 % less new erosions in the new drug group and when expressed in absolute terms, it surely is not impressive at all. On the other hand, if we start out with 20 patients with erosions in either group and end up with 10 new patients with erosions in the new and 20 with in the old treatment groups, the difference in efficacy between the two groups is still 50 %, but the results are surely more meaningful.

In this example one should also be very careful if we are comparing the number of new erosions in one group versus the other or the number of patients with new erosions in either group. It is quite common that drugs are more effective in certain members of the population and in our example if one evaluates the outcome based on the total number of erosions in one group vs. the positive findings in a few patients with relatively large number of erosions might bias the results.

The limits of biological variability in the parameter being studied is yet another point to consider. An illustration of this is found in the reported significant beneficial effect of anti-TNF agents on erosions in rheumatoid arthritis. When we analyzed their effect in absolute numbers on a real scale of the total number of erosions a person with rheumatoid arthritis could develop, the claim that anti- TNF agents significantly decreased the development of new erosions in RA compared to methotrexate became uniformly less impressive for all agents under consideration [37].

While it has been well recognized that the controlled clinical trial has important limitations in reporting especially rare adverse effects (see chapter "Limitations of traditional randomized controlled clinical trials in rheumatology"), to designate any randomized controlled trial also as a safety trial has almost become a cliché [38]. By the time a new agent comes to Phase III in drug development the more common adverse events are mostly recognized and the remainder usually emerge in Phase IV. The main purpose of the Phase III randomized clinical trial is to confirm the efficacy of the new agent and often compare the degree of this efficacy over the traditional agent (s). The whole hypothesis, design, methodology, and most importantly the power considerations are geared to that. A controlled clinical trial is almost never powered for detecting adverse events. This being the case, it is at least not good science to co-name it a safety trial. Even a further unpleasantness is to find in the results and/or the discussion the declaration that "No significant side effects were observed" without what we consider the ethically compulsory next sentence to the effect that "But the reader should not forget that there was little likelihood that any side effect that occurs in less than 1 % of the patients could have been be apparent in this trial since there were 200 patients in each arm." At least 300, 3 x projected rate [39] event free patients have to be observed to conclude with 95 % confidence that the projected rate of any event is about 1 % or less. Even in the most read rheumatology journals, randomized controlled trials are frequently also dubbed safety trials but their sample size, which is too low to come to sound conclusions, is rarely discussed [40]. Another sobering point is that little attention is paid to the timing of adverse events. While this timing is obviously central to conclude causality, only a small fraction of the manuscripts reported the time of onset of even severe adverse events. Finally, the use of patient-years, useful only when the event rate is rather constant in time, is commonly and incorrectly utilized [40].

There are many ways to mesmerize by science. One effective way of doing it is to dazzle the reader with displays of graphs, figures or tables the visual and verbal content of which are "mesmerizingly unfriendly" to the reader. Common examples are amino acid sequences of various probes used or the photographs of immunology blots or microchips which 9/10 times are non-contributory to methodology, results or discussion. Mesmerizing by science happens not only in basic science. In our best clinical journals, like the The New England Journal of Medicine, one regularly comes across p values near, or even at, actual unity. We feel it a direct confrontation with the cognitive abilities of any reader of this reputed journal when we read a statement like "At 28 days, there was no significant difference in mortality between patients in the two study groups who did not have a response to corticotropin (39.2 %/36.1 %, $p=0.69$) or between those who had a response to corticotropin *(28.8 % /28.7 %, p = 1.00)* (italics ours) [41].

There are many other gambits in the statistical foot play. In an attempt to reduce the *apparent* variability of observations authors sometimes report SEMs (standard error of the mean) instead of SDs (standard deviation). Since arithmetically the SEM equals $SD/\sqrt{n}$, it is, by definition a smaller number and as such might suggest less dispersion of the raw data around the mean. In fact, often there is quite some confusion between SEM and SD and it is not recognized that the former is a measure of precision (reproducibility) with which the mean is estimated. A survey of the frequency of this type of mesmerization can be found in the urology literature [42].

Multiple comparisons of two treatment groups by exploring various subgroups, or comparing several treatment groups without correcting for multiple comparisons increase the likelihood of chance finding. In chapter "A review of statistical approaches for the analysis of data in rheumatology" it is shown that the probability of finding an unduly significant result (when $\alpha=0.05$) reaches 1 when twenty of such comparisons are made. There are several ways of properly and honestly handling such multiple comparisons as we have seen in chapter "A review of statistical approaches for the analysis of data in rheumatology".

Post Hoc Data Analysis

Post hoc data analyses are a related issue. A proper study design surely includes well defined endpoints and how they will be analyzed. Also, quite often these endpoints are in hierarchy coined as primary or secondary. Power analyses are also based on precise definitions of these endpoints. Surely it is tempting for the investigators to do further analyses after (post hoc) the data become available. Usually such analyses are discouraged with the broad statement they were not in the primary and secondary outcomes of the study design. We have perhaps a more balanced viewpoint and suggest the following:

1. If unforeseen significant results emerge and their significance remains robust after rigorous correction for multiple comparisons then they should surely be reported. Note that the consideration that the study was not powered for these unforeseen results does not hold here since we take that the results are shown to be statistically significant after correction for multiplicity. Nevertheless, any conclusions derived should only be considered as hypothesis generating and this should also be clearly highlighted in the discussion.

2. Negative, post hoc results should be treated with much more caution. Here we should look for the presence and the adequacy of post hoc power analyses.
3. Finally an ethically healthy rule of the thumb is, feel free to do and surely bring up the results of post hoc analyses if the analyses and/or findings are in the direction of falsifying your hypothesis but try to refrain from them if they are potentially confirmatory.

The Discussion Section

The discussion section of any article is, or should be, nothing more or less than an honest re-account of your hypothesis, a summary of your results, what they indicated in the light of their internal and external validity, the main strengths and especially weaknesses of your work and finally a recap of your main message.

It is to be noted that a careful reader should be able to anticipate the contents of the discussion section before even starting to read it. However, the weaknesses of the work stand alone. It has been said that the discussion section should be curtailed as much as possible but for the study weaknesses [43]. This is so for two main reasons. First, it is usually nobody but the authors themselves who really know what the weaknesses to their work were, including such diverse items as changes in the sources of the animals, chemicals or probes used, the number of patients who refused to enter a particular drug study etc. which might have all affected the study results. The second important reason is simply and directly related to research ethics best verbalized by Feynman in his famous Cargo Cult address [32] which we already quoted in this chapter. As others have also rightfully emphasized [43] his last lines which also we now quote here are most instructive. In order to best explain what he means by self-criticism in scientific writing he chooses a counter example and says: "The easiest way to explain this idea is to contrast it, for example, with advertising…" [32]. That a scientific article is no advertisement is such superb advice.

We recently set out to quantify the degree of self-criticism in three better read journals of rheumatology. Not that this information was not available for rheumatology journals in particular – while its relative paucity had already been noted in scientific literature in general [44]- we hypothesized that our colleagues in basic science give less importance to self-criticism than those in clinical sciences. A survey, both by electronic and traditional reading by 2 independent observers, showed significant differences in the frequency of self-criticism in the discussion sections of the original articles in Annals of the Rheumatic Diseases, Arthritis and Rheumatism and Rheumatology (Oxford). In brief, the frequency of any form of self-criticism was around 75 % among the clinical and 25 % among the basic science articles [45]. It was also indeed rather surprising that when one of us asked a basic science editor why this was so during a recent American College of Rheumatology meeting, the answer was that the journals which mainly publish basic science articles do not highlight self-criticism in their authorship guidelines. This is disconcerting and surely deserves a "no wonder."

References

1. Gewirtz P , "On 'I Know It When I See It'", *Yale LJ* 1996, 105: 1023–47.
2. Basu P. Where are they now? *Nature Medicine* 2006, 12: 492–3
3. Sugarman J, Bingham CO 3rd Ethical issues in rheumatology clinical trials. Nat Clin Pract Rheumatol. 2008, 4:356–63.
4. Pope JE, Tingey DP, Arnold JM, Hong P, Ouimet JM, Krizova A. Are subjects satisfied with the informed consent process? A survey of research participants. J Rheumatol. 2003; 30:815–24.
5. TaylorGJ,WainwrightP.Openlabelextensionstudies:researchormarketing?BMJ.2005;10:331–
6. Abbasi K. The drugs industry: a bad product well marketed.J R Soc Med. 2012 ;105(7):275. doi: 10.1258/jrsm.2012.12k048.
7. Yazici Y, Yazici H. Trial of etanercept and methotrexate with radiographic and patient outcomes two-year clinical and radiographic results: Comment on the article by van der Heijde et al. Arthritis Rheum. 2006;54:3061–2.
8. van der Heijde, D. and Klareskog, L.Reply to letter by Yazici and Yazici commenting on the two-year report on the trial of etanercept and methotrexate with radiographic and patient outcomes. 2007 Arthritis Rheum, 56: 1031–32.
9. Becker MC, Wang TH, Wisniewski L, Wolski K, Libby P, Lüscher TF, Borer JS, Mascette AM, Husni ME, Solomon DH, Graham DY, Yeomans ND, Krum H, Ruschitzka F, Lincoff AM, Nissen SE; PRECISION Investigators. Rationale, design, and governance of Prospective Randomized Evaluation of Celecoxib Integrated Safety versus Ibuprofen Or Naproxen (PRECISION), a cardiovascular end point trial of nonsteroidal antiinflammatory agents in patients with arthritis. Am Heart J. 2009;1574:606–12.
10. Macdonald TM, Mackenzie IS, Wei L, Hawkey CJ, Ford I; SCOT study groupcollaborators. Methodology of a large prospective, randomised, open, blindedendpoint streamlined safety study of celecoxib versus traditional non-steroidal anti-inflammatory drugs in patients with osteoarthritis or rheumatoid arthritis: protocol of the standard care versus celecoxib outcome trial (SCOT). 2013 BMJ Open; 29;3(1) 2013.
11. Lenzer J. Truly independent research? BMJ. 2008;337:a1332.
12. Yazici Y Yazici H. Informed consent: time for more transparency. Arthritis Res Ther. 2010;12:121.
13. Sox HC, Rennie D. "Seeding trials: just say "no"". *Ann Intern Med.* 2008; 149: 279–80.
14. Esen F, Schimmel EK, Yazici H, Yazici Y. An audit of Behcet's syndrome research: a 10-year survey. J Rheumatol. 2011;38:99–103.
15. Little J, Higgins JP, Ioannidis JP, Moher D, Gagnon F, von Elm E, Khoury MJ, Cohen B, Davey-Smith G, Grimshaw J, Scheet P, Gwinn M, Williamson RE, Zou GY, Hutchings K, Johnson CY, Tait V, Wiens M, Golding J, van Duijn C, McLaughlin J, Paterson A, Wells G, Fortier I, Freedman M, Zecevic M, King R, Infante-Rivard C, Stewart A, Birkett N. STrengthening the REporting of Genetic Association Studies (STREGA): an extension of the STROBE statement. PLoS Med. 2009;6:e22.
16. The International FMF Consortium. Ancient missense mutations in a new member of the RoRet gene family are likely to cause familial Mediterranean fever. *Cell* 1997; 90: 797–807.
17. The French FMF Consortium ONSORTIUM. A candidate gene for familial Mediterranean fever. *Nat Genet* 1997; 17: 25–31FMF French consortium.
18. Kirino Y, Zhou Q, Ishigatsubo Y, Mizuki N, Tugal-Tutkun I, Seyahi E, Özyazgan Y, Ugurlu S, Erer B, Abaci N, Ustek D, Meguro A, Ueda A, Takeno M, Inoko H, Ombrello MJ, Satorius CL, Maskeri B, Mullikin JC, Sun HW, Gutierrez-Cruz G, Kim Y, Wilson AF, Kastner DL, Gül A, Remmers EF. Targeted resequencing implicates the familial Mediterranean fever gene MEFV and the toll-like receptor 4 gene TLR4 in Behçet disease. Proc Natl Acad Sci U S A. 2013;110:8134–9.
19. Ocak Z, Ocak T, Duran A, Ozlü T, Kocaman EM. Frequency of MEFV mutation and genotype-phenotype correlation in cases with dysmenorrhea. J Obstet Gynaecol Res. 2013;39:1314–8.

20. Marek-Yagel D, Berkun Y, Padeh S, Abu A, Reznik-Wolf H, Livneh A, Pras M, Pras E. Clinical disease among patients heterozygous for familial Mediterranean fever. Arthritis Rheum 2009;60:1862–6.
21. Esen F Yazici H The use of diseased control groups in genetic association studies. Clin Exp Rheumatol 2009;27(2 Suppl 53):S4–5.
22. Yazici H, van der Linden S. The case-control study and its potential biases.Clin Exp Rheumatol 1996;14:355–8.
23. Masuda K, Nakajima A, Urayama A, Nakae K, Kogure M, Inaba G. Double-masked trial of cyclosporin versus colchicine and long-term open study of cyclosporin in Behçet's disease. Lancet 1989;1:1093–6.
24. Weinblatt ME, Kavanaugh A, Genovese MC, Musser TK, Grossbard EB, Magilavy DB. An oral spleen tyrosine kinase (Syk) inhibitor for rheumatoid arthritis. N Engl J Med 2010 30;363:1303–12.
25. AMBITION referansı Jones G, Sebba A, Gu J, Lowenstein MB, et al. Comparison of tocilizumab monotherapy versus methotrexate monotherapy in patients with moderate to severe rheumatoid arthritis: the AMBITION study. Ann Rheum Dis. 2010 ;69:88–96.
26. Burmester G, Rigby W, van Vollenhoven R, Kay J, Rubbert-Roth A, Kelman A, Dimonaco S, Mitchell N. Tocilizumab in combination and monotherapy versus methotrexate in MTX-naïve patients with early rheumatoid arthritis: Clinical and radiographic outcomes from a randomized, placebo-controlled trial. (presented at EULAR 2013; OP0041)
27. Whitley I , Ball J. Statistics review 4: Sample size calculations. Critical Care 2002;6:335–41.
28. Fries JF, Krishnan E. Equipoise, design bias, and randomized controlled trials: the elusive ethics of new drug development. Arthritis Res Ther. 2004;6:R250–5.
29. Felson DT, Glantz L. A surplus of positive trials: weighing biases and reconsidering equipoise. Arthritis Res Ther 2004;6:117–9.
30. Saxman B. Ethical considerations for outcome-adaptive trial designs: A clinical researcher's perspective.Bioethics 2014; doi: 10.1111/bioe.12084. [Epub ahead of print]
31. Horgan J. Profile: Karl R. Popper – The Intellectual Warrior, Scientific American 1992; 267: 38–44.
32. Feynman R. Cargo Cult Speec. ttp://neurotheory.columbia.edu/~ken/cargo_cult.html Speech. accessed 28.03. 2014
33. Pearce N, Crawford-Brown D. Critical discussion in epidemiology: problems with the Popperian approach. J Clin Epidemiol 1989;42(3):177–84.
34. Glass DJ. A critique of the hypothesis, and a defense of the question, as a framework for experimentation. Clin Chem. 2010;56:1080–5.
35. ICMJE The Recommendations for the Conduct, Reporting, Editing, and Publication of Scholarly work in Medical Journals.at http://www.icmje.org/roles_a.html. Accessed 29.01.2014.
36. Flaherty DK. Ghost- and guest-authored pharmaceutical industry-sponsored studies: abuse of academic integrity, the peer review system, and public trust. Ann Pharmacother. 2013;47:1081–3.
37. Yazici Y, Yazici H. Tumor necrosis factor inhibitors, methotrexate or both? An inquiry into the formal evidence for when they are to be used in rheumatoid arthritis. Clin Exp Rheumatol. 2008;26:449–52.
38. Yazici Y, Adler NM, Yazici H. Most tumour necrosis factor inhibitor trials in rheumatology are undeservedly called 'efficacy and safety' trials: a survey of power considerations. Rheumatology (Oxford). 2008;47:1054–7.
39. Yazici H, Biyikli M, van der Linden S, Schouten HJ. The ‘zero patient design to compare prevalences of rare diseases. Rheumatology (Oxford) 2001; 40 121–2.
40. Yazici Y, Yazici H. A survey of inclusion of the time element when reporting adverse effects in randomised controlled trials of cyclo-oxygenase-2 and tumour necrosis factor alpha inhibitors. Ann Rheum Dis. 2007;66:124–7.

41. Sprung CL, Annane D, Keh D, Moreno R, Singer M, Freivogel K, Weiss YG, Benbenishty J, Kalenka A, Forst H, Laterre PF, Reinhart K, Cuthbertson BH, Payen D, Briegel J; CORTICUS Study Group. Hydrocortisone therapy for patients with septic shock. N Engl J Med 2008 10;358:111–24.
42. Nagele P. Misuse of standard error of the mean (SEM) when reporting variability of a sample. A critical evaluation of four anaesthesia journals. Br J Anaesth. 2003 ;90:514–6.
43. Puhan MA, Akl EA, Bryant D, Xie F, Apolone G, ter Riet G. Discussing study limitations in reports of medical studies - the need for more transparency. Health Qual Life Outcomes 2012;10:23e6.
44. Ioannidis JPA. Limitations are not properly acknowledged in the scientific literature. J Clin Epidemiol 2007;60:324–9.
45. Yazici H, Gogus F, Esen F, Yazici Y. There was less self-critique among basic than in clinical science articles in three rheumatology journals. J Clin Epidemiol 2014. 67: 654–7.

Future Directions

Hasan Yazici, Yusuf Yazici, and Emmanuel Lesaffre

We would like to finalize our work with some take home messages. "What it is" is surely important but "What it ought to be", is perhaps more important in Understanding Evidence Based Rheumatology, as our title reads.

We first have to realize that many of our diseases are still constructs and as such they need continuous clinical and scientific scrutiny. In this context the rather slow materialization of "The Human Phenome Project" should gain speed as we consider it at least as important as the long time finished The Human Genome project. On hindsight, we reflect that it would have been much more scientifically fruitful had the ubiquitous genetic association studies in every conceivable *construct – disease* we read during the last several decades had paid more attention to the phenotypes of the constructs they were studying. This wish of more emphasis on the phenotype applies both to the biomedical and the bio-psychosocial models of approach to better understand our diseases.

In the Preface we have jokingly said that the authors to the statistics chapter (see chapter "A review of statistical approaches for the analysis of data in rheumatology") were instructed to avoid the integral sign in their manuscript, to be better understood. On the other hand perhaps this is not what it ought to be. As we have tried to underline, a sound grasp of methodology, which in turn requires at least a familiarity

H. Yazici, MD (✉)
Division of Rheumatology, Department of Medicine, Cerrahpasa Medical Faculty, University of Istanbul, Istanbul, Turkey

Y. Yazici, MD
Division of Rheumatology, NYU Hospital for Joint Diseases, New York University, New York, USA

E. Lesaffre, Dr, Sc
Department of Biostatistics, Erasmus MC, Rotterdam, The Netherlands

L-Biostat, KU Leuven, Leuven, Belgium

H. Yazici et al. (eds.), *Understanding Evidence-Based Rheumatology*,
DOI 10.1007/978-3-319-08374-2_12

with basic arithmetic and probability theory is a must for being a better clinician and/or a better investigator. A good clinician and/or investigator should surely also be able to recognize, appreciate and avoid many of the cerebral forms of ethical transgressions (see chapter "Ethical issues in study design and reporting") and this is only possible with a sound insight into scientific methodology. The investigators should learn to invite the help of a statistician right from the start of their work, seeking advice not only on best methodology to prove themselves right but more importantly how to falsify their hypotheses and on many occasions even come up with new hypotheses. As a corollary, statisticians should no longer be content with their current role of the Wizard of Oz and should be right at the bed side or bench of any investigation before the investigator goes astray, both inadvertently and, on occasion, intentionally. In brief we should make research methodology and statistical thinking integral parts of teaching, practice and research. The more and more widely available software packages for statistical calculations are both marvellous and to be cursed. They, very often, do not help us to understand what we do. It is to be noted that the p value tells us only how surprising the obtained result is if the null hypothesis were true. Taking a randomized controlled trial as an example, assume we have reason to believe a new drug causes a cure 9 times more than the old drug. We design a controlled study and find out a p value of 0.001 related to the difference in outcome between the two arms of our trial. This p value is nothing more than the probability of observing a difference in the disease outcome between the two arms of the study at least as big as what was actually observed, if all what we observed was due to chance. It does not however tell us that our drug will work 9 times better. The investigator actually is surely more interested in the probability of the stated hypothesis being true (9:1 odds in our example). Confidence intervals and perhaps even more the Bayesian methodology are of more helpful here (see chapter "A review of statistical approaches for the analysis of data in rheumatology"). Specifically we should make every effort to be more knowledgeable about what the Bayesian approach with its conditional probabilities is, how it can be very helpful to us both in decision making and setting up and interpreting drug studies.

All constructs need precise definitions. We are afraid that our disease criteria have not been very successful thus far. We underline some thought barriers for this in chapter "Disease classification/diagnosis criteria". We propose that future disease criteria will be much more useful if they are tailored to the conditional probabilities of the disease in the populations these criteria would be used. Note that Bayesian conditional probabilities are very relevant here, as well. Furthermore the artificial designation of disease criteria as classification versus diagnostic should be abandoned. The understandable strive to have good biomarkers to identify rheumatologic diseases, to assess their severity, prognosis, outcome and tailor therapy should continue. However what we have warned about the importance of the phenotype for the genetic association studies equally applies for every other biomarker, as well. Those of us keen to develop such biomarkers should be aware that this is both a money and time expensive undertaking almost akin to developing a new drug as emphasized in chapter "Biomarkers, genetic association, and genomic studies". Perhaps the more successful future biomarkers will be those that combine both genetic and immunologic/biochemical markers and as the current evidence suggests, that ACCP negative rheumatoid arthritis might well be one disease construct in which such efforts might be more helpful. However, we need to have a frank discussion about the very real possibility that there may be no biomarkers, or genetic profiles that will be useful in individual patients. These however are the main concern of doctors making treatment plans, predicting disease response and assessing the overall prognosis.

Clinical outcome measures are all important not only in assessing the outcomes of clinical trials but also in daily care of patients. As such they should be as simple as possible and yet have useful discriminating value. As our chapter "Outcome measures in rheumatoid arthritis" emphasizes the patient reported outcomes are becoming much more popular and this is rightfully so. Needless to say that we will see more and more emphasis on patient reported outcomes in the years to come and we must also underline that this is very gratifying not only from the scientific/methodological angle but from its most useful humanistic message. The doctors are giving more and more importance to what the patient says.

We all like to say that world has become too small and indeed it has in many ways. On the other hand it is curious how comparatively little we utilize the enormous opportunities we now have in specimen and data collection on a global scale. There surely are many reasons behind this lagging behind. One important reason is the investigator ego. It is quite understandable that an investigator can shy away from global data collection so as not to share or give away his/her "dear" hypothesis. However we propose that the vast scientific opportunities such joint global work will bring to each participant will convince everybody to suppress his/her ego and get started in this sharing of opportunities. The trick is to put everybody's share of work and opportunity on the agenda from the start. A similar concern holds true for data repositories of any sort, ranging from blood or tissue banks to administrative data bases. Each participant will need to be assured and feel convinced that he/she will have just his/her share eventually.

Once the pinnacle of evidence based medicine, the controlled clinical trial is having hard times. Evidence for drug efficacy is being sought more and more in observational data. As we try to bring up in chapters "The randomized controlled trial: methodological perspectives", "Limitations of traditional randomized controlled clinical trials in rheumatology", and "Systematic reviews and meta-analyses in rheumatology" either modality is and should be complimentary to the other. With our current sophisticated technological capabilities of both storing and analysing data we should be able to solve many of our management problems with ease and precision. In this line we look forward to more sophisticated studies based on patient repositories and administrative data bases free as much as possible from inherent, but more and more better recognized, biases of such work. We also predict that more and more drug efficacy studies will utilize adaptive and Bayesian methods (which allows including historical information) especially considering the monetary and time pressures in drug development. Ethical considerations are obviously all important in any rapidly changing human activity and we surely and luckily, have abundance of that in rheumatology. There is little doubt that drug industry has immensely contributed to our truly spectacular performance in handling our diseases today. On the other hand there is also little doubt that today's main ethical transgressions in research and practice of medicine frequently have their roots, again in the drug industry.

We do not think that the solution to such transgressions lies in what we like to call the Queen Gertrude, "The lady protests too much, me thinks." approach. Meaningless ethical husbandry like declaring conflicts of interest in small letters or limiting meeting support to pencils and notepads or friendly drug representative's visit to 20 dollars' worth of coffee and doughnuts has not and will not solve these important ethical transgressions. Much more of consequence are unnecessary seeding trials, mesmerizing by science or statistics and informed consent forms of, by and for the lawyers. We surely hope more transparency of the right kind will soon prevail while we use more and more of today's very sophisticated technical know-how in accessing and disseminating truth.

We finally should also point out that journals along with their editors have very important responsibilities in the current and future quality of our research. There are lots of journals around and their number is ever increasing. They, like any other business venture, are after material gain. These factors along with the well-recognized pressure on the researcher to publish for his/her subsistence, produces a lot of low quality work [1]. This final point should probably be the foremost concern of all authors, readers and practitioners of evidence based rheumatology now and in the near future.

Reference

1. Ioannidis JP. Why most published research findings published are false. PLoS Med 2005; 2: e124.

Index

A

ACPA. *See* Antibodies to citrullinated protein antigen (ACPA)
ACR. *See* American College of Rheumatology (ACR)
Actemra *versus* Methotrexate double-Blind Investigative Trial In monotherapy (AMBITION study), 253
Agreement
  Bland-Altman plot, 37–38
  Cohen's kappa, 38, 39
  intra-class correlation, 37
  weighted kappas, 38
Alpha-fetoprotein (AFP), 82
Alpha spending approach, 170
American College of Rheumatology (ACR)
  ACR 20, 50, and 70 responses, 129
  MTX monotherapy and tocilizumab, 253
  vasculitis criteria, 66
ANA. *See* Antinuclear antibodies (ANA)
Analysis of variance (ANOVA) test
  one-way ANOVA test
    categorical measurements, 32–33
    continuous measurements, 30–32
  two-way ANOVA analysis, 33–35
Ankylosing spondylitis, 90, 230, 252
Antibodies to citrullinated protein antigen (ACPA), 91–92
Anti-carbamylated protein (anti-CarP), 92
Anti-cyclic citrullinated protein (anti-CCP), 91
Antinuclear antibodies (ANA), 4, 68–69, 180
Anti-tumor necrosis factor (anti-TNF), 110, 219
Arthrotec compared to acetaminophen (ACTA), 199
Association, 35–36
Authorship, 256–257

B

Bar chart, 15
Bayes' theorem (BT), 70, 176, 266
  vs. classical frequentist approach, 60–61
  hypothesis, 59
  Markov chain Monte Carlo sampling techniques, 61
  RA, prevalence of, 59–60
Behçet's syndrome (BS)
  constructs, 67
  control group, 251, 252
  ISGC and ICBD criteria, 70–72
  meta-analysis, 231
Beta-Blocker Heart Attack Trial (BHAT) study, 191–192
Biomarkers, 266
  ACPA antibody, 91–92
  alpha-fetoprotein, 82
  analytical validity, 85–86
  anti-CarP antibodies, 92
  carcinoembryonic antigen, 82
  clinical utility determination
    area under ROC curve analysis, 87–88
    calibration, 88
    OR/relative risk, 87
    risk prediction, 87–88
    risk reclassification, 88–89
  clinical validity, 86

H. Yazici et al. (eds.), *Understanding Evidence-Based Rheumatology*,
DOI 10.1007/978-3-319-08374-2

Biomarkers (*cont.*)
definition of, 82
for diagnosis, 102, 104–105
discovery phase, 84–85
disease activity assessment
genetic markers, 106–108
index of, 105–106
MBDA score, 108, 110
nongenetic markers, 108, 109
disease susceptibility
epigenetic markers for, 100–103
GWAS, 83, 92–100
failures, types of, 89–90
gold standard, 1–2
MammaPrint, 82
MBDA test, 135
OMERACT validation criteria, 90–91
prostate-specific antigen, 82
replication, 85
risk factors, 83–84
treatment response and outcome
abacavir, carbamazepine and allopurinol, 110
anti-TNF treatment, 111–113
leflunomide and sulfasalazine, 111
matrices, 111
methotrexate, 111
personalized medicine, 110
types of, 83
uses of, 82–83
Biomedical model, 5–6
Biopsychosocial model
vs. biomedical model, 6
breast cancer, in C3H mice, 7
rheumatic disease, 6–7
Bland-Altman plot, 37–38
Body mass index (BMI), 106, 108
Bonferroni correction, 25
BT. *See* Bayes' theorem (BT)

C

Carcinoembryonic antigen (CEA), 82
Carry-over effect, 168
Categorical data, 15, 57
CDAI. *See* Clinical disease activity index (CDAI)
Cerebral and Pudendal ethical transgressions, 247, 248
Censoring, 17
Chapel Hill Consensus Conference (CHC) criteria, 66
Chi-square test, 28–29
Clinical disease activity index (CDAI), 2, 106, 128, 131–132
Cochrane conditions, 29
Cohen's kappa, 38–39
Confidence interval (CI), 266
of absolute risk reduction, 29
age and gender, 34
Bayesian approach, 60
geometric means, ratio of, 28
for HAQ, 17
for hazard ratio, 49
intra-class correlation, 37
NEJM guidelines, 24
odds ratio, 46
one-sided and two-sided interval, 22
Pearson correlation, 36
vs. P-value, 24
of survival function, 30
true and sample mean, 19
Congestive heart failure (CHF), 3
Consolidated Standards of Reporting Trials (CONSORT), 61–62
Continual reassessment method (CRM), 171
Control group
AMBITION study, 253
Behçet's syndrome, 251, 252
biomarker, 251
FMF, 251
hypercoagulability, 250
litmus test, 250
MTX, 253
osteoarthritis, 251
pyrin (MEFV) mutations, 251
STREGA, 251
traditional medication, 252–253
Coronary artery disease (CAD), 72
Cox regression model
frailty model, 58
hazard function, 47–48
proportional hazards (PH) assumption, 48–49
Cross-over effect, 168

D

Data and Safety Monitoring Board (DSMB), 169–170
Data Monitoring Committee (DMC), 169
Degrees of freedom *(df)*, 21, 30, 32
Diagnostic criteria, 266
2010 ACR/EULAR criteria, 77–76
ACR vasculitis criteria, 66
Behcet's disease criteria, 66
CHC criteria, 66
circular logic, definition of, 73
circular manner *vs.* reasoning, 73
vs. classification criteria, 73–74

constructs, 67–68
family history, 77
Jones criteria, rheumatic fever, 66
pretest and likelihood ratios probability
Bayes' theorem, 70, 73
Behcet's syndrome, ISGC/ICBD criteria, 70–72
clinical prediction rue, 71
coronary artery disease, 72
positive and negative predictive value, 71
reasons for, 67
sensitivity and specificity
confidence intervals, 69, 77
ROCs, 69–70
SLE patients, ANA test, 68–69
Disease criteria. *see* Diagnostic criteria
Disease-modifying antirheumatic drugs (DMARDs), 110, 111, 182, 187

E

Epigenetics, 100–103
Error bar plot, 16, 17
Erythrocyte sedimentation rate (ESR), 2, 106, 130, 180
Ethical issues
pudendal and cerebral forms, 247–248
in reporting
authorship, 256–257
data presentation, 258–259
post hoc data analyses, 259–260
self-criticism, 260
in study design
control group (*see* Control group)
equipoise, 254–255
informed consent forms, 248–250
Popper's falsification, 254–255
power calculations, 254
Evidence-based medicine (EBM), rheumatology
biomedical model, 5–6
biopsychosocial model (*see* Biopsychosocial model)
emergence of, 9
gold standard biomarker, absence of, 1–2
histopathology, limitations of, 5
imaging, limitations of, 5
indices, 3
laboratory findings, limitations of, 4
limited money/resource concern, 9–10
patient history and physical examination, 3–4
pooled indices, 2–3
randomized controlled clinical trial, limitations of, 7–8

F

Factorial designs, 35
Familial Mediterranean fever (FMF), 8, 251
F-distribution, 30
Fibroblast like synoviocytes (FLS), 102
Fisher's exact test, 29
Fixed effects model, 167
Frailty model, 58
Frequentist approach, 24, 176
Futility analysis, 170

G

Gaussian distribution, 17, 40, 41
Generalized estimating equations (GEE) approach, 57
Generalized linear mixed model, 56–57
Genetic markers
advantages, 106
disease activity assessment, 106–108
for disease susceptibility, 92–100
Genome-wide association studies (GWAS)
ACPA-positive and negative RA, 92, 98
meta-analysis of, 93–99
Ghost authorship, 257
Gold standard, 1–2
Gouty arthritis, 72

H

Health Assessment Questionnaire (HAQ), 14, 16–17, 28, 35–36, 134, 150

I

Inflammatory arthritis, 5, 75, 102
Informed consent, 248–250
Intention-to-treat (ITT) analysis, 172–173
Interactive voice response system (IVRS), 167
Interquartile range (IQR), 16–17
Interstitial lung disease (ILD), 216
Interval censoring, 17
Intra-class correlation (ICC), 37

K

Kaplan–Meier survival curve, 18, 30
Kappa coefficient, 38–39
Kruskal–Wallis test, 31

L

Last-observation-carried-forward (LOCF) approach, 52, 173
Leflunomide, 111, 216
Left censoring, 17
Likelihood ratio (LR)
  Bayes' theorem, 70, 73
  Behcet's syndrome, 70–72, 77
  clinical prediction rue, 71
  coronary artery disease, 72
  positive and negative predictive value, 71
Linear mixed model (LMM), 52–56
Linear regression models
  multiple linear regression, 41–43
  simple linear regression, 39–41
Logistic random effects model, 56
Logistic random intercept model, 56–57
Logistic regression model
  fictive preclinical study, 44–45
  generalized linear models, 46
  ordinal logistic regression model, 46
  probit and complementary log–log regression model, 46
  simple linear logistic model, 44
  tREACH study, 45–46
Lognormal distribution, 30
Log-rank test, 168

M

Magnetic resonance imaging (MRI), 5
Major adverse cardiac events (MACE), 165
MammaPrint test, 82
Mann–Whitney U test, 27
Mantel-Haenszel-type test, 167
Manual of Procedures (MOP), 173–174
McNemar test, 29
Meta-analyses and systematic reviews
  confidence intervals, 236
  data extraction, 233–234
  dichotomous outcome variable, 236
  EULAR recommendations, 230
  extracted data, 236
  fixed-effect analysis, 239–240
  heterogeneity, 241
  inclusion/exclusion criteria, studies selection, 232
  logarithmic scale, 238
  publication bias and funnel plot, 243–244
  quality of studies, 233
  QuantiFERON, 230
  random-effect analysis, 241–243
  reporting results, 235
  research question, formulation of, 231–232
  risk ratio, 238
  search strategy development, 232
  Stata, 236
  statistical methods, 244–245
  summarizing data, 235
Methotrexate (MTX), 74–76, 111, 253
Missing at random (MAR), 50, 51
Missing completely at random (MCAR), 50, 51
Missing data, 50–51
Missing not at random (MNAR), 50, 51, 58
MTX. *See* Methotrexate (MTX)
Multi-biomarker disease activity (MBDA), 108, 110, 135
Multidimensional health assessment questionnaire (MDHAQ), 132, 134
Multiple imputation (MI) approach, 52
Multiple linear regression model, 41–43
Multiple testing problem, 25
Multivariate ANOVA (MANOVA), 51

N

National Institutes of Health (NIH), 160, 188
Non steroidal anti-inflammatory drugs (NSAIDs), 249

O

Odds ratio (OR), 26, 29, 36, 44, 46, 83–84, 87
Ordinal logistic regression model, 46
Osteoarthritis, 76, 164, 168, 252
Outcome Measures in Rheumatoid Arthritis Clinical Trials (OMERACT)
  biomarkers, validation criteria for, 90–91
  RA, outcome measures in, 127–128

P

Paired *t*-test, 27
Patient global assessment of disease status (PGADS), 164
Pearson correlation coefficient, 36, 37, 41
Per-protocol (PP) analysis, 172
Pretest probability (PrP)
  Bayes' theorem, 70, 73
  Behcet's syndrome, 70–72, 77
  clinical prediction rue, 71
  coronary artery disease, 72
  positive and negative predictive value, 71
Progression-free survival (PFS), 165
Prospective Randomized Evaluation Of Celecoxib Integrated Safety vs Ibuprofen Or Naproxen (PRECISION), 249

Prostate-specific antigen (PSA), 82, 89
Protein tyrosine phosphatase non-receptor 22 (PTPN22) gene, 99
P-value
  Bayesian approach, 60
  Bonferroni correction, 25
  chi-square test, 28–29
  data dredging, 25
  Fisher's exact test, 29
  F-ratio, 31
  F-tests, 34
  multiple comparison tests, 32
  multiple testing problem, 25, 43
  null hypothesis, 20–21, 38
  one-sided and two-sided tests, 22–23
  one-way ANOVA, 32
  opportunistic testing, 25
  Pearson correlation, 36
  Popper's falsification, 255
  posterior probability, 24
  of regression coefficient, 42
  surprise index, 21
  Wilcoxon rank-sum test, 27

Q
the Queen Gertrude approach to ethical transgessions, 267

R
RA. *See* Rheumatoid arthritis (RA)
Randomized controlled trials (RCTs), 266
  adaptive designs, 160
  antitumor necrosis factor (TNF) drugs, 209
  Bayesian approach, 176
  biomarkers, 180
  blinding, 167
  British Medical Research Council trial, 159
  confirmatory trials, 160
  definition, 159
  dysregulatory diseases, 180
  endpoints
    average profiles, 165
    binary, 164–165
    composite, 165
    hard, 164
    patient-centered, 165
    soft, 164
    surrogate, 165
  equivalence test, 163
  infectious diseases, 179
  informed consent form, 174
  intervention/control treatment, 162
  intrinsic limitations, 181, 182
    adverse event effects, 199–200
    control group inclusion, 197–198
    crossover clinical trial, 199
    placebo effects, 200
  ITT analysis, 172–173
  learning/exploratory phase trials, 160
  limitations, clinical care, 7–8
  LOCF approach, 173
  Medical Ethical Committee/Institutional Review Boards, US, 174
  Mesmerize by science, 258
  MOP, 173–174
  non-inferiority trial, 163–164
  observational study designs, 175–176
    anti-TNF drugs, 213
    "at-risk" period, 218
    Bayesian models, 212
    belimumab, 211
    channeling bias, 215–216
    clinical setting, 211
    confounding, indication, 213–215
    external validity, 211
    geographic setting, 211
    immortal time bias, 216–217
    limitations, 210, 212
    open-label extension studies, 211–212
    RA biologics and malignancies, 218–221
    registry and administrative database research, 221–223
    robust methodology, 210
    systemic sclerosis, 212
  patient history information, 181
  pharmacoepidemiological approaches, 209
  population, 161–162
  postmarketing surveillance study, 160
  PP analysis, 172
  pragmatic limitations, 181, 182
    adverse events, 196–197
    BHAT study, 191–192
    disease-modifying antirheumatic drugs, 182, 187
    enhanced statistical power, 190–191
    inclusion and exclusion criteria, 188–189
    inflexible and flexible dosage schedules, 193
    long time frame, 187–188
    NSAIDs, 189–190
    observational study, 185
    SLE nephritis, 190–191
    standard composite treatment effect, 183, 184
    strategy trials, 193–195
    surrogate markers and indices, 193, 195–196

Randomized controlled trials (RCTs) (*cont.*)
  preclinical phase, 160
  primary scientific question, 161
  radiographic outcomes in, 135–136
  randomization technique, 166–167
  sample size calculation, 171–172
  SAP, 174
  secondary scientific question, 161
  study designs
    adaptive design, 171
    cluster-randomized, 169
    factorial designs, 168–169
    group sequential, 169–170
    parallel-group *vs.* cross-over, 168
    single-center *vs.* multicenter, 167
  superiority trial, 163
  technical report, 174–175
  translational research, 160
  types, 160
  unpaired *t*-test, 174
RAPID3. *See* Routine assessment of patient index data 3 (RAPID3)
Rasch model, 57
RCTs. *See* Randomized controlled trials (RCTs)
Receiver operating characteristic (ROC) curve analysis, 69–70, 84, 87–88
Regression models
  Cox regression model
    frailty model, 58
    hazard function, 47–48
    proportional hazards (PH) assumption, 30, 48–49
  logistic regression model
    fictive preclinical study, 44–45
    generalized linear models, 46
    ordinal logistic regression model, 46
    probit and complementary log–log regression model, 46
    simple linear logistic model, 44
    tREACH study, 45–46
  multiple linear regression, 41–43
  simple linear regression, 39–41
Repeated significance testing approach, 51
Rheumatic fever, 66
Rheumatoid arthritis (RA)
  biologics and malignancies
    anti-TNF drugs, 220
    cytokine pathways, 219
    indications, 220
    infliximab and adalimumab data, 219
    lymphoproliferative cancers, 219
    risks, 218
  biomarkers (*see* Biomarkers)
  diagnostic criteria (*see* Diagnostic criteria)
  fictive study
    Bland-Altman plots, 38
    Cohen's kappa, 38–39
    intra-class correlation, 37
    logistic models, probability morbidity, 44–45
    one-way ANOVA test, 31–33
    survivor function, Kaplan–Meier curve of, 17–18, 48–49
    two-way ANOVA analysis, 34
  gold standard biomarkers, 1
  histopathology, limitations of, 5
  imaging, limitations of, 5
  laboratory findings, limitations of, 4
  laboratory tests, 127
  outcome measures in, 267
    ACR 20, 50, and 70, 129
    ACR/EULAR remission criteria, 133–134
    CDAI, 131–132
    composite indices, 128
    Core Data Set measures, 128–129
    DAS, 129–130
    DAS28, 130–131
    HAQ, 134
    MBDA test, 135
    OMERACT, 127–128
    patient-reported outcomes, 128
    radiographic joint damage, 135–136
    RAPID3, 132–133
    SDAI, 131
    "treating to target," concept of, 128
  patient history and physical examination, 4
  pooled indices, 2–3
  RAPPORT study, 14
    categorical data, 15
    convenience sample, 19–20
    counts, and continuous data, 15
    frequencies of patients, 28–29
    histograms, 15–17
    SEM and CI, 19
    statistical inference, 20–21
  rheumatoid factor, 1
  tREACH study
    DAS28 and HAQ, Spearman correlation of, 35–36
    DAS and RADAI, Pearson correlation, 35–36
    LMM analysis, 54–56
    logistic models, bDAS, 45–46
    multiple linear regression, DAS, 42–43
    simple linear regression, DAS, 39–41

Rheumatology research project
algorithm, 142
case–control studies, 146–147
data analysis, 153–154
data collection tools and manual
information bias, 151
measurement and misclassification, 151
observational biases, 151
primary data collection, 150
questionnaires, 150
secondary data collection, 150, 151
study/field manuals, 152
effect modification, 145
ethical considerations and approval, 152–153
exposure variable, 144
measurement devices/criteria, 145
multidisciplinary study team, 143
outcome variables, 144
potential confounders, 144
protocol components
abstract/executive summary, 155
aims, 155
background section, 155–156
budget, 156
human subjects, 156
research design and methods, 156
research question, 143–144
sample size calculation, 147–149
study population, 145–146
timeline and budget, 153
Right censoring, 17–18
Ritchie Articular Index (RAI), 130
Routine assessment of patient index data 3 (RAPID3), 2–3, 106, 132–133

S

Sharp–van der Heijde method, 111
Simple linear regression model, 39–41
Simplified disease activity index (SDAI), 106, 131
Spearman rank correlation, 36
Standard Care Versus Celecoxib Outcome Trial (SCOT), 249
Standard deviation (SD), 16–17
Standard error of the mean (SEM), 19
Statistical analysis plan (SAP), 174
Statistical inference
Bayesian approach, 24
confidence interval (*see* Confidence interval (CI))
frequentist approach, 24
posterior probability, 24
power of test, 23
P-value (*see P*-value)
sample and population, 19–20
tools for, 20–22
Type I error, 23–24
Type II error, 23
Statistical tests
comparison of more than two groups
categorical measurements, 32–33
continuous measurements, 30–32
two-way ANOVA analysis, 33–35
comparison of two groups
binary data, 28–29
continuous data, 27–28
factors, 22, 26–27
survival time, 29
Strengthening the Reporting of Genetic Association Studies (STREGA), 251
Strengthening the Reporting of Observational Studies in Epidemiology (STROBE), 251
Student's *t*-test, 21
Sulfasalazine, 111, 183–185
Surveillance, Epidemiology, and End Results (SEER) database, 219
Survival time
Cox regression, 46
hazard functions, 47–48
PH assumption, 30, 49
frailty model, 58
interval censoring, 17
left censoring, 17
right censoring, 17–18, 30
survival function, Kaplan–Meier curve of, 18, 30, 49
Systemic lupus erythematosus (SLE)
antinuclear antibodies, 68–69
control group, 252
epigenetics, 101

T

T-cell receptor (TCR), 100
Tetrachoric correlation, 36
Time-dependent regressors, 49
Time-to-event data, 17–18
Time-weighted average (TWA), 164
Tukey multiple comparison test, 32
Tumor necrosis factor-alpha-induced protein 3 (TNFAIP3), 99
Two-sample *t*-test, 21
Type I error, 23–24
Type II error, 23

U
Ultrasound, 5

W
Weibull distribution, 30, 48
Weighted kappas, 38
Welch test, 27
Wilcoxon rank-sum test, 27
WOMAC pain subscale (WOMACPA), 164
WOMAC physical function subscale (WOMACPH), 164
Working correlation matrix, 57

Printed by Printforce, the Netherlands